Culture and Medicine

Culture and Medicine

Critical Readings in the Health and Medical Humanities

Edited by
Rishi Goyal and Arden Hegele

BLOOMSBURY ACADEMIC
LONDON • NEW YORK • OXFORD • NEW DELHI • SYDNEY

BLOOMSBURY ACADEMIC
Bloomsbury Publishing Plc
50 Bedford Square, London, WC1B 3DP, UK
1385 Broadway, New York, NY 10018, USA
29 Earlsfort Terrace, Dublin 2, Ireland

BLOOMSBURY, BLOOMSBURY ACADEMIC and the Diana logo are trademarks of Bloomsbury Publishing Plc

First published in Great Britain 2023
Paperback edition published 2024

Copyright © Rishi Goyal, Arden Hegele, and contributors 2023, 2024

The editors and contributors have asserted their right under the Copyright, Designs and Patents Act, 1988, to be identified as Authors of this work.

For legal purposes the Acknowledgments on pp. viii–ix constitute an extension of this copyright page.

Cover design: Rebecca Heselton
Cover image: 'In transition' / drawing by Samanta Batra Mehta, 2018

All rights reserved. No part of this publication may be reproduced or transmitted in any form or by any means, electronic or mechanical, including photocopying, recording, or any information storage or retrieval system, without prior permission in writing from the publishers.

Bloomsbury Publishing Plc does not have any control over, or responsibility for, any third-party websites referred to or in this book. All internet addresses given in this book were correct at the time of going to press. The author and publisher regret any inconvenience caused if addresses have changed or sites have ceased to exist, but can accept no responsibility for any such changes.

A catalogue record for this book is available from the British Library.

A catalog record for this book is available from the Library of Congress.

ISBN: HB: 978-1-3502-4861-8
PB: 978-1-3502-4865-6
ePDF: 978-1-3502-4862-5
eBook: 978-1-3502-4863-2

Typeset by Newgen KnowledgeWorks Pvt. Ltd., Chennai, India

To find out more about our authors and books visit www.bloomsbury.com and sign up for our newsletters.

Contents

List of Figures	vii
Acknowledgments	viii
Introduction *Rishi Goyal and Arden Hegele*	1
Part 1 Identities/Institutions	19
1 Reproducing Horror: Nineteenth-Century Vampires and Twenty-First Century Megasellers *Livia Arndal Woods*	23
2 Postpartum Exhaustion in William Shakespeare's *The Winter's Tale* *Alicia Andrzejewski*	39
3 Medical and Military Transitions in *Anatomy of a Soldier* *Kristina Fleuty*	57
Part 2 Practices	71
4 On the Record: What Physician Texts Reveal about Physician Identities and the Electronic Health Record *Kamna S. Balhara*	75
5 Mixed Feedback: The Promise of Structural Competency Education *Joshua Franklin*	93
6 The Perceived Freedom of the Visual Analogue Scale *Gabi Schaffzin*	105
Part 3 Contingencies	125
7 Toward a Crip Medical Humanities *Travis Chi Wing Lau*	129

8 *Tales of the City* as Historical Document: HIV/AIDS, Serialization, Urban Landscapes, and Sexuality 141
   John A. Carranza

9 The Suffering Caregiver: Toward an Embodied Experience of End-of-Life Pain through Literature 161
   Benjamin Gagnon Chainey

Part 4   Alternatives 177

10 Against "Endochronology": Hormonal Rebellion and Generic Blending in *Confessions of the Fox* 181
    Diana Rose Newby

11 Whose Dystopia? 197
    Anna Fenton-Hathaway

Coda 211
Roanne Kantor

References 215
List of Contributors 239
Index 243

Figures

6.1	Graphic rating report on workers	107
6.2	Graphic scale for executives, department heads, foremen, and supervisors	109
6.3	Graphic Rating Scale	110
6.4	Intercorrelations of average ratings	111

Acknowledgments

We write with profound appreciation for all those who have supported this book.

First and foremost, we wish to thank the writers of *Synapsis: A Health Humanities Journal*, the digital publication where many of these ideas were first germinated in short form. As founders and editors of *Synapsis*, we are indebted to all our writers for their exceptional intellectual generosity and collaborative attitudes. We wish to thank both the contributors to the volume, whose essays here represent some of the best intellectual work done at the journal in its inaugural years, and also the many other writers-in-residence at *Synapsis* who have offered brilliant commitments to advancing the attitudinal orientations of the medical humanities that we chart in this volume.

We owe a great debt of gratitude to our student editors—Liz Bowen, Kimberley Gani, and Molly Lindberg—for their indefatigable help in assisting with the preparation of this volume. Assembling the collection would not have been possible without their savoir faire. At *Synapsis*, we are also grateful to have had the editorial assistance of Danielle Drees and Lilith Todd, who have served as assistant editors; of Naazanene Vatan, Radhika Patel, Malvika Jolly, Kimia Heydari, and Angelica Modabber, who have served as social media/copy editors; of Lan A. Li, who designed the site; and of Matthew Cappetta, the developmental editor.

We have been fortunate to have had a strong institutional support of the medical humanities at Columbia University, including from the medical humanities major at the Institute for Comparative Literature and Society, the Department of Medical Humanities and Ethics at the Columbia University Irving Medical Center, and the Society of Fellows and Heyman Center for the Humanities. Lydia Liu and Anupama Rao, Rita Charon, and Eileen Gillooly have offered remarkable counsel, support, and wisdom from their unique vantages. Sarah Monks has provided sustained administrative support to our work. We are grateful, too, for the support of our respective departments: Emergency Medicine and English and Comparative Literature. And we are indebted to the Dean of Humanities and the Provost for their enthusiasm for the growth of medical humanities in the arts and sciences at Columbia. We are grateful, too, to Columbia World Projects and the Center for the Study of Social Difference for supporting individual initiatives within the medical humanities, and to the Center for Science and Society for helping us by sponsoring a number of exciting conferences and initiatives. Beyond Columbia, we are grateful to the Consortium of Humanities Centers and Institutes' Health and Medical Humanities Network for the collegial community of scholars who have brought writers together with other leading-edge thinkers and practitioners worldwide to *Synapsis*.

Friends and colleagues, who are too many to list here, have lent encouragement to our efforts at every stage. We would particularly like to thank our students at Columbia, especially the students (RG) in "Risk, Illness Narratives, and the Contemporary Novel," "Marginalization in Medicine," "Literature, Medicine, and Technology," "Imagining Illness," and "Foundations of Clinical Medicine," and (AH) in "Literature and the Health Humanities," "Medical Fictions," "Contradictions of Care," "Pandemic Fictions," and the "Graduate Symposium in Medical Humanities." Finally, we wish to thank our families, who have lent us unconditional encouragement in this work and in every professional pursuit.

Introduction

Rishi Goyal and Arden Hegele

This book engages with the question of how biomedical knowledge is constructed, negotiated, and circulated as a cultural practice. It is also an attempt to illustrate the possibilities and contours of the emerging disciplines of medical and health humanities. These distinct but related fields recognize disease as a sociocultural *and* a biomedical phenomenon. They approach medicine through a critique of ideology, class, gender, and race-based assumptions with an appreciation for the constructive dimensions of language. The medical and health humanities denaturalize the biomedical sciences without diminishing their power to effect change in the physical and mental world of patients.

The medical and health humanities is a heterogeneous group of methods and ideas that engage the humanities and social sciences disciplines, such as history, language, anthropology, and sociology, alongside scientific disciplines, such as biology, genetics, neuroscience, and biomedical engineering. These diverse fields are marshaled to emphasize a set of common principles that extend across disciplines, including an acknowledgment of the vulnerability of human bodies, an adoption of anti-essentialist approaches to biology, a sensitivity to discursive and rhetorical factors in health, an attention to social justice, and an awareness of the structural determinants of health. Such ways of thinking defend against practices and perspectives that limit inclusivity and diminish health. Political and economic pressures can marginalize and exclude certain kinds of people. Women, black and brown people, migrants, refugees, sex workers, the elderly, the undomiciled, and other abjected peoples have been and continue to be excluded from the benefits of modernity and, at times, from the very definition of the human. By questioning normative assumptions, the medical and health humanities interrupt and interrogate the processes that limit who counts as human.

This book charts shared advances across the medical humanities and health humanities, connecting the biological sciences approaches with the humanities and human sciences. Through a series of essays emerging out of diverse fields—from literary studies and medical anthropology to neurology and emergency medicine—this collection illustrates how the methods and orientations of medical and health humanities might be constructively juxtaposed and potentially bridged.

This collection explores a shared problem for medical practice and humanities scholarship: how are biomedical ideas about the body constituted, circulated, and settled? While biomedicine often aspires to be a positivist science, it is, explicitly and implicitly, in constant negotiation with other domains of culture. Medical science shapes a set of normative cultural practices that define the limits of health and the body, from the body's place and trajectory in the world, to how bodies relate to one another, to what counts as health and illness. Aging is both a medical reality and a social condition; sex is a biological act inseparably tied to cultural ideas of affect, desire, and beauty. This volume examines how these and other concepts are shaped through traffic between medico-scientific knowledge and ways of knowing derived from other domains, and it interrogates how biomedical frameworks become settled forms for a broader cultural understanding. The borders of health and illness, like the normal and the pathological, are fragile—new illnesses appear and old illnesses disappear as a result of epistemic shifts and drifts.

Drawn from short articles by new and emerging scholarly voices first published in our digital journal, *Synapsis: A Health Humanities Journal*, the essays in this volume apply the decentering critical perspectives of the humanities to a diverse array of medical objects, ideas, and practices. These range from literary texts and historical evidence to artifacts more squarely situated within hospitalist contexts, such as the norms of medical education and the electronic health record. Institutionally, the collection aspires to be a "Department without Walls," allying critical viewpoints that are often siloed by disciplinary divisions. The volume's inclusion of perspectives from both health professionals and humanities scholars is intended to spark a generative conversation that advances thought in the medical and health humanities.

Why "medical and health humanities"? The fields are both interwoven and distinct. As scholarly domains, they operate in concert and in tension, adopting common aims and practices but sometimes taking opposite perspectives vis-à-vis the institutions of medicine. One of our aims in this volume is to reveal the shared values that underpin the medical humanities and health humanities despite different perspectives, critical stances, and methods. This reconciliation is essential for medical and health humanities to make authentic contributions to the pressing problems of the present day, such as exposing the communication patterns of science denialism or revealing the structural racism in the industry of "essential work" and caregiving. The medical humanities and health humanities need not be antagonistic, either disciplinarily or professionally. If the field is to make tangible interventions into real-world problems—as it must—it needs flexibility and openness to perspectives from inside and outside the clinic.[1]

At the outset, then, a few definitions: *medical humanities*, the more established of the two fields, is "an inter- and multi-disciplinary field that explores contexts, experiences, and critical and conceptual issues in medicine and health care, while supporting professional identity formation," particularly around physician education.[2] Scholarship in the medical humanities is concerned with surveying and critiquing the disciplinary norms of the medical and healthcare context while also training physicians and other health professionals in approaches related to and/or derived from the humanities (for instance, in bioethics and narrative medicine). In its focus on practical training, medical humanities tends to emphasize educating health professionals in what Andrea Charise has labeled the "god terms"—"empathy, listening, moral imagination, and self-reflection."[3] As it has matured, the field has adopted a critical perspective more aligned with cultural critique in the humanities in order to consider "the social, the political, even the economic" factors that shape medical encounters and institutions.[4] The "critical medical humanities," for example, adopts a decentering attitude that is reminiscent of the health humanities (see below) as it applies a self-conscious perspective to the implicit assumptions that structure

---

[1] We are not the first to comment that a professional opposition between medical humanities and health humanities is "conceptually questionable." See Sarah Atkinson, Bethan Evans, Angela Woods, and Robin Kearns, "'The Medical' and 'Health' in a Critical Medical Humanities," *Journal of Medical Humanities* 36, no. 1 (2015): 71–81.

[2] Thomas R. Cole, Ronald A. Carson, and Nathan S. Carlin, *Medical Humanities: An Introduction* (Cambridge: Cambridge University Press, 2014), ix. This definition is further quoted in Olivia Banner, "Introduction: For Impossible Demands," in *Teaching Health Humanities*, ed. Olivia Banner, Nathan Carlin, and Thomas R. Cole, 1–18 (New York: Oxford University Press, 2019)..

[3] Banner, "Introduction: For Impossible Demands," 5; for a more extensive discussion of "god terms," see Andrea Charise, "Resemblance, Diversity, and Making Age Studies Matter," in *Teaching Health Humanities*, ed. Olivia Banner, Nathan Carlin, and Thomas R. Cole (New York: Oxford University Press, 2019), 188–206.

[4] Banner, "Introduction: For Impossible Demands," 3.

the medical field.[5] While still engaging directly with medicine, new work in the medical humanities seeks to attend more sensitively to the hidden biases that a biomedical context imposes on the field, particularly its capacity for ideological and political critique.

Health humanities, meanwhile, is more difficult to pin down in a singular definition. While Therese Jones, Delease Wear, and Lester D. Friedman argued in *The Health Humanities Reader* (*HHR*, 2014) for a replacement of the term "medical" with "health" humanities in describing the field, over time the "medical" and "health" domains have evolved into distinct and sometimes rival spheres.[6] In response to the perceived limitations of the "medical humanities" (with its focus on the more narrow notion of "disease" rather than the expansive concept of "health"), health humanities scholars suggest that a health humanities approach looks both at and beyond medicine to critique its influence over cultural norms.[7] More often situated in humanities departments than in clinical spaces, and introducing the creative arts as well as traditional analytical disciplines, health humanities adopts the characteristic attitudes of the study of humanities—inclusivity, diversity, and intersectionality, among others—to an applied critique of the frameworks and institutions that govern healthcare and its effects on culture. Health humanities is concerned with broad contexts, prioritizing a view beyond the medical humanities' narrower frame of reference by considering the authority and identity formation of patients, caregivers, and allied health professionals. Health humanities scholarship addresses a broad array of objects of study: rich areas of exploration include topics such as disability, bias and exclusion, structural inequality, aging, grief, suffering, and death. In addition to this diversity in its objects of study, health humanities also draws on a capacious set of methodological tools adapted from an array of humanities disciplines—close reading, historiography, qualitative assessment—to offer a critical commentary on the influence of medicine and healthcare on human experience.

---

[5] Anne Whitehead et al., eds., *The Edinburgh Companion to the Critical Medical Humanities* (Edinburgh: Edinburgh University Press, 2016).

[6] Felice Aull, "Health Humanities Reader," *LitMed: Literature, Arts, Medicine Database* (October 30, 2014), accessed July 20, 2021, https://medhum.med.nyu.edu/view/15463. See also Banner's account of the rivalry between disciplines throughout "Introduction: For Impossible Demands."

[7] Therese Jones, Delese Wear, and Lester D. Friedman, *Health Humanities Reader* (New Brunswick, NJ: Rutgers University Press, 2014); Paul Crawford et al., *Health Humanities* (New York: Palgrave Macmillan, 2015); see also Banner et al., Teaching Health Humanities. See further Albert Howard Carter, III, "Health Humanities," *LitMed: Literature, Arts, Medicine Database* (October 20, 2016), accessed July 20, 2021, https://medhum.med.nyu.edu/view/16593.

Placing the Intervention

Health professionals and humanities scholars working in these fields share, to a certain degree, common goals. Both seek to apply the methods of humanities to medicine, whether through practice or through critique, and both strive to understand the cultural norms wrought by medicine and its institutions. As health professionals seek to deepen their disciplinary self-understanding and enrich their practice with methods foraged from the humanities, scholars in traditional humanities and social sciences fields (e.g., literature, history, sociology, anthropology) are producing critiques of the biomedical models that permeate culture beyond the institutions and practices of medicine. Both approaches tend to destabilize authority, provide self-reflection, increase intersubjectivity, and critique dominant ideological structures. In light of the shared aims of these diverse professional identities, this collection bridges the fields of medical humanities and health humanities by focusing on biomedicine as a cultural practice. Rather than collapsing the distinction between medical humanities and health humanities, the collection instead models a collaborative form of knowledge that adopts the disciplinary competencies cultivated both inside and outside clinical spaces: an intervention that has the capacity to transform the practices of medical humanities and health humanities scholars alike.[8]

Situated at the crossroads of health humanities and medical humanities, the essays in this volume join other works of contemporary scholarship as they characterize the contours of the fields. Critical work in the medical and health humanities, taken together, tends to fall methodologically into three categories, all of which find their voices in this collection. The first group of studies takes the medical and/or health humanities as a conceptual approach and applies it to a specific domain of humanities scholarship, such as history or literary studies. Landmark examples in this vein from the field of literary

---

[8] For a compelling and clear account of the "humanistic competencies" that might be imported from the humanities into medicine, see Sari Altschuler, *The Medical Imagination: Literature and Health in the Early United States* (Philadelphia: University of Pennsylvania Press, 2018). For a discussion of competency-based education in medical training, see Jonathan M. Metzl and Helena Hansen, "Structure Competency: Theorizing a New Medical Engagement with Stigma and Inequality," *Social Science & Medicine* 103 (February 1, 2014): 126–33, https://doi.org/10.1016/j.socscimed.2013.06.032. See also Arno K. Kumagai, "From Competencies to Human Interests: Ways of Knowing and Understanding in Medical Education," *Academic Medicine* 89, no. 7 (2014): 978–83, and Jason R. Frank et al., "Competency-Based Medical Education: Theory to Practice," *Medical Teacher* 32, no. 8 (2010): 638–45, https://doi.org/10.3109/0142159X.2010.501190. See also Chapter 5 in this volume, by Joshua Franklin, for a critique of "structural competency" education.

studies include Erika Wright's *Reading for Health: Medical Narratives and the Nineteenth-Century Novel* (2016) and Anne Whitehead's *Medicine and Empathy in Contemporary British Fiction: An Intervention in Medical Humanities* (2017). Sari Altschuler's *The Medical Imagination: Literature and Health in the Early United States* (2018) is a particularly nuanced example of how literary studies might make an intervention in medical knowledge, as it charts how eighteenth- and nineteenth-century American fiction transposed epistemological attitudes from literature into medicine. Several chapters in our volume take a similar approach by considering aesthetic objects, such as literary texts, through the lens of the medical and health humanities in order to mine a corpus of seemingly nonmedical work for its insights into the poetics of communicating lived bodily experience.

A second group of studies takes a reverse methodology by applying an analytical lens from the medical and health humanities to problems within medicine and healthcare. Many works grapple, for instance, with the ethical status of physician empathy, which has recently come under critical and popular scrutiny from a health humanities perspective—most compellingly, perhaps, in Leslie Jamison's *The Empathy Exams* (2015) and in Kate Polak's *Ethics in the Gutter: Empathy and Historical Fiction in Comics* (2017). The essays in this volume are interested in expanding the purview of the medical humanities—which, some scholars have claimed, is too narrowly focused on cultivating an empathetic medical practice through the study of patient testimony—by arguing for the relevance of disability activism, illness memoirs, and testimonies of the end of life to the defamiliarization of biomedical cultural norms such as a teleology toward a "cure." The collection considers instead how medicine and its institutions operate as practices of culture, discourse, and representation. This widening scope makes the volume an apt complement to the *Health Humanities* manifesto (2015), which desires to extend health humanities "beyond Medical Humanities to advance the inclusion and impact of the arts and humanities in healthcare, health and well-being."[9]

Finally, a third group of studies, focused on pedagogical approaches, frames the medical and health humanities in their range of institutional contexts, whether in medical schools or humanities departments. This collection is formally and conceptually similar to collections in health humanities, including *HHR* (2014) and *Teaching Health Humanities* (2019), and to volumes in medical humanities,

---

[9] Charley Baker, Victoria Tischler, and Brian Adams, *Health Humanities* (London: Palgrave Macmillan, 2015).

such as *The Edinburgh Companion to the Critical Medical Humanities* (2016) and *The Principles and Practices of Narrative Medicine* (2016). The *Edinburgh* volume resembles ours in its critical stance toward an increasingly institutionalized "medical humanities." Our editorial orientation as literary scholars has shaped the objects of study in the volume: we are particularly alive to how fiction finds powerful forms of expression for changing ways of life, and our collection includes a robust selection of literary criticism in particular. Meanwhile, our work is aligned disciplinarily with the central tenets of *HHR* while adopting quite a different temporal orientation: *HHR* provides an overview of the past several decades of medical humanities scholarship, while our work emphasizes the field's present and future possibilities, cultivating a scholarly conversation between the practice of medicine and the study of medicine's cultural roles.

Our essays' various positions on a spectrum from clinical practice to literary and cultural criticism, as well as their engagement with pressing contemporary questions in health humanities and medical humanities, invite a broad audience. Modeling how the approaches of health humanities and medical humanities are distinct but complementary, the collection treats the perspectives of both the clinic and the humanities department as valid in the broader critical examination of biomedicine's cultural influence. This collection posits a set of shared ideational *values* that sustain the medical and health humanities alike.

Attitudinal Orientations

The essays in this volume are illustrative of a range of interdisciplinary methodologies at work in the medical and health humanities while articulating the values that shape the medical and health humanities as a field. Taking the language of "orientations" from phenomenology, we explore how the medical and health humanities cultivates a set of attitudinal orientations across the various contrasting disciplines invested in the progress of the field.[10] Our volume trains readers in the medical and health humanities to appreciate and become sensitized to the attitudes and outlooks that implicitly shape their scholarship. Medical and health humanities are interwoven, we argue, through our shared orientations toward three fundamental values, which unite all our contributions and buttress our understanding of the medical and health humanities.

---

[10] See, most importantly, Sara Ahmed, "Orientations: Toward a Queer Phenomenology," *GLQ: A Journal of Lesbian and Gay Studies* 12, no. 4 (2006): 543–74.

The first is ethical value. By ethics, we do not mean a traditional deontological approach, but rather ethics as a support to human life and well-being through discovery. Work in the medical and health humanities must acknowledge suffering and marginalization and act to alleviate both. The various lenses of the humanities disciplines make new insights visible, fortifying scientific research and clinical activity. By situating the work within a matrix of scientific, social, and political transformation, we enframe the human and historical dimensions of health and illness. The medical and health humanities illuminate unacknowledged areas of bias, exclusion, or inequality as they relate to what health is and how we achieve it. As we examine how the technological and political management of bodies privileges some bodies over others, we actively adopt feminist, antiracist, and anti-essentialist critical stances. And, as we consider how the aspects of life are medicalized in the past and the present, we also imagine ways in which institutions and practices could become more inclusive and just in the future.

Our second fundamental value is the importance of critique. In a humanist enlightenment tradition, critique might be defined as a systemic inquiry into the limits of a totalizing idea, practice, or governing principle; this application of a method of radical doubt is at the heart of many scholarly practices that fall under the umbrella of the humanities, and it is central to our approach. Critique is powerful, we argue, not only in its ability to identify lacunae and inadequacies but also in its capacity to articulate alternatives to the institutional status quo. These capacities have become urgently important in the present day for their ability to counter antiscientific thinking. Rather than aiming to undercut medicine as a good, we argue, the critical value of the medical and health humanities might also be to strengthen biomedical progress with multiple perspectives and to contest a global epidemic of science denialism. While pursuing a critical eye toward ideological concepts and hierarchies masquerading as science, we can use the critical reasoning of the humanities to understand and emphasize the role of ideologies and cultural assumptions in the production of medical knowledge.

Our final fundamental value is a sensitivity to style. Interdisciplinary work can be stymied through an insistence on jargon and closed vocabularies. We strive to reach across disciplines through clear communication, without sacrificing meaning and nuance. We break down institutional siloes by actively rejecting jargon that is restricted to specific communities or disciplines while also examining how language is used to circulate information about the body. As far as possible, we promote accessible and ordinary language while retaining scholarly rigor and specificity. These values, we believe, are essential to interdisciplinary scholarship in the medical and health humanities. They operate beyond specific thematic concerns or disciplinary conventions to unify all our chapters and, we believe, a considerable body of scholarship beyond this collection. By articulating these values in our volume, we make explicit a vision of the medical and health humanities linked not so much by their interdisciplinary approaches but by their collective attitudes, which is portable beyond this book.

An Anatomy of the Volume

The essays in this collection offer a window into the state of scholarship in the medical humanities and health humanities while also showing how these fields can work together, and they offer a useful model for students new to the fields, in addition to being relevant for scholars well versed in these conversations. Even as they model the orientations underpinning interventions in the medical and health humanities, they also thematically consider the shared problem with which we began this introduction: how are biomedical ideas about the body constituted, circulated, and settled? Together, our essays consider how the institutions, power structures, and professional norms of biomedicine work on a cultural level that can be analyzed through the critical perspectives of the humanities. Our theoretical framework for medico-scientific knowledge draws on the historian of science Steven Shapin's account of science as a set of practices within culture:

> There was [no] singular and discrete event, localized in time and space, that can be pointed to as "the" Scientific Revolution. [Nor was] there any single coherent cultural entity called "science" ... to undergo revolutionary change. There was, rather, a diverse array of cultural practices aimed at understanding, explaining, and controlling the natural world, each with different characteristics and each experiencing different modes of change.[11]

Whether investigating how medicalizing forces shape identity, gender, and sexuality, how the carceral system influences aesthetics, or how disability narratives are pressured to conform to linear trajectories, the essays in this collection exceed the usual divides to consider the cultural ramifications of medico-scientific knowledge across a wide range of exemplary objects.

---

[11] Steven Shapin, *The Scientific Revolution*, 2nd ed. (Chicago: The University of Chicago Press, [1996] 2018), 3.

The book is structured in four thematic parts, each with a brief critical introduction to the problem under consideration. The first part, "Identities/Institutions," considers the role of historical and contemporary biomedical institutions in shaping literary bodily identities, including postpartum bodies in Shakespeare, and pregnant bodies in contemporary bestsellers. The second part, "Practices," explores the cultural conditions that produced familiar humanities-informed practices within medicine—structural competence education and empathy training—and, in turn, the corresponding influence of such practices on aesthetic objects, including graphic novels and the analogue pain scale. The third part, "Contingencies," examines instances in which a biomedical cultural framework breaks down when it collides with bodily realities that challenge linearity, such as disability, chronic illness, and death. This part attends particularly to how biomedicine engenders notions of bias and marginalization in its assumption of cultural authority. Finally, the fourth part, "Alternatives," imagines creative possibilities that challenge our contemporary reality of biomedicine's cultural influence. Speculative and dystopian fictions offer particularly rich sites for experimentation for writers and thinkers seeking compelling alternatives to the biomedical institutions and practices that govern our cultural perceptions of illness and health. The Coda reflects on the influence and legacy of medico-scientific knowledge practices. Even as they delve deeply into distinct exhibits, case histories, and literary texts whose historical range spans from the early-modern period to the twenty-first century, the essays in this volume all engage with the present power of biomedicine to act as a shaping cultural force. Situated at the crossroads between health and medical humanities, the collection aims to provide a synoptic view of the norms of medico-scientific knowledge.

The first part, "Identities/Institutions," takes a health humanities approach to the analysis of literary artifacts. The introduction reveals the influence medical frameworks can have on knowledge in other spheres of human activity. The three chapters that follow chart how historical and contemporary biomedical institutions shape literary and bodily identities. The first two chapters examine the individual construction of a biomedical bodily self, while the last turns to a nonmedical institution—the army—that serves as a purveyor of medical cultural practices in its regulation of individual life.

The first chapter, "Reproducing Horror: Nineteenth-Century Vampires and Twenty-First Century Megasellers" by Livia Arndal Woods, reads the Victorian texture of depictions of pregnancy in two related contemporary bestsellers, Stephenie Meyer's 2008 *Breaking Dawn* and E. L. James's 2012 *Fifty Shades*

Freed, and the film adaptations of both novels. Woods puts Victorian narrative conventions for the literary treatment of pregnancy in conversation with the specter of reproductive trauma in Victorian vampire fiction, most notably Sheridan Le Fanu's *Carmilla* and Bram Stoker's *Dracula*, to argue that the *Twilight* and *Fifty Shades of Grey* series draw on a tradition of moralization about women's reproductive bodies that positions pregnancy as the ultimate danger, and the reader in the uneasy position of an arbiter of the degree to which that danger is self-inflicted.

Turning from pregnancy to childbirth, the literary horrors of reproduction are taken up from a more distant historical vantage in Chapter 2, "Postpartum Exhaustion in William Shakespeare's *The Winter's Tale*," by Alicia Andrzejewski. This chapter finds that Hermione's denied "lying-in" rights in the first act of *The Winter's Tale* set the play's larger concern with bodies and worlds that are exhausted—weary, precarious, and abandoned—in motion. In many ways, *The Winter's Tale* is a tale about exhaustion, retreat, and death, all of which are inextricably tied to the pregnant and postpartum body. The chapter begins with a historical overview of the "child-bed privilege" that Hermione declares is "denied [for] her": the early-modern practice of "lying-in" for about a month postpartum. From there, the work attends to exhaustion as an atmosphere throughout *The Winter's Tale* in order to think through the play's age-old critical question: the reason for Hermione's sixteen-year-long retreat and resurrection. The chapter situates contemporary performances of *The Winter's Tale* within the current postpartum care crisis in America.

Like Andrzejewski's essay, the third chapter, "Medical and Military Transitions in *Anatomy of a Soldier*" by Kristina Fleuty, is interested in what the narrative points of view of marginal or even inanimate figures in the text might have to say about contemporary states of health and illness. Exploring medical and military transitions, Harry Parker's semi-autobiographical novel *Anatomy of a Soldier* parallels two important life transitions, from able-bodied to amputee, and from soldier to veteran. Existing academic enquiry into limb loss focuses mostly on the etiology of limb loss or the practical aspects of recovery. Using inanimate objects (especially medical objects) as narrators, *Anatomy of a Soldier* recognizes these practical aspects while exploring how the individual comes to terms with the loss of their limb and the gain of a prosthetic. In a military context, this medical transition is complicated further by a change of identity, as a soldier becomes a veteran and civilian. And while the current focus on military transition prioritizes supporting the practical aspects of transition, such as relocating or finding a job, this chapter embodies the emotional experience of these transitions. As a whole, the chapters in this part attend to how the narrative allows for a humanistic rather than scientific focus on the medical experience.

The second part, "Practices," treats the medical humanities as a tool for the dissemination of medico-scientific frameworks. The introduction considers how conventional practices in medical humanities, designed to "humanize" medical care, can themselves propagate the norms of biomedical culture. The three chapters that follow reveal the cultural conditions that produced humanities-informed practices within medicine—structural competence education and empathy training—and they critique the value and effectiveness of such practices. The chapters also present medicine as a cultural practice shaping the aesthetic objects used in the field, such as the electronic health record and the analogue pain scale.

The fourth chapter in the volume, Kamna S. Balhara's "On the Record: What Physician Texts Reveal about Physician Identities and the Electronic Health Record," explores the narrative affordances and the practical impact of computational record-keeping. Balhara traces how the medical record has undergone numerous transitions in response to political, legal, bureaucratic, and technological forces. Its most recent iteration, the electronic health record (EHR) has attracted significant conversation and controversy as it has come into widespread use in the United States after President Obama's 2009 Health Information Technology for Economic and Clinical Health Act. A decade after its adoption across the United States, the EHR remains linked with physician dissatisfaction and burnout. Common refrains populate physicians' complaints about the EHR, including erosion of the doctor–patient relationship, degradation of bedside skills, loss of autonomy, and encroachment into time away from work. This chapter argues that the root of physician resistance to the EHR may also lie in the fundamental changes and perceived threats to physician identity wrought by the EHR. While some of these changes are emblematic of the larger commodification and corporatization of medicine, this chapter demonstrates that such changes are occurring from the "inside out," via the very structure and form of the EHR itself.

Taking up the question of how artifacts imported from humanities are currently shaping physician education and practice, Joshua Franklin's "Mixed Feedback: The Promise of Structural Competence Education," the fifth chapter in the volume, describes how medical schools have organized their efforts to foster critical consciousness about the social and cultural context of medicine. Names for these projects have shifted from "cultural competence" to "structural competence," incorporating new ways of thinking about social inequality, cultural meanings, power, violence, and care in health professions. Because questions of social justice are understood to draw from knowledge and experience outside of the domain of biomedicine, these initiatives provide a unique opportunity for students to lead the conversation, resulting in novel forms of collaboration with the faculty. The chapter focuses on the experience of one such program at the author's home institution, the University of Pennsylvania, to examine what happens when frameworks based on reflection and critical consciousness are deployed in a context where students are subject to established educational requirements but are also able to transform their curriculum through an essentially consumer logic of feedback. Drawing from the work of theorist Lauren Berlant, Franklin argues that disciplinary knowledges such as medical anthropology become objects of "cruel optimism"— places where we are able to displace our anxieties and concerns about the unfinished ethical work of medicine and sustain our hope for their resolution.

The sixth chapter in the collection, Gabi Schaffzin's "The Perceived Freedom of the Visual Analogue Scale," explores the concealed capitalist underpinnings of a tool used ubiquitously in today's clinical trials and doctors' offices from an art-historical perspective. The Visual Analogue Scale (VAS) emerged from the work of the Walter Dill Scott Company, a management consultancy, in 1920. Following a path through industrial and behavioral psychology, the scale was eventually adopted by researchers studying the levels of pain in their subjects. This chapter traces the history of the VAS, especially as the field of clinical pain studies turned from small-n-"objective" pain research to large-n-"subjective" studies after the First World War—studies funded and operated under the auspices of corporations developing newly emerging synthetic opiates. At stake here is a recognition that subjects in pain are stand-ins for the micromanaged laborers of early twentieth-century Taylorist fantasies.

The collection's third part, "Contingencies," turns to the limitations of medical knowledge by demonstrating instances in which a biomedical framework for knowledge collapses when it comes into contact with bodily realities that challenge linearity, such as disability, chronic illness, and death. The introduction applies the critical tools of health humanities to areas of ambiguity and uncertainty in medical (and medical humanities) practice. The three chapters that follow offer innovative models, derived from a broader, more inclusive perspective, for changing medical practice and perception. This part attends particularly to how biomedicine engenders notions of bias and marginalization in its assumption of cultural authority, and the positive function of health humanities in challenging these forces.

Chapter 7, "Toward a Crip Medical Humanities" by Travis Chi Wing Lau, makes a case for thinking about how the activist history and scholarly approaches of disability studies can shift the ways in which we teach and understand the medical humanities as a field. The chapter takes up both Diane Price Herndl's assessment that the formation of medical humanities within medical schools renders it less critical of the practice of medicine at large, and Otniel E. Dror's assertion that the medical humanities "suppresses those dimensions of the humanities that can most significantly contribute to medicine."[12] Disability studies rejects the ideas that disability is an individual defect and that it should be under the purview of health professionals. It is a field that has exposed the ways in which medicine has historically held the institutional and cultural power to determine what is normal, what is healthy, and what is to be done with those falling out of these categories. By refusing the typical linear trajectory of diagnosis, treatment, and cure, disability troubles the conventional narratives of medical progress that continue to persist in medical education. Echoing Sari Altschuler's call for a more robust medical humanities that extends beyond cultivating empathy and attending to patient narratives, this chapter argues that disability studies offers the conceptual tools and different critical objects that can be used to reorient medicine in a set of traditions, practices, and values with histories still understudied in medical education.

By considering another context in which bodily realities trouble the governing structures of biomedicine, John A. Carranza's "*Tales of the City* as Historical Document: HIV/AIDS, Serialization, Urban Landscapes, and Sexuality," the eighth chapter in the collection, asks: "What can the reader learn from the intersections of literature and history?" To answer this methodological question, Carranza considers how Armistead Maupin's *Tales of the City* series is not just an engaging piece of fiction, but is also a first-hand account of the HIV/AIDS crisis of the 1970s and 1980s. The chapter takes an unconventional interdisciplinary approach by treating these fictional sources as historical documents. Carranza argues that *Tales of the City* is a unique primary source for historians as manuscript evidence of the HIV/AIDS epidemic. Written in a serial format, Maupin's instalments document real-time events that he witnessed. To this end, Carranza's examination of the literary series treats it

---

[12] Otniel E. Dror, "De-medicalizing the Medical Humanities," *European Legacy* 16, no. 3 (2011): 317–26, abstract.

as an archive that can be mined for a first-hand account of the arrival of HIV/AIDS in the American consciousness. The HIV/AIDS epidemic is taken up again through a different lens in the book's ninth chapter, by Benjamin Gagnon Chainey, titled "The Suffering Caregiver: Toward an Embodied Experience of End-of-Life Pain through Literature."

Gagnon Chainey begins his analysis with a provocation from the French writer Hervé Guibert: "Is the experience of pain preferable to the annihilation of experience?" Guibert's question resounds from the darkest point of his terminal phase: the writer died in 1991 at the apex of the Western AIDS epidemic. By extending Guibert's question to debates about the end of life, Gagnon Chainey reaches to the heart of contemporary debates over physician-assisted dying, which consider the patient's experience of "intolerable and irreversible pain"— physical or psychological—as a ticket to this "ultimate form of care": that of a "chosen and dignified death." As medical and legal discourses dominate physician-assisted death, it appears that many physician-caregivers working in end-of-life care find the task difficult. Rather than demanding that patients clearly express their pain within the bounds of medical and legal discourses for the physicians to assess it, Gagnon Chainey asks, could we instead conceive of modes of experiencing pain that would break free from such limiting forms of expression? Could a more attentive ear to the words of patients like Guibert provide a path toward a more resolutely empathetic experience? Beyond the alleviation of an emotional burden on providers, this kind of experience could reveal meaningful facets of pain endured by both patient and caregiver in their end-of-life relationship.

The volume's fourth and final part, "Alternatives," imagines new possibilities through cultural and aesthetic objects that contest biomedicine's dominant structures. This part offers compelling alternatives to the medical frameworks for knowledge that shape the world we live in today. The introduction details how creative writing and thought transcend the institutions and practices that govern our immediate perceptions of illness and health to imagine other ways of thinking about health and well-being. The two chapters that follow explore creative models of health in literary fiction that differ from conventional notions of health. The part presents speculative and dystopian fiction (and their analysis) as rich sites for experimentation.

Chapter 10, "Against 'Endochronology': Hormonal Rebellion and Generic Blending in *Confessions of the Fox*" by Diana Rose Newby, argues that Jordy Rosenberg's 2018 novel offers a creative inquiry into democratizing the consumption of hormones such as testosterone, imagining the possibilities for getting beyond the reductive logics of "endochronology," the "progress narrative of the alignment of sex hormones and subjectivity." Although sex hormones have been traditionally recruited by essentialist narratives of human behavior and identity, their actual activity tends to undermine those narratives: in its material expression, testosterone blurs the binary division of sex that Western culture and medicine have labored to uphold. Rosenberg's figurations of hormonal rebellion situate his novel at the intersection of contemporary hormone studies, gender and sexuality studies, and the new materialisms, a critical juncture where scholars have theorized not only bodies but also sex hormones themselves as "material-semiotic actors" that play a complex and critical role in the biomedical and political maintenance of sexual difference. The chapter suggests that Rosenberg's novel draws a through-line between its characters' hormonal rebellion and the novel's own formal insurgency. Attentive to the complicity of literary and disciplinary conventions with the often-violent management of biological sex, *Confessions* blends a variety of formal structures and styles in ways that complicate not only the novel's classification generically but also its designation as a novel at all.

The question of generic classification is taken up again by Anna Fenton-Hathaway in the volume's final chapter, "Whose Dystopia?" In a 2014 TEDx talk, Dr. Leana Wen described China's healthcare system as a "dystopia" and warned her American audience that they needed to act collectively to avoid recreating that dystopia at home. Fenton-Hathaway finds that such overt call to action is a feature of what Rob McAlear calls the "rhetorical model of dystopia," and her chapter asks: Is this rhetorical model useful for bioethicists? Or for the general public? In addition to Wen's talk, Fenton-Hathaway examines two other contexts in which the rhetorical model of dystopia has been applied to contemporary end-of-life policy concerns. These examples suggest that a dystopia is not an imaginary place of malevolence and suffering, as it is typically described, but rather a form of description, one that could be (and increasingly is) applied to mostly any place. The chapter concludes with a discussion of the imaginative limitations of "dystopian" writing and a call to reconsider the teaching of "dystopia" in the medical and health humanities.

The book's Coda, by Roanne Kantor, reflects on the problem of medico-scientific knowledge operating as a cultural practice. Such a framework for knowledge might be critiqued and challenged, or alternatively harnessed toward different aims. Kantor finds that the literary analyses that appear in many of the volume's chapters "shake up [our] doxa" about the function and effect of a hermeneutic analysis, especially in relation to the reading of the body. Kantor speculates about the future directions of interdisciplinary scholarship in the medical and health humanities. The critical orientation of the humanities might allow for a new compatibility with medicine's urgent temporal demands. Kantor's Coda, in dialogue with all the essays in this volume, invites us to reflect anew on how the medical and health humanities raise pressing questions that impinge on the body, politics, aesthetics, and the social world. Collectively, our writers interrogate how forms of representation and interpretation work to disseminate the influence of biomedicine—whether in a literary text, in an institutional setting, or even in an empathetic exchange. By taking seriously the question of how our ways of knowing in and experiencing the world are shaped by a hegemonic medicalized framework, their chapters urge us to examine how such a framework can teach us about human experience in the past and the present.

Part 1
Identities/Institutions

Introduction

This part addresses the multiple roles institutions (medical and otherwise) play in shaping an individual's sense of identity and belonging. Taking a literary approach, Livia Arndal Woods, Alicia Andrzejewski, and Kristina Fleuty read novels and plays to denaturalize biomedical knowledge and expand the layers of identity. Investigating a variety of texts along these themes, this part spans a wide historical period and a range of genres—from William Shakespeare's *The Winter's Tale* (1611) to Stephenie Meyer's *Twilight* (2005) and Harry Parker's *Anatomy of a Soldier* (2016)—and medical topics from postpartum exhaustion to prosthetic limbs. These multiple contexts manifest the role institutions play in shaping our understanding of illness and health. Taken together, the chapters point to the relevance of literary analysis as a hermeneutic mode for examining the historical and contemporary interplay between institution and identity. While indebted to Michel Foucault's critiques of the institutions that discipline bodies, these essays depart from that register to instead stress rhetorical and figurative devices that sustain power relations.

These chapters demonstrate the ethical and critical values that are shared by all contributions to the volume. By questioning the relationship between identity and institution—from the hospital to the military—the authors ask readers to think creatively with them about the literary devices that might support a disciplinary function. By being attuned to the presence and power of such devices, the chapters offer critical training both in how to communicate medical realities within and outside institutions and in how to analyze institutional rhetoric to uncover hidden areas of exclusion or bias. In their attention to mass communication (for instance, in Woods's analysis of modern megasellers), the chapters extend the purview of rhetorical analysis to widely disseminated forms and genres, a democratizing impulse that also points to an individual's sense of belonging to a community of readers.

The first two chapters illustrate both the lasting institutional problems that women face with respect to their reproductive health, and persistent collisions between female reproductive systems and the cultural and social mores in which they live. Chapter 1, by Woods, finds that nineteenth-century works by Samuel Taylor Coleridge and Sheridan Le Fanu employ tropes of vampirism and imprisonment in relation to pregnancy and childbirth that persist and flourish in twenty-first century bestsellers by Stephenie Meyer and E. L. James. Female vampirism, Woods argues, affords a compelling metaphorical register, in the nineteenth century and now, for engaging with the horrors of childbirth that contemporary medical practice has defamiliarized for us. Meanwhile, carceral and medical institutions figure in the representation of the pregnant female body, which in this genre becomes a "little prison." The transhistorical circulation of tropes that Woods traces offers a sharp commentary on the horrors of childbirth that bestselling fiction makes both invisible and "hypervisible."

The visibility of the gestating body and its encounter with (and against) the medical establishment is taken up again in Chapter 2 as it considers Shakespeare's "problem play," *The Winter's Tale* (1611). This chapter focuses on how the "dominant ideologies of chastity, companionate marriage, and motherhood fail women in the early modern period" through a close literary analysis of Shakespeare's late drama. The "lying-in rights" denied to Shakespeare's protagonist, Hermione, become a rallying point for a consideration of the absence of appropriate postpartum care denied to women in the present day, particularly women of color who are marginalized by the institutions of medicine. In keeping with the volume's stylistic value of clarity and rigor, the essay models the insertion of a forward-looking first-person perspective, even as it offers a fresh reading of some of Shakespeare's most enigmatic, unresolved scenes.

Further investigating the intersections between medical and nonmedical institutions in framing notions of health and illness, Chapter 3, by Fleuty, takes a narratologic approach to Harry Parker's novel *Anatomy of a Soldier* (2016), which adopts an unconventional narrative strategy—a point of view that inhabits the objects that the protagonist soldier encounters as he experiences wartime injury and civilian recovery. Parker's narrative redefines the boundaries between human self and object other (including a prosthetic limb, which blurs those boundaries) while also exploring the porous distinction between military and civilian life, and abled and disabled bodies. As with other chapters,

Fleuty's work finds in rhetorical and figurative experimentation new strategies for pursuing the ethical value of this collection—to enframe the human and historical dimensions of illness and health. Reading these texts in their contexts, the chapters in this part expose stereotypes, injustices, and the need for changes in institutions that frequently fail the people they are made to serve.

1

Reproducing Horror: Nineteenth-Century Vampires and Twenty-First Century Megasellers

Livia Arndal Woods

Reproduction has always been laced with horror. Conception, pregnancy, childbirth, and the postpartum periods can be magical, transcendent, and empowering, of course. But they *will* be uncertain, bloody, and risky. Humans in modernity have increasingly tried to distance themselves from the risks of reproduction by turning to medicine. When someone seeks out a licensed provider for prenatal care or childbirth, they express a connection to a particular medical history of obstetrics and gynecology that traces back about three hundred years. In the mid-twentieth century, the advances in this field began—almost miraculously—to obscure the ever-present horror of death in life that has always been with us. (Or, rather, these medical developments often obscured that horror for privileged persons.) But the horror remains; it is a legacy that will not be suppressed, a threat that cannot die, a violence that always stalks maternity.

In some ways, the stories Anglo-American literary traditions tell about reproductive horror have shifted over time. But—despite changes in reproductive care that would have been unimaginable even a century ago, not to mention three—these stories retain striking similarities. This chapter compares the specter of reproductive horror in nineteenth-century vampire tales to graphic depictions of pregnancy and childbirth in twenty-first century megaselling fiction to explore both the shifts and similarities. I gloss nineteenth-century

This chapter extends upon and draws from shorter pieces published by the author in *Synapsis: A Health Humanities Journal*, namely "Mothers, Memoir, and Medicine" (Woods, 2019), "Vampire Dearest: Maternal Bodies and the Female Vampire" (Woods, 2018), and "Mrs. Grey Will See You Now: The Legacy of Victorian Pregnancy" (Woods, 2018).

literary conventions for the treatment of reproductive bodies and read those conventions in conversation with Samuel Taylor Coleridge's 1816 "Christabel," Sheridan Le Fanu's 1872 *Carmilla*, and Bram Stoker's 1897 *Dracula*. Though sexuality, pregnancy, childbirth, and nursing are figurative rather than literal in these texts, all play against the general tendency of nineteenth-century realist fiction to avoid the depiction of reproductive bodies.

In the nineteenth century, the vampire emerges as an increasingly articulable nightmare of the repressed maternal body. It is the persistence of that nightmare in an era less shocked by female sexuality and more free from reproductive danger that makes readings of Stephenie Meyer's 2008 *Breaking Dawn* (the fourth and final book in her *Twilight* series) and E. L. James's 2012 *Fifty Shades Freed* (the third and final installment in her *Fifty Shades* trilogy) in conversation with these nineteenth-century texts interesting. These books are connected to the nineteenth century in part by *Twilight*'s engagement with the vampire literary tradition and *Fifty Shades*'s origin as *Twilight* fan-fiction. But *Twilight* and *Fifty Shades of Grey* are also connected to the nineteenth century and to one another by their explicit and repeated references to Victorian fiction. These twenty-first century megasellers draw on a tradition of horror centered on women's reproductive bodies. At a moment in which reproductive options and bodies are more varied and visible than at any other point in human history, and in which a concomitant reproductive literary explosion of sorts has occurred, it is particularly important to identify and critique familiar gothic patterns for articulating pregnancy and childbirth in climates of fear.

Representing Reproductive Bodies in Nineteenth-Century Literature

Just as nineteenth-century literature—especially literature of the Victorian period—tends to avoid representing sexuality explicitly, so does it tend to avoid representing reproductive bodies as bodies rather than as metaphors, acts, or social roles (like that of a "nursing mother").[1] This is perhaps most notable in the disinclination of nineteenth-century literature to name or depict pregnancy.[2]

---

[1] My use in this chapter of reproductive bodies to mean bodies during conception, pregnancy, childbirth, and the postpartum/nursing draws on Cristina Mazzoni's working definition of maternity in *Maternal Impressions: Pregnancy and Childbirth in Literature and Theory* (Ithaca, NY: Cornell University Press, 2002), 2.

[2] For more on this tendency, see Cynthia Northcutt Malone, "Near Confinement: Pregnant Women in the Nineteenth-Century British Novel," *Dickens Studies Annual* 29 (2000): 367–85; Clare Hanson,

When pregnant women *are* represented as having expanding bodies with particular sensations and needs, this representation serves as a kind of narrative punishment, an exposure of women who have erred or fallen. Unsurprisingly, pregnancy in the Victorian novel is a marker of moral (mis)development often figured as physical death, maternal failure, or miscarriage. Think of Cathy Linton's death in childbirth delivering a preterm daughter in Emily Brontë's 1847 *Wuthering Heights*, the failure of Hetty Sorrel to develop a meaningful maternal instinct in George Eliot's 1859 *Adam Bede*, or the miscarriage of Rosamond Lydgate's pregnancy in Eliot's 1871 *Middlemarch*, for example.

Plenty of babies were born in the nineteenth century (birth rates were high[3]), and plenty of babies are born in nineteenth-century literature. When these babies are born to characters who conform to Victorian expectations about femininity, their arrival is generally a soft-focus surprise, largely unanticipated by any explicit mentions of pregnancy. Insofar as pregnancy is mentioned in such cases, it is treated euphemistically, as an "interesting condition" or "indisposition," perhaps. Consider, for example, Dora's pregnancy and miscarriage in Charles Dickens's *David Copperfield* (1850):

> Dora was not strong. I had hoped that lighter hands than mine would help to mould her character, and that a baby-smile upon her breast might change my child-wife to a woman.
>
> It was not to be. The spirit fluttered for a moment on the threshold of its little prison, and, unconscious of captivity, took wing.[4]

Dora's pregnancy and miscarriage here is a bird, a "wing[ed]" "spirit" briefly "captive[e]" in a "little prison." That little prison is, of course, the body, but the body sketched at a remove. There is no morning sickness, no expansion, no blood, no pain. Dora may be silly, but she is not disobedient or immoral, and so the text veils her pregnant and miscarrying body with metaphor. That David had hoped—in much more bodily language—that a "baby-smile upon her breast" would "mold" Dora is an indication of the much easier depictions

---

A Cultural History of Pregnancy: Pregnancy, Medicine, and Culture, 1750–2000 (New York: Palgrave Macmillan, 2004), Livia Arndal Woods, "Now You See It: Concealing and Revealing Pregnant Bodies in 'Wuthering Heights' and 'The Clever Woman of the Family,'" *Victorian Network* 6, no. 1 (May 3, 2015): 32–54, https://doi.org/10.5283/vn.54, and "'Mrs. Grey Will See You Now': The Legacy of Victorian Pregnancy," *SYNAPSIS*, February 13, 2018, https://medicalhealthhumanities.com/2018/02/13/mrs-grey-will-see-you-now/.

[3] See Kaara L. Peterson, *Popular Medicine, Hysterical Disease, and Social Controversy in Shakespeare's England*, Literary and Scientific Cultures of Early Modernity (Burlington, VT: Ashgate, 2010).

[4] Charles Dickens, *David Copperfield*, ed. Nina Burgis, The Clarendon Dickens (Oxford: Clarendon Press, [1850] 1981), 596.

of breastfeeding in nineteenth-century literature. Such candor is particular to breastfeeding among embodied reproductive conditions, in part because it can fall under the protective umbrella of "nursing," which can refer to a host of different care acts.

Childbirth can be narrated more directly, but from a great distance. It occurs behind closed doors, between chapters, right before the beginning of a novel. *David Copperfield* once again offers a relatively paradigmatic example of the hazy distance from which childbirth is articulated:

> Whether I shall turn out to be the hero of my own life, or whether that station will be held by anybody else, these pages must show. To begin my life with the beginning of my life, I record that I was born (as I have been informed and believe) on a Friday, at twelve o'clock at night. It was remarked that the clock began to strike, and I began to cry, simultaneously.[5]

As the famous opening lines of the novel indicates, this is a story about the past being told in the present. The birth with which *Copperfield* opens is chronologically distant from the narrative setting. The syntactic hemming and hawing of "begin my life with the beginning of my life" creates another layer of distance, a thick coat of language between the reader and the birth made more marked by the parenthetical that follows shortly after. "As I have been informed and believe" certainly doesn't frame this event as untrue, but it does present the birth as strangely subjective, a little distant from the sort of pure fact of a life beginning. Finally, it is never articulated to whom the remark of the passive "it was remarked" belongs. A statement about the exact moment of David's birth floats free from direct attribution, distanced from the characters we soon come to know. In nineteenth-century fiction, childbirth is salient enough to plot that it cannot be avoided as assiduously as can pregnancy, but it is treated from a narrative remove rather than as an embodied moment.

Pregnancy, childbirth, and even nursing tend to function more explicitly as narrative markers for something, anything other than the physical experiences they also are. This tendency makes textual representations of reproductive bodies mutable, more expressive of the priorities and anxieties of a given culture than of, say, the likelihood that pregnant bellies will expand or nursing breasts will leak. Narrative convention for the representation of vampires is, of course, very different than these conventions for the representation of reproductive bodies. (I assume, for example, that literal, humanoid vampirism isn't a fact of

[5] Ibid., 1.

lived experience the way that reproduction is.) But nineteenth-century vampire narratives, which increasingly focus on the reproduction of the monstrous condition, have much in common with nineteenth-century depictions (or lack thereof) of reproduction. These are commonalities, moreover, that converge explicitly in the twenty-first century. Vampires are often read—perhaps most notably by Nina Auerbach in *Our Vampires, Ourselves*—as shifting ciphers for the desires and fears of a particular cultural-historical moment. Furthermore, vampiric bodies often express the fears about reproduction that realist nineteenth-century narratives struggle to depict directly: fears about the traumas of violation and sexuality, the dangers of heritability, the degree to which bodies exceed medical control. Auerbach's title is a play on this tendency, evoking the 1970 women's health classic *Our Bodies, Ourselves*. This intersection between reproduction and vampire narrative is particularly legible in notable nineteenth-century depictions of female vampires in Coleridge's "Christabel," Le Fanu's *Carmilla*, and Stoker's *Dracula*.

The Nineteenth-Century Female Vampire and the Reproductive Body

Among the immutable hallmarks of the vampire myth is disordered reproduction; vampires—as any child can explain—breed by biting. But as Auerbach observes, the bite as a hallmark of the vampire myth wasn't common until well into the nineteenth century as these tales gained popularity in English.[6] While they suck the life-energy from their victims, early nineteenth-century vampires neither bite nor reproduce—though, to be fair, early nineteenth-century vampires are sometimes not even referred to as vampires. Such is the case with Geraldine in Coleridge's poem "Christabel," likely written in 1798 and 1800 despite its 1816 publication. That Geraldine is a kind of parasite is clear enough, but Geraldine has no fangs, sucks no blood, and makes no "children." This makes the reproductive texture of her depiction particularly relevant evidence of an insistent intersection between narratives of vampires and narratives of (or avoidant of) reproduction.

"Christabel" relates a tale of sexual violation followed sometime later by a complicated, painful, and embodied "maternity" that makes manifest the vampire's relationship to her victim. Geraldine enters the poem as the result of

---

[6] Nina Auerbach, *Our Vampires, Ourselves* (Chicago: University of Chicago Press, 1995), 13.

an abduction from her father's home at the hands of "five warriors [who] seized [her and] … choked [her] cries with force and fright."[7] Here is a transgression of the boundaries between public and private, male and female, meant to "protect" women from danger. Geraldine cannot, however, articulate any sexual trauma in recounting this transgression, but, rather, performs a repetitive recoiling and weakening at intervals after her "rescue" by Christabel. These repetitions are triggered by the crossing of boundaries (the gates to the castle and the doorway into Christabel's chamber) and reach their apex in a bedroom. It is here that Geraldine discloses her physical trauma to Christabel:

> Then drawing in her breath aloud,
> Like one that shuddered, she unbound
> The cincture from beneath her breast …
> Behold! Her bosom and half her side—
> A sight to dream of, not to tell![8]

The alliterative emphasis in this scene of revelation falls on a "b" sound that highlights "breast" and "bosom." But these are only the body parts that can be named; this passage also locates something that cannot be named ("A sight to dream of, not to tell") along Geraldine's "side," or torso. That unnamable thing—suggestive of the inarticulable pregnant bellies of much nineteenth-century literature—exerts its power via silence. Geraldine's body, particularly her breasts and "side," reveals and is marked by her sexual trauma in ways that are suggestive of the reproductive body. Geraldine articulates her body as her "shame":

> In the touch of this bosom there worketh a spell,
> Which is lord of thy utterance Christabel!
> Thou knowest tonight, and wilt know tomorrow,
> This mark of my shame, this seal of my sorrow;
> But vainly thou warrest,
> For this is alone in
> Thy power to declare …[9]

Geraldine passes this mesmerizing "spell" to Christabel via the breast, the "touch of this bosom."[10] This "bosom" repeats from the passage above, emphasizing

---

[7] Samuel Taylor Coleridge, "Christabel," in *Norton Anthology of English Literature*, ed. Stephen Greenblatt, 10th ed., vol. 2 (New York: W.W. Norton, [1816] 2018), ll. 79–81.
[8] Ibid., ll. 247–53.
[9] Ibid., ll. 267–72.
[10] It is helpful to note Auerbach's observation that the site of Vampire contagion moves upward from the breast to the neck over the course of the nineteenth century. *Our Vampires, Ourselves* (Chicago: University of Chicago Press, 1995), 52–3.

this as a scene of nursing inverted: Geraldine's breasts are sucking words from Christabel's mouth ("Lord of thy utterance") rather than offering sustenance. Having already shaken off the spirit of the mother who died giving birth to Christabel, Geraldine establishes a distorted maternal relationship to Christabel by some "spell" in her body, a generative spell that cannot be named.

The relationship between "Christabel" and Le Fanu's *Carmilla* has been recognized by literary critics since at least Arthur H. Nethercot's "Coleridge's 'Christabel' and Le Fanu's 'Carmilla'" (1949), in which the critic traces the many similarities between the two texts. Nethercot notices that "the antagonists in both stories ... are female vampires; and female vampires are comparatively rare ... More than this, the main victims ... are women; and such restriction of sex—women to women—is even rarer."[11] Though Nethercot addresses and dismisses lesbian readings of these similarities, this connection and its sexual texture have been a common thread in criticism on the two texts ever since. What has been less common is a focus on the particularly *reproductive* texture of the sexualized female bodies in "Christabel" and *Carmilla*.

As in "Christabel," in *Carmilla* the eponymous vampire relates a trauma that signals the transgression of sexual boundaries. Explaining her odd habit of sleeping with the bedroom door locked (with additional meanings related to the necessities of her life as a vampire), Carmilla tells her prey/lover Laura: "I was all but assassinated in my bed, wounded here," she touched her breast, "and never was the same since."[12] The terror of this attack haunts Carmilla, and she repeats the circumstances of it again and again: stealing into the bedrooms of unsuspecting women and violating them. But Carmilla also forms a maternal bond with her special victims, like the motherless Laura to whom she declares, "I live in your warm life, and you shall die—die, sweetly die—into mine."[13] The nestling qualities of this description call to mind a twisting of both the relationship of pregnant mother to fetus and the relationship of nursing mother to child. This is an implication heightened by the location of Carmilla's bites on Laura's breast. The first instance of such a wound occurs in Laura's bedroom when she is six years old:

> I saw a solemn, but very pretty face looking at me from the side of the bed. It was that of a young lady who was kneeling, with her hands under the coverlet.

---

[11] Arthur H. Nethercot, "Coleridge's 'Christabel' and Lefanu's 'Carmilla,'" *Modern Philology* 47, no. 1 (1949): 32.
[12] Joseph Sheridan Le Fanu, "Carmilla," in *In a Glass Darkly*, ed. Robert Tracy, Oxford World's Classics (Oxford: Oxford University Press, [1872] 1999), 276.
[13] Ibid., 263.

I looked at her with a kind of pleased wonder, and ceased whimpering. She caressed me with her hands, and lay down beside me on the bed, and drew me towards her, smiling; I felt immediately delightfully soothed, and fell asleep again. I was wakened by a sensation as if two needles ran into my breast very deep at the same moment, and I cried loudly.[14]

This "young lady" (Carmilla) takes an embodied and maternal stance with the motherless Laura, climbing into her bed and "caress[ing]" and "sooth[ing]" her. But the seemingly maternal body reveals itself to be horrific when, instead of offering Laura sustenance, it draws sustenance—not milk but blood—from her breast.

Bram Stoker's *Dracula* differs from "Christabel" and *Carmilla* in many ways. Here, the most notable is that the central, eponymous vampire of *Dracula* is male. Auerbach notes that, "in nineteenth-century iconography, male vampires are allies of death who end their narratives by killing or dying, but females are so implicated in life's sources that their stories overwhelm closure."[15] And, indeed, Dracula's death concludes Stoker's tale relatively tidily. Insofar as a record of his gothic threat survives, it survives in the reproductive body of Mina, his not-quite-vampire victim: her son—given the names of all the men who fought against Dracula—is born on the anniversary of Dracula's death, and "this boy will some day know what a brave and gallant woman his mother is. Already he knows her sweetness and loving care; later on he will understand how some men so loved her, that they did dare much for her sake." Though "every trace of all that [time] had been blotted out," it will survive in the memory of Mina's child in his understanding of her as his endangered mother.[16]

But perhaps more paradigmatic of the female vampire's "implicat[ion] in life's sources" is the character of Lucy Westenra, who is turned into a vampire by Dracula before being destroyed by the men who desired her when she was alive. Consider the scene in which the undead Lucy first appears. As Leslie Anne Minot notes, this scene and others like it have primarily been of interest to critics writing on "mothering and 'bad mothers.'"[17] Minot is interested in

---

[14] Ibid., 246.
[15] Auerbach, *Our Vampires, Ourselves*, 50.
[16] Bram Stoker, *Dracula*, ed. Nina Auerbach and David J. Skal (New York: W.W. Norton, [1897] 1996), 326.
[17] Leslie Ann Minot, "Vamping the Children: The 'Bloofer Lady,' the 'London Minotaur' and Child-Victimization in Late-Nineteenth-Century England," in *Victorian Crime, Madness and Sensation*, ed. Andrew Maunder and Grace Moore, The Nineteenth Century Series (Aldershot: Ashgate, 2004), 207.

the overt sexuality of these scenes, especially the ways in which we can read them as reflections on child abuse. I am most interested in the implications of the sexual and the reproductive body—especially, again, the breast—in these scenes. Lucy is holding a small child "strenuously to her breast," not to nourish it but to take her nourishment from it. Once sweet and virginal, Lucy is now "unclean and full of hell-fire ... blaz[ing] with unholy light, and ... wreathed in a voluptuous smile."[18] Lucy—once haunted by barely remembered nocturnal bedroom attacks—is now "voluptuous," actively enjoying her body. This voluptuous Lucy is referred to by the children on whom she preys as a "bloofer lady,"[19] "a demonic mother-parody, taking nourishment from children instead of giving it," and evoking cultural anxieties about the power and danger of women's reproductive bodies.[20]

Throughout *Dracula*, Lucy is characterized by a sexualized hypervisibility typified in the three marriage proposals she receives on the same day and in the "bloofer lady" into which she is transformed. Whereas nineteenth-century texts actively avoid focusing the narrative gaze on reproductive bodies, there's a pulsing visibility about the bodies of all the female vampires this chapter reads. Their bodies are seen as bodies rather than as soft-focus expressions of feminine souls. This flirtation with seeing reproductive embodiment via the sexualized hypervisibility of female vampires is a sharp point of connection between the nineteenth-century and Meyer's early twenty-first century *Breaking Dawn*. What I'm referring to as the "hypervisibility" of bodily horror—whether vampiric, reproductive, or both—is one of the central connections I draw between the Victorian period and our own in this chapter. In Victorian vampire literature, the supernatural female body pulses with power. In contemporary megasellers, the reproductive body takes on this spotlit position. In *Breaking Dawn*, the horror of reproduction explodes into the vampire narrative explicitly rather than implicitly. The *Twilight* series—in turn—produces its own (horrible) child in James's *Fifty Shades of Grey*. Contrary to Victorian literature, in which sexuality and the reproductive body are often repressed, James's novels repress the figure of the vampire and express the dangers women face through a literal visualization of the fetus.

---

[18] Stoker, *Dracula*, 227.
[19] Ibid., 160.
[20] Gail B. Griffin, "'Your Girls That You All Love Are Mine': 'Dracula' and the Victorian Male Sexual Imagination," *International Journal of Women's Studies* 3, no. 5 (September 1, 1980): 460.

Reproductive Horror in *Twilight* and *Fifty Shades of Grey*

Connections between Stephanie Meyer's *Twilight* series and nineteenth-century literature range from Meyer's naming preferences (she chose Edward as a name for her protagonist because of inspiration from "Charlotte Bronte's Mr. Rochester and Jane Austen's Mr. Ferrars") to Bella's compulsive reading of *Wuthering Heights*.[21] A more explicit connection to the nineteenth-century vampiric tradition is that Meyer's vampires aren't vulnerable to the sun (except insofar as it reveals their otherness). As Auerbach notes, being destroyed by the sun is a twentieth-century addition to the vampire myth.[22] Though all the "vamping" scenes of "Christabel," *Carmilla*, and *Dracula* I've read here occur at night, the sun isn't an existential threat to the Victorian vampire. Neither is the danger the light poses to Meyer's vampires existential: Meyer's vampires sparkle in the sun. It renders them hypervisible, not dead. And insofar as vampires figure anxieties about reproductive horror, that horror itself becomes hypervisible in *Breaking Dawn*.

The *Twilight* series follows Bella Swan on her path toward becoming a vampire wife and mother. Bella moves to Forks, Washington, as a teenager. There, she meets the Cullens, a family of "vegetarian" vampires living off the blood of animals.[23] At first, the overwhelming scent of Bella's blood threatens to drive Edward Cullen to break his diet, but in the end, Edward masters his desires enough to have a relationship with Bella, whom he must constantly remind of the danger he poses to her. As a result of that "danger," they maintain a chaste relationship until after their marriage in *Breaking Dawn*. Again and again over the course of the quadrilogy, Edward emphasizes the inherent threat of any physical interaction with the human Bella, establishing sexual contact between the two as inescapably violent. Once married, Edward and Bella do have sex, but Edward is unable to avoid leaving Bella bruised, sore, and pregnant with his inhuman spawn. The message is that sexuality between a vampire and a human can only ever be traumatic, and this trauma possesses Bella's body fully and quickly. Bella experiences an accelerated pregnancy in which she is battered from the inside by her half-vampire fetus; its kicks and movements break her ribs. Although Edward declares that "in myths ... other monsters like this would chew their way out of their own mothers," this fear proves only partially correct.[24] ella's labor is triggered

---

[21] Stephenie Meyer, "The Story of Twilight & Getting Published," *Stephenie Meyer* (blog), accessed February 5, 2021, https://stepheniemeyer.com/the-story-of-twilight-getting-published/.
[22] Auerbach, *Our Vampires, Ourselves*, 74.
[23] Stephenie Meyer, *New Moon* (New York: Little, Brown Books for Young Readers, 2006), 188.
[24] Stephenie Meyer, *Breaking Dawn* (New York: Little, Brown, 2008), 307.

by the fetus's surge toward a cup of "dark red blood spilling out onto the pale fabric" of a living room carpet.²⁵ There is "the strangest muffled sound from the center of her body," and then Bella passes out, never to regain full consciousness during labor or what remains of her human life.²⁶

What happens next is an explosion of the terrible reproductive possibilities that stalk the edges of the vampiric narratives in "Christabel," *Carmilla*, and *Dracula*. Bella gives birth to a half-vampire child and she is herself reborn as a vampire all in the space of one extended, drugged, partially conscious episode marked by explicitly embodied references to blood and pain. "The pain," during Bella's lucid moments, is "bewildering."²⁷ Her skin is "red with blood—the blood that had flowed from her mouth, the blood smeared all over the creature, and fresh blood welling out of a tiny double-crescent bite mark just over her left breast."²⁸ This "tiny bite mark just over her left breast" is a wound inflicted on Bella by her vampire baby, an evocation of the nineteenth-century insistence of the breast and the bosom as the site of female vampiric focus. Another evocation of the nineteenth century occurs in the effect pain management has on Bella: "I hadn't guessed," she says, "that the morphine would have this effect—that it would pin me down and gag me."²⁹ Bella's silencing here recalls the silencing of Christabel, for example, but also the silencing of the reproductive body in nineteenth-century literature more generally.³⁰

That what silences Bella is the administration of a drug, though, speaks to the shifts in the medicalization of reproduction that occurred between the nineteenth and twenty-first centuries. A very real awareness of the deadly possibilities of reproduction in the nineteenth century runs alongside the period's unwillingness to represent pregnant and birthing bodies in fiction. Though medicine didn't bring its significant (though always inequitable)

---

[25] This cup of blood had been prepared for Bella herself. Her pregnancy triggers a previously dormant appetite. Emma Dunn's "Good Vampires Don't Eat: Anorexic Logic in Stephanie Meyers *Twilight* Series" notes that "the scenes in which Bella does eat can be divided into two categories: those in which she eats because she must, which occur throughout the series, and those in which Bella eats for pleasure, which occur primarily in *Breaking Dawn*, during her pregnancy" (*Jeunesse: Young People, Texts, Cultures* 10, no. 1 [June 22, 2018]: 116). This suggestion of pregnancy as a condition embodied by appetitiveness (and physical expansion) calls to mind Susan Bordo's work in *Unbearable Weight: Feminism, Western Culture, and the Body* (Berkeley: University of California Press, 1993) on the Victorian roots of anorexic logic. In the critical conversation on appetite and appetite suppression in the *Twilight* series, then, we see another connection to the nineteenth century.

[26] Meyer, Breaking Dawn, 346.
[27] Ibid., 369.
[28] Ibid., 353.
[29] Ibid., 377.
[30] This *Twilight* birth similarly recalls the effects of the Twilight Birth or Twilight Sleep drug cocktail administered to women for much of the mid-twentieth century, though a closer reading of this is not possible in the scope of this chapter.

declines in maternal and fetal mortality to Britain and America until the twentieth century, the nineteenth century saw the widespread establishment of obstetric and gynecologic study and training, maternity wards in hospitals, the administration of pain medication during labor, and the understanding of germ theory that preceded those declines. While medicine was creating itself as a field that could look pregnancy and childbirth in the face and battle the death it saw there, Anglo-American literary cultures looked politely away. By the end of the twentieth and beginning of the twenty-first centuries, medicine had created the impression of a safe distance between birth and death. From this seemingly safe distance, we started to stare: "In just a couple of decades" reproductive bodies went from "shameful and hidden to sexy and spectacular."[31] Compare, for example, the billowing cut of maternity wear common into the early 1990s with the form-fitting styles more popular in this century. Bella may be silenced by the drugs she's given during birth, but her body is rendered hypervisible by a medical context that enables us to see both her sexual awakening during her honeymoon and the resulting reproductive gore.

* * *

Like the *Twilight* series, the *Fifty Shades of Grey* trilogy evokes the nineteenth century explicitly and implicitly throughout.[32] But where the nineteenth-century vampire as a nightmare of the maternal body becomes a waking—if fevered—reality in *Twilight*, it recedes into the unspoken recesses of *Fifty Shades*. Though E. L. James's novels can see and name the sexuality and reproductive bodies that nineteenth-century narratives cannot, the vampire just under the surface of the text cannot be articulated. This present-absence is, of course, the result of the *Fifty Shades* origin story: E. L. James's novels began as fanfiction retellings of Stephanie Meyer's stories, and their publication depended on a careful excision of anything directly attributable to the *Twilight* universe. The books themselves are not unlike the undead: strange reproductions sucking life from another source. Furthermore, as Sara Upstone has noted,

---

[31] Kelly Oliver, *Knock Me Up, Knock Me Down: Images of Pregnancy in Hollywood Films* (New York: Columbia University Press, 2012), 2.

[32] See, for example, Amy Billone's exploration of the nineteenth-century texture of both books in *The Future of the Nineteenth-Century Dream-Child*: "Just as it reads as fanfiction of Stephanie Meyer's *Twilight* series, the hugely popular *Fifty Shades* series reads a fanfiction of Thomas Hardy's *Tess of the d'Urbervilles*, a novel with which E. L. James's characters are obsessed." *The Future of the Nineteenth-Century Dream-Child: Fantasy, Dystopia, Cyberculture*, Children's Literature and Culture (New York: Routledge, 2016), 115.

Fifty Shades as "mommy porn" "draws heavily from Meyer in the pregnancy sections."[33,34]

Twilight's hypervisual expression of the vampire as narrative vector for reproductive anxiety is perhaps most apparent in the film adaptation of *Breaking Dawn*. When the movie was released in 2011, a spate of popular pieces on the graphic horror of the pregnancy and birth scenes was published.[35] Similarly, the narrative work of pregnancy as an expression of danger and fear in James is perhaps most accessible in the trailer for the 2018 film adaptation of *Fifty Shades Freed*, the third and final installment in the *Fifty Shades* series. The trailer reveals heroine Anastasia (Ana) Steele's pregnancy as a kind of narrative "twist" in its final seconds. It starts with a montage of clips spanning the first meeting of Christian Grey and Ana to their engagement, wedding, scenes of Ana's newfound empowerment as Mrs. Grey, the mansion Christian buys, and a dream vacation reached via private plane. This celebration of heteronormative capitalism is all interspersed with (mostly vanilla) sex scenes. At the 1:10 mark, though, conflict emerges: Ana's abusive former boss, Jack, seems to have gone from bad to murderous worse; we get a glimpse of Christian's own abusive past, of Christian and Ana's BDSM sex life, of Ana getting herself a gun, and Ana meeting Jack face to face as the thumping rhythm of Bishop Briggs's remix of "Never Tear Us Apart" crescendos and dovetails with a breathy sigh from Ana and the instruction that the viewer shouldn't "miss the climax." Cue title. And then, in the final five seconds, a close-up on Ana's shocked face and a voice on the other side of camera: "It seems you're pregnant, Mrs. Grey."[36]

This revelation revises the scenes of sexualized danger, simulated and real, that precede it. It posits a specific reproductive future and, in so doing, positions the murderous ex-boss, the gun, getting tied up and whipped as threats to that

---

[33] Sara Upstone, "Beyond the Bedroom: Motherhood in E. L. James's *Fifty Shades of Grey* Trilogy," *Frontiers: A Journal of Women Studies* 37, no. 2 (2016): 162, https://doi.org/10.5250/fronjwomestud.37.2.0138.

[34] Much of the popular and scholarly conversation around *Fifty Shades* has revolved around the perceived feminism or antifeminism of the series. In this context, Upstone (2016, p. 139) offers a particularly focused analysis of this "mommy-porn" descriptor and "the novels' positioning of women in terms of one contested and dominant social role—motherhood" rather than the more intuitive sex-object.

[35] See, for example, Jen Chaney, "The Pregnancies in 'Breaking Dawn' and 'American Horror Story': A Comparative Study," *Washington Post*, November 22, 2011; Katherine Don, "Bringing Up Baby: The Terrifying, Transformational Birth Scene Showdown: *Twilight* vs. *Game of Thrones*," *Bitch Media*, November 22, 2011; or Dana Stevens, "*Twilight: Breaking Dawn*, Part I Is One Seriously Sick Little Blockbuster," *Slate Magazine*, November 18, 2011, for a few examples.

[36] James Foley, *Fifty Shades Freed Trailer 3* (KinoCheck International, 2018).

future, threats to the lineage-bearing "Mrs. Grey" as much as to Ana herself. In both the film adaptation and the book, the scene in which Ana's pregnancy is discovered is followed by a very early ultrasound during which Ana is able to see "a little blip"[37]:

> It's a little blip. There's a tiny little blip in my belly. Tiny. Wow. I forget my discomfort as I stare dumbfounded at the blip … The little blip is a baby. A real honest to goodness baby. Christian's baby. My baby. Holy cow. A baby![38]

From this point on, Ana thinks of this pregnancy as a "little blip" for much of the novel. The visual image of the embryo becomes the text's shorthand for the pregnancy. Where Bella's pregnancy is hypervisible because it develops at an exaggeratedly fast pace and literally explodes in and on the body, Ana's pregnancy is figured in a hypervisible vocabulary that expresses a sea change in the way we manage reproductive bodies. For all of human history until the twentieth century, pregnancy was visible only insofar as its embodied indicators were visible. Even these cues (such as an enlarged belly, for example) weren't conclusive so much as indicative. The widespread availability of ultrasound technology in the final decades of the twentieth century radically revised the ways in which we understand pregnancy and its dangers.[39]

This shift in pregnancy from a primarily interior, hidden state to a condition that can be externalized and made visible seems to echo the work *Fifty Shades* does as fan-fiction: pulling a possibility from the realm of the minor, the unspoken, or the interpretive into the light. A dismissive attitude about the literary value of fan-fiction evokes the anxieties about disordered reproduction familiar to scholars of vampire literature. In reading *Fifty Shades Freed*, this chapter returns full-circle to a vampire narrative that eschews the word "vampire"—and yet, like vampire stories, *Fifty Shades* is a misbegotten child able to locate certain cultural pulses that remain inaccessible to much of the literary landscape.

---

[37] Upstone (2016, p. 162) notes that James's "use of 'blip' for Ana's fetus is a reworking of Bella's designation of her unborn child as a nudge; likewise Bella's protective instinct against Edward's wish for her to abort their unborn child is extremely similar to James's storyline."

[38] E. L. James, *Fifty Shades Freed* (New York: Vintage, 2012), 411.

[39] For more on this, Lisa Meryn Mitchell, *Baby's First Picture: Ultrasound and the Politics of Fetal Subjects* (Toronto: University of Toronto Press, 2001); Janelle S. Taylor, *The Public Life of the Fetal Sonogram: Technology, Consumption, and the Politics of Reproduction*, Studies in Medical Anthropology (New Brunswick, NJ: Rutgers University Press, 2008); Julie Roberts, The Visualised Foetus: A Cultural and Political Analysis of Ultrasound Imagery, Theory, Technology and Society (Abingdon: Routledge, 2012); and Emelie Egger's two-part blog post: "Five Decades of 'Semiotic' Fetal Imagery in the US: Parts 1 and 2," *SYNAPSIS*, 2019.

Conclusion

Reproduction is terrifying and it always has been; centering danger on the reproductive body isn't a pathology of a literary tradition so much as an expression of reality. To associate horror with reproduction is, especially in the broad arc of human history, good sense. The degree to which these dangers are understood to be articulable as the embodied realities of women, however, varies. Nineteenth-century literature tended to avoid such articulations, and some of the most embodied reproductive narratives aren't explicitly reproductive at all. Yet, literature found symbolic and indirect ways to represent implicit cultural fears. The vampire emerges as a figure for the expression of nineteenth-century anxieties ranging from nonnormative sexuality to nationalism. This chapter has demonstrated the ways in which female vampires reflect anxieties about maternal embodiment in literature of this period. And though we may not now be Foucault's "Other Victorians" (if ever we were), so many of the stories we tell and sell about women's reproductive lives rely on the specters of Victorian threats for narrative traction.[40] Such a reliance is particularly evident in the *Twilight* and *Fifty Shades* series, as perhaps in genre literature more generally. As this chapter has demonstrated, the final installment of each megaselling series transforms the nineteenth-century game of reproductive peek-a-boo into an explosion of the visible.

But the contemporary turn toward explicit textual representations of reproductive bodies is hardly limited to the novels of Stephanie Meyer and E.L. James. Picking up on a recurring reproductive thread—perhaps best typified by Margaret Atwood's 1985 *The Handmaid's Tale* (airing as a visually striking, critically lauded Hulu series at the time of writing)—dystopian literature has increasingly imagined worlds made horrible for women on the basis of their reproductive capacity (or lack thereof). And the last decade saw a glut of memoirs grappling with what it means to navigate fear and the reproductive body. Eula Biss's *On Immunity* (2014), Maggie Nelson's *The Argonauts* (2015), Ariel Levy's *The Rules Do Not Apply* (2017), and Angela Garber's *Like a Mother* (2018) are all notable examples. As our abilities to shape and control reproduction increase at dizzying speeds, contemporary literature is asking insistent questions about the relationship between danger and conception, pregnancy, childbirth, and early maternity. *Breaking Dawn* and *Fifty Shades Freed* offer particularly clear examples of the ways these questions work in conversation with longer literary traditions.

---

[40] Michel Foucault, *The History of Sexuality*, first American ed. (New York: Pantheon Books, 1978).

2

Postpartum Exhaustion in William Shakespeare's *The Winter's Tale*

Alicia Andrzejewski

Introduction

In William Shakespeare's *The Winter's Tale* (c. 1609–11), Hermione is dragged to court by her husband, King Leontes, a few days postpartum to defend herself against accusations of infidelity. In the scenes prior, Leontes descends into the "diseased opinion" that Hermione is carrying his friend's child—and his subjects "must believe" him.[1] Because of her husband's cruelty and his male subjects' complicity, Hermione gives birth to her daughter, Perdita, in a jail cell. Moreover, Perdita is born "before her time"[2]—a premature delivery attributed to Hermione's "frights and griefs."[3] This child is then taken from her mother and "haled out to murder."[4] Mamillius, Hermione's son, the Kingdom's "greatest promise,"[5] begins to "decline, droop," and languish as Leontes separates him from his mother, blaming Hermione's "dishonor" for their son's illness.[6] In short, for the "good queen" Hermione, *The Winter's Tale* demonstrates how the dominant ideologies of chastity, companionate marriage, and motherhood fail women in the early modern period.[7]

Once in court, however, Hermione gathers herself together and pleads against Leontes's "immodest hatred" with eloquence and rhetorical skill reminiscent of

---

[1] William Shakespeare, *The Winter's Tale*, ed. John Pitcher and Arden Shakespeare, 3rd ser. (London: Bloomsbury, 2010), 1.2.332, 295.
[2] Ibid., 2.2.31.
[3] Ibid., 2.2.21–3.
[4] Ibid., 3.2.99.
[5] Ibid., 1.2.32.
[6] Ibid., 2.3.12–16.
[7] Ibid., 2.3.57. Leontes retreats from one of the very few normative families figured in Shakespeare's canon, as Stephen Orgel points out, "consisting of father, mother, and children," in William Shakespeare, *The Winter's Tale: The Oxford Shakespeare*, ed. Stephen Orgel (Oxford: Oxford University Press, 2008), 12.

Shakespeare's earlier courtroom heroines.[8] While doing so, Hermione meditates being denied the "child-bed privilege":

HERMIONE
                    which 'longs
To women of all fashion; lastly, hurried
Here to this place, i' the open air, before
I have got strength of limit.[9]

The "child-bed privilege" Hermione describes in these lines is the early modern practice of "lying in" for about a month postpartum, concluded by a churching ceremony to symbolize the new mother's reentry into the social world. Laura Gowing argues that many early modern women did not fully observe the rules of the lying-in period, which included abstaining from sex, household labor, and going to church, yet "the concept of the lying-in month was still a powerful one."[10] By arguing that the lying-in period belongs to women "of *all* fashion," Hermione highlights Leontes's insensitive demand that she defend herself in public during a private time, by adopting a "strength" she has not yet recovered in order to accommodate his fantasies. She reminds audiences that no woman—chaste or otherwise—deserves the abuse she endures.

Hermione's argument, that all pregnant people deserve to rest after giving birth, is one that we—postpartum bodies—are still making in the face of exhausting conditions. In a gynecological manual written centuries after *The Winter's Tale*, *Obstetrics: Normal and Problem Pregnancies* (2017), the postpartum period, or *puerperium*, is defined as the 6–12 weeks after the delivery of the placenta. The authors also note, however, that many cardiovascular changes and psychological changes "persist" for many more months, often years.[11] The authors go on to say that postpartum care has been shaped by traditions, superstitions, and rituals as opposed to science: "For example, the 6-week postpartum check-up approximates the end of the 40 days of rest and sexual separation required in traditional societies."[12] These historical touches across time—these articulations of postpartum care—are most vivid in the *lack of care* faced by people in both "traditional societies," a gesture to the society Hermione finds herself in, perhaps,

---

[8] *WT* 3.2.100.
[9] *WT* 3.2.101–4.
[10] Laura Gowing, *Common Bodies: Women, Touch and Power in Seventeenth-Century England* (New Haven, CT: Yale University Press, 2003), 172.
[11] Steven G. Gabbe et al., *Obstetrics: Normal and Problem Pregnancies*, 7th ed. (Philadelphia, PA: Elsevier, [1986] 2017), 498.
[12] Ibid., 499.

and our own. In short, Hermione's courtroom speech is harrowing not only because of the abuse she endures but also because pregnant people must still navigate a world that offers lip-service, at best, when it comes to postpartum care.

Although Hermione argues that lying-in rights *belong* to all women, hers are denied by her husband, in particular. Leontes's treatment of his wife as both a husband and king, and his rapid descent into madness in the early acts of the play, has puzzled early modern scholars. On the one hand, in many ways, his "diseased opinion" that Hermione is unfaithful defies "the canons of 'realistic' psychological portraiture, even in early modern drama."[13] On the other hand, early modern drama offers us many iterations of the same story—pregnant people are threatening in their ability to body forth the future. As Beatrice Bradley and Tanya Pollard observe, Leontes's "anxiety about his wife's reproductive powers" leads to the violence that ensues.[14] The anxiety medical professionals then and now feel about the power pregnant people have to shape unborn children leads to unnecessary and violent intervention by authority figures.

Despite Hermione's persuasive argument that she has done nothing to deserve this treatment, as well as an oracle that affirms her innocence, Leontes is not convinced she is chaste until his son, Mamillius, is declared dead. Mamillius's name and subsequent death is a clear reference to Leontes's disregard of motherhood, infancy, and nursing in the play.[15] Similarly, Leontes orders that Perdita, his newborn infant, be plucked from her mother's breast shortly after birth, with "the innocent milk" still in her "most innocent mouth"—according to Hermione in her courtroom speech.[16] It is not puzzling, then, if one considers the nonsensical dismissal, policing, and hypocrisy pregnant people have faced across time, that Leontes exhausts Hermione as a mother, pregnant person, and someone who has just given birth. If Leontes is exhausted, it's an exhaustion of his own making.

---

[13] Gail Kern Paster, *The Body Embarrassed: Drama and the Disciplines of Shame in Early Modern England*, illustrated ed. (Ithaca, NY: Cornell University Press, 1993), 266.

[14] Paige Martin Reynolds, among others, observes that "Leontes could also be reacting to his wife's pregnancy not only of evidence of infidelity, but as a signifier of her sexuality in general," in "Sin, Sacredness, and Childbirth in Early Modern Drama," *Medieval & Renaissance Drama in England* 28 (2015): 40. In other words, pregnant women in the period disrupted the dichotomy of virgin and mother, a liminal and thus threatening bodily state. See also, Beatrice Bradley and Tanya Pollard, "Tragicomic Conceptions: *The Winter's Tale* as Response to Amphitryo," *English Literary Renaissance* 47, no. 2 (March 1, 2017): 255, https://doi.org/10.1086/693893.

[15] For an extended consideration of Mamillius's name and death, see Susan Snyder's "Mamillius and Gender Polarization in *The Winter's Tale*." Of note, Snyder argues that Hermione's restoration "operates like a long-delayed churching ceremony," but argues that "the concluding ritual ends a sexual separation inscribed on a whole society": *Shakespeare Quarterly* 50, no. 1 (1999): 8.

[16] *WT* 3.2.98.

In light of all Leontes puts Hermione through, however, it is unsurprising that her denied lying-in rights have not garnered as much critical attention. As Kaara Peterson observes, rarely "have the more *localized* early modern stories about revivification come to our awareness or their immediate contexts."[17] In other words, Hermione's revival after the sixteen years she is presumed dead by Leontes lends itself to rigorous critical inquiry, while an aside in a larger attempt to argue for her life seems less important, or simply unrelated. It is also the case, however, that postpartum recovery is obscured from our current cultural imagination as a crucial part of pregnancy and motherhood narratives. *The Winter's Tale* is part of this long legacy of how we imagine pregnancy and the postpartum period today—and attending to this legacy informs the immediate early modern contexts Peterson describes. Moreover, Shakespeare's play is just one example of how works of fiction grant glimpses into the medical histories embedded in our collective imaginings; in this case, the histories that narrate the relationship between the postpartum period and our understanding of exhaustion, burnout, and revival. In *Exhaustion: A History*, Anna Katharina Schaffner meditates on this relationship between works of fiction and medicine, the affective and physical state of exhaustion, and the diagnoses that accompany it.[18] These interdisciplinary relationships undoubtedly inform Shakespeare's representations of pregnant people—Hermione's treatment and postpartum revival, in particular.

For these reasons, I argue that Hermione's denied "lying-in" rights in the first act of William Shakespeare's *The Winter's Tale* set in motion the play's larger concern with bodies and worlds that are exhausted—weary, precarious, and abandoned. The demands of pregnancy and motherhood are central to *The Winter's Tale*'s inciting incident, and Hermione's trajectory after she is abused postpartum makes clear that this "sad tale ... best for winter" is about exhaustion, retreat, and emergence only after the promise of something better.[19] As Schaffner argues, "Exhaustion is related to some of our darkest primordial fears: decay, illness, aging, waning of engagement, death."[20] In *The Winter's Tale*, these fears,

---

[17] Kaara L. Peterson's reading of Hermione's postpartum experience is that "Shakespeare's portrayal in *The Winter's Tale* of Hermione's tragic postpartum death, 16-year absence, and reanimation pointedly mirrors the hibernating hysteric and probably accounts for the title of the play": *Popular Medicine, Hysterical Disease, and Social Controversy in Shakespeare's England*, Literary and Scientific Cultures of Early Modernity (Abingdon: Routledge, 2010), 145–6, https://doi.org/10.4324/978131 5601373<<<REFC>>>. See particularly p. 147.
[18] Anna Katharina Schaffner. *Exhaustion: A History* (New York: Columbia University Press, 2016), 13.
[19] *WT* 2.1.33–4.
[20] Schaffner, *Exhaustion*, 13.

and their relationship to exhaustion, are inextricably tied to the pregnant and postpartum body.

* * *

Hermione's refused lying-in ceremony becomes the catalyst for her collapse, supposed death, and sixteen-year retreat, as evidenced by early modern gynecological manuals as well as the play-text. In *The Winter's Tale*, exhaustion and collapse are highlighted as part of Hermione's narrative, as well as of pregnancy and childbirth more broadly (let alone motherhood). By focusing on what Hermione's body must weather, I center bodies that *bear* children, these people's burdens, and the rituals that both deplete and revive them. By the end of Act 3, Scene 2, both Mamillius and Hermione are declared dead. Sicilia is barren. After "Time" comes onstage and announces the passing of sixteen years, audiences travel to Bohemia where they meet Hermione's daughter, Perdita, who survives despite being left for dead. Hermione does not appear again until the final scene of the play, revived by her friend Paulina, and tells Perdita that she "preserved" herself in the hopes she was alive. Whether or not Hermione is magically resurrected in the final act of the play, as some scholars argue, she *stops* for sixteen years.[21] During this period of retreat and preservation, Hermione stops participating in many of the roles assigned to her as an early modern woman—much like new mothers lying in. Reading *The Winter's Tale* as a narrative of exhaustion illuminates Hermione's metaphorical death as a period of recovery, alternatively—a rejection of the exhausting standards to which she and other pregnant and postpartum people are held, then and now.

Dragged out into the "open air" by her husband, emboldened by a culture in which adulteresses could be put on trial, Hermione watches her world grow colder and colder in minutes. *The Winter's Tale* is, as the title suggests, a tale about frigidity and barrenness, most notably Leontes's part in constructing a cold or even barren womb. In the early modern period, notably, fertility was tied to warmth. During the lying-in period, midwives and physicians prescribed hot foods and spices in order to raise the heat of the body and to combat "the devastating effects of frigidity which, through coldness, robbed

---

[21] While I and many other scholars are convinced that Hermione retreats and returns to see her daughter, there is a breadth of early modern scholarship that argues she is resurrected through Paulina's magic. J. A. Bryant, Jr., argues in "Shakespeare's Allegory: 'The Winter's Tale,'" for example, that Hermione's return is a "gratuitous miracle so completely arresting that it overshadows everything that has gone before": *Sewanee Review* 63, no. 2 (1955): 203.

the body of its ability to experience sexual pleasure and its ability to conceive."[22] It was widely believed that the body was more open and porous after giving birth and that cold air might enter the body and cause a range of illnesses, as alluded to in Herimone's reference to the "open air" Leontes subjects her to postpartum.[23] This belief informed the medical advice to "lie in" after giving birth, so as to not expose the body to external elements that would imbalance the postpartum body's humors—an imbalance that could lead to illness and exhaustion.

Hermione's reference to the "open air" in her courtroom monologue, then, gestures not only to her postpartum body but also toward medical beliefs in the period about one's postpartum humoral composition.[24] An imbalance of the humors could cause a whole host of mental and physical health problems. As Schaffner observes, in "Galen's writings, we encounter exhaustion primarily in the guise of lethargy, torpor, weariness, sluggishness, and lack of energy."[25] In the early modern period, the humors played a part in the recognition that rest and rejuvenation was needed postpartum. A reparative reading of the belief that women's bodies were more "open" during this period, and therefore less efficient, would be the realization, or acknowledgment, that they are particularly vulnerable after giving birth—in need of rest and recovery.

As is the case in so many of Shakespeare's plays, *The Winter's Tale* offers Hermione, and audiences, an alternative course of action. This alternative exists, as Valerie Traub would say, *behind the seen*[26]; as Theodora Jankowski argues, in "the lesbian void"[27]; and, as I argue, in a sixteen-year lying-in ceremony that revives and then "preserves" Hermione.[28] Before the eighteenth century, the birthing chamber—where a woman gave birth and spent much of her postpartum recovery—was a space filled with women, midwives, neighbors, and relatives who had given birth. A male physician or husband was called only in the direst circumstances. As the historians Jacques Gélis and Rosemary

[22] Jennifer Evans, "'Gentle Purges Corrected with Hot Spices, Whether They Work or Not, Do Vehemently Provoke Venery': Menstrual Provocation and Procreation in Early Modern England," *Social History of Medicine: The Journal of the Society for the Social History of Medicine* 25, no. 1 (February 1, 2012): 7, https://doi.org/10.1093/shm/hkr021.
[23] *WT* 3.2.112.
[24] *WT* 3.2.103.
[25] Schaffner, *Exhaustion*, 16.
[26] Valerie Traub, *The Renaissance of Lesbianism in Early Modern England*, Cambridge Studies in Renaissance Literature and Culture 42 (Cambridge: Cambridge University Press, 2002), 69.
[27] Theodora A. Jankowski, "… in the Lesbian Void: Woman-Woman Eroticism in Shakespeare's Plays," in *A Feminist Companion to Shakespeare*, ed. Dympna Callaghan (Chichester: John Wiley & Sons, 2016), 306, https://doi.org/10.1002/9781118501221.ch16.
[28] *WT* 5.3.127.

Morris write, "Childbirth was women's business. Usually it was female relatives, neighbors or friends that surrounded the woman in labor," and this extended to postpartum rituals and care.[29] The alternative course of action when faced with patriarchal tyranny, as demonstrated in *The Winter's Tale*, is love and care between women—Hermione and Paulina. This love and care allows Hermione to endure her violent experience of bearing and birthing a child, a time "fraught with obstacles and dangers from beginning to end" in general in the early modern period.[30]

Paulina's initial decisions and actions after Hermione collapses and is declared dead reflect these cultural practices. Leontes's response to the "dire situation" of Hermione's postpartum condition is not helpful and does not suggest the death of his son has, in fact, made him "a man of truth, of mercy" as he claims.[31] After he denounces the oracle, Mamillius dies, and Hermione collapses; Leontes quickly notes, "She will recover," then continues to lament the destruction his "bloody thoughts" has wrought for twenty-some lines.[32] When Paulina returns and "swears" that Hermione is dead, she tells Leontes:

PAULINA
> go and see. If you can bring
> Tincture or lustre in her lip, her eye,
> Heat outwardly or breath within, I'll serve you
> As I would do the gods.[33]

Leontes chooses not to, but these lines gesture toward the care Hermione would've received from Paulina in the early days of her revival. Early modern gynecological manuals written for midwives offer clues as to what might have happened as Paulina nursed Hermione back to health. There are particular remedies for bringing back color—bringing back heat—to the postpartum body. In the few days following birth, a piece of dry cloth, folded in two or in four and warmed up, was put at the opening of the womb, called a "blocker" or "warmer," because it stopped the air and cold from entering what was perceived as a vulnerable, open body. Manuals advised this cloth must not be too tight,

---

[29] Jacques Gélis, *History of Childbirth: Fertility, Pregnancy, and Birth in Early Modern Europe*, trans. Rosemary Morris (Cambridge, MA: Polity Press, [1991] 2005), 99.
[30] Linda A. Pollock, "Embarking on a Rough Passage: The Experience of Pregnancy in Early-Modern Society," in *Women as Mothers in Pre-Industrial England*, ed. Valerie Fildes (London: Routledge, 1990), 40.
[31] *WT* 3.2.154.
[32] *WT* 3.2.156.
[33] *WT* 3.2.204

however, or it might stop the flow of the cleansings and cause fainting due to the vapors that would then be unable to escape.[34]

These intimate exchanges might have set the tone for the following sixteen years, as some scholars suggest. Theodora Jankowski, for example, argues that Paulina's affections for Hermione inform her revival in the final scene of the play. For Jankowski, Paulina and Hermione develop a spousal relationship over the course of sixteen years that reflects the supposed "invisibility" of lesbian relationships in the period.[35] I add to Jankowski's instructive reading that the medical techniques used to revive postpartum people in the period are all techniques associated with heat, friction—and thus generation. Hermione and Paulina fashion a space of healing outside of a world where men face few consequences for their violence, one that allows them to rest in the hope Perdita will return. Paulina's ability to nurse Hermione back to health postpartum suggests a familiarity with gynecological knowledge, as well as a space—however invisible—of love, warmth, heat, and friction.

Not surprisingly, Paulina's on- and off-stage attempts to love, heal, and protect Hermione from Leontes's cold wrath earn her the titles of "mankind witch," "intelligencing bawd," and "callet" or strumpet,[36] all descriptors that gesture to the anxiety-producing relationship between witchcraft and gynecological knowledge in the period. Leontes's accusations attempt to demonize Paulina's ability to care for Hermione. Kirstie Gulick Rosenfield points out, however, that every primary female character in *The Winter's Tale* is figured as a witch at some point—is "accused of this specifically female crime."[37] Hermione is first "contained" as an accused witch, and even Perdita is deemed a "fresh piece / Of excellent witchcraft" by Polixenes.[38] For Rosenfield, *The Winter's Tale* "identifies female vocality, sexuality, maternity, and midwifery with the witch and then reveals those associations as accusations designed to contain the threat of the transgressing woman."[39] And, as Mario DiGangi contends, the "gruesome associations" leveled at Paulina are meant to delegitimize her testimony and her intimacy with Hermione, yet end up exposing the "tendentiousness" of Leontes's classifications instead.[40]

---

[34] Gélis, *History of Childbirth*, 179.
[35] Jankowski, "… in the Lesbian Void," 320.
[36] *WT* 2.3.84–5, 116.
[37] Kirstie Gulick Rosenfield, "Nursing Nothing: Witchcraft and Female Sexuality in *The Winter's Tale*," *Mosaic: An Interdisciplinary Critical Journal* 35, no. 1 (March 2002): 95.
[38] *WT* 4.4.428–9.
[39] Rosenfield, "Nursing Nothing," 96.
[40] Mario DiGangi, *Sexual Types: Embodiment, Agency, and Dramatic Character from Shakespeare to Shirley* (Philadelphia: University of Pennsylvania Press, 2011), 84.

These early associations with witchcraft, in fact, foreshadow Paulina's ability to revive, heal, and care for Hermione postpartum.[41] While Gervase Markham's *The English Husbandman* (1613) posits that a husband is "the Maister of the earth, turning sterrillitie and barrainesse, into fruitfulnesse and increase,"[42] Jennifer Munroe argues that *The Winter's Tale* demonstrates that a husband only achieves this transformation by "deferring authority," by "being made subject both to woman and to the natural world."[43] Paulina revives the womb in *The Winter's Tale* through warmth and intimacy, bringing figurative fruits and flowers back to life.

Not surprisingly, then, the lying-in ceremony was not popular among men writing about it in the early modern period. The husband was required to facilitate the lying-in period financially as the host of the "gossips" or female friends—in other words, "contributing household resources to festive lying-in celebrations, during which the community can witness his appreciation of his wife, their child, and the women who assisted in the birth."[44] The dramas of the period demonstrate that *some* men saw this as a lavish, unnecessary expense, and they resented the gossips' presence and consumption of resources, as well as being required to play the good host. In Thomas Middleton's *A Chaste Maid in Cheapside* (c. 1613), for example, a christening feast is depicted that perpetuates misogynistic stereotypes about the birthing room and the female communities present—the gossips tell each other secrets, get tipsy on wine, and overturn stools—doing literal damage to Mr. Allwit's home.[45] All the while, the audience knows the child is not even his, but the result of an affair. In short, lying-in periods were not just a source of financial anxiety for husbands, but also anxiety over paternity.

In this way, Hermione and Paulina create an invisible space of recovery from exhaustion, one that is not under the scrutiny and control of men. The early

---

[41] Mario DiGangi has also argued that, in Paulina's attempts to protect Hermione from Leontes's cold-wrath, her monikers of "mankind witch," "intelligencing bawd," and "callet" or strumpet are all sexual types that, in early modern drama, "pursue illicit bodily intimacy with other women": ibid., 84.

[42] Gervase Markham, *The English Husbandman: The First Part: Contayning the Knowledge of the True Nature of Euery Soyle Within This Kingdome: How to Plow It; and the Manner of the Plough, and Other Instruments Belonging Thereto. Together with the Art of Planting, Grafting, and Gardening after Our Latest and Rarest Fashion. A Worke Neuer Written before by Any Author: And Now Newly Compiled for the Benefit of This Kingdon* (London: Thomas Snodham, 1613), 4.

[43] Jennifer Munroe, "It's All about the Gillyvors: Engendering Art and Nature in *The Winter's Tale*," in *Ecocritical Shakespeare*, ed. Lynne Bruckner and Dan Brayton (Farnham: Routledge, 2011), 145.

[44] Sara D. Luttfring, *Bodies, Speech, and Reproductive Knowledge in Early Modern England*, Routledge Studies in Renaissance Literature and Culture 26 (New York: Routledge, 2016), 134.

[45] Gail Kern Paster argues Mr. Allwit's anxiety evidences that "the men of the play must unite to conserve … an economic and sexual substance that the appetite of woman and her conspicuous lack of self-control threaten to destroy": *The Body Embarrassed: Drama and the Disciplines of Shame in Early Modern England*, illustrated ed. (Ithaca, NY: Cornell University Press, 1993), 57.

acts of the play suggest the necessity of this space—indeed, audiences watch Hermione pushed past her limits well before the courtroom scene. "Take the boy to you," she tells her ladies in waiting of Mamillius—"He so troubles me/ 'Tis past enduring."[46] In one of the first moments audiences witness women speaking to each other in *The Winter's Tale*, they are negotiating the burden of motherhood. In the same scene, one of Hermione's ladies in waiting observes of the queen's pregnant body: "She is spread of late / Into a goodly bulk: good time encounter her!"[47] The brief reference, the wish, for "good time" stands in stark contrast to the asynchrony of Leontes's rapid descent into a jealous rage, as well as Mamillius's treatment of not only his mother but also the ladies who wait on him—"I'll none of you," he tells them after his mother departs.[48] These lines, and the community of women who speak them, conjure private chambers of being and belonging between women—the birthing chamber, a space Leontes transforms into a literal prison. Although Hermione returns to Mamillius in this scene, telling him "I am for you again," her only request after Leontes acts on his jealous fantasies, when pushed past endurance over and over again, is that "my women may be with me."[49]

Shakespeare's bereft, bleeding Hermione—dragged to court and exonerated by her son's death, which Leontes interprets as his punishment for rejecting the oracle—is quite different from Middleton's depiction of an extravagant lying-in ceremony and clueless Mr. Allwit. Both plays, however, demonstrate anxieties around paternity and midwifery. Leontes's intrusions into "women's business" however—separating Mamillius from his mother and attempting to put his supposedly illegitimate newborn daughter to death—are not only wildly unsuccessful but also cause notable harm to his family and kingdom. In this respect, Paulina knows Leontes and his apologies cannot revive Hermione. In *The Winter's Tale*, then, "good time" for reproductive bodies looks quite different from Hermione's experience. It is not until Hermione is in Paulina's care that this good time occurs over sixteen years—a gap of time audiences are not privy to.

After this gap of time, and Perdita's return to court, Hermione is revived by Paulina and emerges to reunite with her daughter, the only family member she speaks to at the play's end—despite the fact Leontes is desperate for Paulina to make Hermione "speak as move."[50] As I've suggested, some scholars believe that

---

[46] *WT* 2.1.1–2.
[47] *WT* 2.1.19–20.
[48] *WT* 2.1.5.
[49] *WT* 2.1.29, 117.
[50] *WT* 5.3.93.

Hermione does, in fact, die in the courtroom scene and is resurrected by Paulina through magic sixteen years later. Richard McCoy, for example, argues that the "miracles in these late plays are not gifts from the gods but result instead from families reuniting and comforting one another."[51] Theatergoers must, as Paulina argues in the final scene, "awake their faith" in order to suspend their disbelief and allow for this miracle.[52] Although these readings offer an important perspective, it is clear to me that, in *The Winter's Tale*, the "gap of time" that Hermione and Paulina spend together is an arrangement made possible by pregnancy and the lying-in ceremony in early modern England. Hermione's pregnancy comes to fruition sixteen years late, after she is revived by Paulina's care and reunited with her daughter. For these reasons, I read Hermione's silence at the play's end as a step toward reclaiming the dignity, strength, and sexual freedom "which 'longs / To women of all fashion.'"[53]

In the lines she does speak, however, Hermione does not address Leontes. Instead, she addresses Perdita as "mine own," a notable address considering the play's ongoing investment in the threatening power of the pregnant body and female alliances.[54] Just moments before this line, Leontes conjures the Aristotelian model of generation when he first sees Polixenes's son, Florizel: "Your mother was most true to wedlock, prince, / For she did print your royal father off, / Conceiving you."[55] That Hermione addresses Perdita as "mine own" is also poignant as this phrase is used by Aaron in *Titus Andronicus* to describe the child his partner, Tamora, sent away to be murdered: "Tell the empress from me I am of age / To keep mine own, excuse it how she can."[56] In both cases, parents claim a child left for dead—forming nonnormative families. It is no accident, then, in my mind, that Paulina tells Hermione after she descends the staircase and returns to her family—"*our* Perdita is found."[57]

When put in conversation with the history of obstetrics and gynecology, *The Winter's Tale* resonates to this day because most people find themselves, like Hermione, "hurried" to various places, institutions, before they have fully recovered their "strength of limit."[58] For many people who have given birth

---

[51] Richard C. McCoy, *Faith in Shakespeare* (Oxford: Oxford University Press, [2013] 2015), 115.
[52] *WT* 5.3.95.
[53] *WT* 3.2.101–2.
[54] *WT* 5.3.124.
[55] *WT* 5.1.123–5.
[56] William Shakespeare, *Titus Andronicus*, ed. Jonathan Bate and Arden Shakespeare, 3rd ser. (London: Bloomsbury, 1995), 4.2.106–7.
[57] *WT* 5.3.152.
[58] *WT* 3.2.104.

today, postpartum recovery means healing after a major surgery—for instance, as Meaghan O'Connell describes in her memoir, being unable to "stand up and go to the bathroom without searing pain and the feeling of my guts threatening to come pouring out of my C-section incision."[59] For others, like Molly Caro May, postpartum recovery means years of incontinence. In her memoir, May describes how birth rendered her "unable to do anything but care for Eula. Not cook. Not clean. Not even put a respectable outfit on my body … [making] literal movement through life difficult."[60] But, like Hermione, people who have just given birth in our era endure incredible institutional violence, working to preserve themselves in whatever ways they can, often depending on the unpaid labor of those who understand how important the right to recover postpartum is.

In *The Winter's Tale*, the fact that Leontes does not allow Hermione to rest and recover postpartum is one of many wrongs she endures at the hands of a tyrant, yet it is important enough to warrant four lines of meditation in a powerful monologue, as well as emphasis in recent productions of *The Winter's Tale*. Kelly Hunter, for the Royal Shakespeare Company (2011), delivered Hermione's monologue "wrapped in bloodstained rags."[61] The American Shakespeare Center (2012) also costumed Hermione so that she looked "bloodied and bedraggled."[62] In Theatre for a New Audience's production (2018), Hermione, performed by Kelley Curran, is brought onstage in a dirty nightgown by two men, struggling to walk, to hold herself upright, eyes wild.

I watched Curran perform Hermione's monologue when I was ten months postpartum. Instantly, her gestures transported me back to the sharp sting of trying to walk after giving birth. Watching Curran hobble onstage, hold on to various structures, and breathe heavily while pleading her case reminded me of when—two weeks postpartum—I put on dress pants and a fresh, supersized pad between my legs, leaving my husband with our newborn baby, to go to a job interview. Still unsure of how I was going to fund the sixth year of my PhD

---

[59] Meaghan O'Connell, *And Now We Have Everything: On Motherhood before I Was Ready*, 1st ed. (New York: Little Brown, 2018), 114–15.
[60] Molly Caro May, *Body Full of Stars: Female Rage and My Passage into Motherhood* (Berkeley, CA: Counterpoint, 2018), loc. 692 of 1696.
[61] Jennifer Farrar, "Tyranny Drives 'Winter's Tale,'" *The Blade*, July 27, 2011, https://www.toledoblade.com/a-e/music-theater-dance/2011/07/28/Tyranny-drives-searing-Winter-s-Tale/stories/201107280029.
[62] Eric Minton, "Trust the Bard, for His Magic Is True," PlayShakespeare: Free Shakespeare Resource, September 11, 2012, https://www.playshakespeare.com/the-winters-tale-reviews/theatre-reviews/trust-the-bard-for-his-magic-is-true.

program, I felt like I didn't have a choice. I sat in a department chair's office, bleeding in a blazer, poised and eloquent. I got the job.

We, postpartum bodies, are *still* exhausted, an embodied experience bound to feelings of abandonment, liminality, numbness, fatigue, and precarity. It is exhausting enough to be pregnant, give birth, and care for a child postpartum—let alone deal with anxious partners' and doctors' respective feelings and beliefs around how to treat people postpartum. Postpartum, parents are expected to have unlimited fumes, heat, and fire to keep going—no matter how exhausting and unaccommodating the world they find themselves in is. Unfortunately, most of us do not have Paulinas to revive us.

In an attempt to address this unconcerned world, the American College of Obstetricians and Gynecologists (ACOG) recently released committee opinion notes acknowledging that 50 percent of pregnancy-related deaths occur after the child is born; in other words, during the postpartum period, a period "devoid of formal or informal maternal support." The council acknowledges that the mother is an afterthought once the child is born, and this lack of care and concern is even more pertinent to working mothers, 45 percent of whom are back at work within forty days. As a solution, however, the new ACOG guidelines recommend that all women should "have contact with a maternal care provider within the first 3 weeks postpartum" and a final postpartum visit that includes "a full assessment of physical, social, and psychological well-being."

While these guidelines attempt to correct the dearth of care that is currently provided to new mothers, there is a more subtle distinction that institutions like the ACOG fail to recognize—that is, between monitoring new mothers and listening to them. I had to stop and catch my breath at the brief's description of trauma, for example. The ACOG writes, "Trauma is in the eye of the beholder, and health care providers should be aware that a woman may experience a birth as traumatic even if she and the infant are healthy."[63] Although this statement suggests it is important to listen to people who have just given birth, the assumption at the heart of this advice is that health is measured by survival, and trauma is a perception that must be acknowledged, however distorted.

The relationship between trauma, survival, and exhaustion is at the heart of *The Winter's Tale*—and how scholars read its ending. By the end of the play,

---

[63] "Optimizing Postpartum Care," Committee Opinion (Washington, DC: American College of Obstetricians and Gynecologists, May 2018), https://www.acog.org/en/Clinical/ClinicalGuida nce/ Committee Opinion/Articles/2018/05/Optimizing Postpartum Care.

Hermione and her daughter are alive—healthy, even. But Mamillius has died, a plot point that scholars have puzzled over.[64] In my mind, the easy reading of the play's end is the reunion of a (now) happy family. In other words, the end of Hermione's extended postpartum period, after she rests, recovers, and reunites with the man who abused her, means she forgives the death of one of her children—and the trauma that accompanies it—in lieu of the survival of another. She must also accept the trauma and sacrifice that led up to her reunion with her surviving child. To assume Hermione is able to forgive and forget mirrors the perspective of *modern* medical advice in chilling ways—advice that centers healthy children and (presumed) happy endings above all else. But, as far too many of us know, healthy endings often come at the cost of someone else's happy ending, and survival is not the same as healing.

Throughout these notes, for example, the ACOG recognizes the disparity between the care white women and women of color receive postpartum, yet argue that "populations with limited resources" do not attend postpartum appointments—a phenomenon that puts their health at risk.[65] In addition to people of color's limited resources and warranted fear of medical establishments, this disparity of care is based on damaging tropes and stereotypes of Black women's reproductive bodies that date back to early modern gynecological manuals and travelogues. In the sixteenth century, easy births without long labors or ceremonial lyings-in were a marker of cultural and social inferiority—a cultural construction at the heart of the lack of care single mothers, people of color, and Black women, in particular, experience while pregnant.[66]

In the early modern period, difficult labor distinguished white women from Black women, Christians from pagans, and virtuous women from whores.[67] As Jane Sharp's *Midwives Book* notes, "If any feel but a little pain it is commonly harlots who are so used to it that they make little reckoning of it, and are wont to fare better at present than virtuous persons do."[68] Womanist and intersectional

---

[64] Some notable scholarship that takes up this plot point includes Janet Adelman's *Suffocating Mothers: Fantasies of Maternal Origin in Shakespeare's Plays, "Hamlet" to "The Tempest"* (New York: Routledge, 1992); Susan Synder's "Mamillius and Gender Polarization in *The Winter's Tale*," *Shakespeare Quarterly* 50, no. 1 (1999); and Thomas Kullmann's "Shakespeare's *Winter's Tale* and the Myth of Childhood Innocence," *Poetica* 46, no. 3/4 (2014).

[65] "Optimizing Postpartum Care."

[66] For a more in-depth study on premodern enslaved women's reproductive lives and the tropes through which these lives were described, see Jennifer L. Morgan, *Laboring Women: Reproduction and Gender in New World Slavery*, Early American Studies (Philadelphia: University of Pennsylvania Press, 2004).

[67] Gowing, *Common Bodies*, 170.

[68] Jane Sharp, *Midwives Book* (London: Simon Miller, 1671), quoted in ibid.

feminist movements have made substantial efforts to highlight the issues that plague reproductive justice for women of color, which expand from the violent histories of gynecological experiments and forced sterilization, to ongoing issues of child displacements (in adoption and foster care as well as immigrant detention centers) and the alarming rate of Black women's pregnancy complications, as well as an overall lack of medical resources.[69]

In short, as Serena Williams's high-profile case demonstrates, dragging women of color, especially Black women, to more appointments with doctors isn't going to change the fact that no one hears them when they're there. As Maya Salam writes in the *New York Times*, Williams's "agonizing postnatal experience" included "an episode in which hospital employees did not act on her concern that she was experiencing a pulmonary embolism, a sudden blockage of an artery in the lung by a blood clot."[70] Williams insisted to her nurse and doctor that she needed care and was ignored. Finally, after many useless tests were performed, the doctor listened to Williams and a CT scan showed several blood clots in her lungs. The institutionalization of childbirth, the "business of being born," hinges on the premise that pregnant people need to be monitored and policed in order to ensure the safety of the child—knowledge of our own bodies is consequently side-lined, and many physicians seem to have little interest in listening to their patients, especially if they are people of color.

In conversation with *The Winter's Tale*, Maya Salam's discussion of Dr. Elizabeth Howell's research on why Black women more commonly suffer from life-threatening complications postpartum is revealing. The answer is not, Howell concludes, access to care—as Williams's case demonstrates and many people assume. Dr. Howell charges physicians to think instead about how "bias shapes the ways we hear our patients."[71] Williams's case is just one contemporary example of how, like Hermione, pregnant people are stripped of bodily knowledge, their narratives dismissed in favor of medical experts'. Without a doubt, the medicalization of childbirth that began in the early modern

---

[69] One of the most notable texts that addresses medical racism in obstetrics and gynecology, in particular, is Dorothy E. Roberts, *Killing the Black Body: Race, Reproduction, and the Meaning of Liberty*, 1st ed., Black Women Writers (New York: Pantheon Books, 1997). Two other key resources are Deirdre Benia Cooper Owens, *Medical Bondage: Race, Gender, and the Origins of American Gynecology* (Athens: University of Georgia Press, 2017) and Harriet A. Washington, *Medical Apartheid: The Dark History of Medical Experimentation on Black Americans from Colonial Times to the Present* (New York: Doubleday, 2006).
[70] Maya Salam, "For Serena Williams, Childbirth Was a Harrowing Ordeal. She's Not Alone," *New York Times*, January 11, 2018, sec. Sports, para. 2, https://www.nytimes.com/2018/01/11/sports/tennis/serena-williams-baby-vogue.html.
[71] Ibid., para. 22.

period, and the developments made by modern medicine, has eased the wild and strange journey of pregnancy for countless people, saved many lives, but what has been lost in this process? The sixteen years that Hermione lives apart from her husband and daughter with another woman—reclaiming her time and strength that "which 'longs / To women of all fashion"—is in so many ways an escape from what José Esteban Muñoz might call a "poisonous and insolvent" present for pregnant people and postpartum bodies—then and now.[72]

In short, requiring nonworking and working mothers alike to attend extra appointments is not the solution to our cultural crisis in postpartum care. Even as a white woman whose reproductive body is privileged, if only for the future of the white child it houses—who has both medical insurance to afford postpartum appointments and a family willing to help—attending my first postpartum appointment three weeks after giving birth was an astounding feat. Although I could physically walk, my partner was already back to work after a "generous" two-week paternity leave, and my breastfeeding baby was literally attached to my body around the clock. My sister came with me—an instance of informal caregiving by another woman that mirrors Gowing's challenge to historians (such as Adrian Wilson) who argue that the social ritual of the lying-in period "could pose a significant, if temporary, threat to male authority" as the woman's needs took precedence within the household.[73] Gowing argues, alternatively, that "rather than an inversion of marital roles, lying-in involved a redistribution of them amongst other women."[74] My sister and I had to stop twice in the half-mile walk to my obstetrician so I could feed my daughter, who was not happy, on strangers' steps. My sister held her in the waiting room, and I was too distracted by the sounds of shrieking babies—maybe my own—to talk seriously with the nurse inquiring about postpartum depression symptoms.

I know I do not speak only for myself when I say I do not dream of more appointments with doctors for postpartum people, or even quicker healing. Inspired by Laura Dorwart's piece, "What the World Gets Wrong about My Quadriplegic Husband and Me," of the future she dreams of for her husband, a quadriplegic man, I dream of a different kind of accommodation. I dream of professionals coming to women's homes, of postpartum labor being distributed fairly among men and women, of people who have not given birth knowing or caring what postpartum people might need, and of postpartum parents feeling

---

[72] *WT* 3.2.30; Muñoz, *Cruising Utopia*, 30.
[73] Adrian Wilson, quoted in Gowing, *Common Bodies*, 173.
[74] Gowing, *Common Bodies*, 173.

more comfortable asking for what they need. As Dorwart says, "In my dreams, I don't watch him walk. I watch him stop being hurt."[75] For Leontes, it takes the perceived death of his wife and daughter, and actual death of his son, to "awake his faith"—to stop hurting and start trusting those he loves—although *The Winter's Tale* offers little evidence he has actually changed.[76]

The state of postpartum care today, alongside Leontes's focus on himself and his male child, is why Hermione's vehement claim to her child-bed rights still feels progressive. Although there were different approaches to postpartum care in the early modern period, depending on class, location, race, and other distinctions between women, Hermione emphasizes that the right to recover after giving birth belongs to "women of all fashion":[77] postpartum bodies of all types of "make, build, [and] shape … manner, mold, and way."[78] Given these differences, Lauren Smith Brody argues that the most important question a person can ask themselves postpartum is, "What do you need right now?"—and then to ask for it.[79] In *The Fifth Trimester*, a book about returning to work after giving birth, Brody argues that if she had even thought to ask herself that question, then perhaps she wouldn't have "spiraled quite as severely."[80] The answer to our postpartum care crisis, as Brody posits, is not to require even more surveillance, but for postpartum people to advocate for themselves in the hopes that institutions will listen. As a start, we might hear Hermione when Leontes refuses to, as well as the voices of people who are speaking out now, so as to begin taking postpartum exhaustion seriously—"to desire differently, to desire more, to desire better" for people who have just given birth.[81]

---

[75] Laura Dorwart, "What the World Gets Wrong about My Quadriplegic Husband and Me," *Catapult*, December 6, 2017, para. 21.
[76] *WT* 5.3.94–5.
[77] *WT* 3.2.102.
[78] "Fashion, n.," in *OED Online* (Oxford University Press), para. 2, accessed March 6, 2021, http://www.oed.com/view/Entry/68389.
[79] Lauren Smith Brody, *The Fifth Trimester: The Working Mom's Guide to Style, Sanity, and Success after Baby* (New York: Doubleday, 2017), 108.
[80] Ibid.
[81] Muñoz, *Cruising Utopia*, 189.

3

Medical and Military Transitions in *Anatomy of a Soldier*

Kristina Fleuty

Harry Parker's novel *Anatomy of a Soldier* (2016) is a fictionalized semi-autobiographical account of Parker's own lived experience of military conflict and traumatic limb loss. Parker, similarly to his protagonist Tom Barnes, served as an officer in the British Army and became a double below-the-knee amputee after stepping on an improvised explosive device (IED) while deployed. The novel explores the aftermath of Tom's injury, his rehabilitation, and his life as an amputee veteran.

This chapter aims to move discussion beyond the etiology of limb loss and the practical aspects of recovery to focus on the embodied experience of losing a limb, as presented in Parker's novel, and explore how Tom as an individual, and as part of family and social groups, comes to terms with this loss and subsequent gain of a prosthetic. This transition from able-bodied to amputee is complicated further by another change of identity for Tom: from soldier to amputee veteran. This chapter will consider Tom's limb loss within the context of his transition from the military back into civilian society, as well as the impact this has on Tom's recovery, rehabilitation, and identities, as he comes to terms with two forced transitions as a result of his injuries.

Parker narrates *Anatomy of a Soldier* through the imagined first-person perspectives of forty-five anthropomorphized objects, each voice of which narrates a chapter of the novel to tell Tom's story. Not all object narrators are involved in communicating Tom's story; some are involved in the stories of other characters. This chapter will focus on the objects significant to Tom's injury on the battlefield, medical treatment, rehabilitation and recovery, and parallel transition into being a veteran.[1]

Transitioning from Military to Civilian

Transition is defined as the period of reintegration into civilian life after leaving the Armed Forces.[2] Research on transition has tended to focus on the practical aspects of leaving the military environment, such as the support an individual might need to find somewhere to live, new employment, managing their finances, gaining further qualifications and adapting to "everyday" life as the civilian world generally understands it.[3] Most people make a smooth and positive transition out of the military.[4] Nonetheless, it is a significant transition in an individual's, and often a family's, life.[5] The process involves coping with complicated psychological and emotional changes, which makes transition worthy of further discussion beyond everyday practicalities. The necessity of having to develop new civilian identities as part of transition will "inevitably be bound up with emotional health,"[6] and some attention has been given to the need for psychological readiness, including consideration of how transition impacts upon an individual's understanding of their own self-identity.[7] The exploration this chapter makes will consider how transition affects identity constructions, including as a result of the changes experienced in social group identification in relation to becoming both an amputee and a veteran.

In *Anatomy of a Soldier*, the navigation of veteran status as part of civilian social identity is informed by Tom's own military legacy. Research has begun to discuss how the military legacy endures, with military culture continuing to shape the individual post-service.[8] Cooper et al. draw attention to the

---

[1] There are fourteen object narrators that are significant to Tom's medical and military transitions: tourniquet, breathing tube, call button, O-positive blood, catheter, razor, photograph, wheelchair, mirror, bed, prosthetic leg, pint glass, electric leg, and running leg.
[2] Forces in Mind Trust, *The Transition Mapping Study* (n.p., 2013).
[3] Ibid.
[4] Lord Ashcroft, *The Veterans' Transition Review* (2014), 12.
[5] Linda Cooper et al., "Transition from the Military into Civilian Life: An Exploration of Cultural Competence," *Armed Forces & Society* 44, no. 1 (2016): 156–77.
[6] Forces in Mind Trust, *The Transition Mapping Study*, 54.
[7] Mary Keeling, "Stories of Transition: US Veterans' Narratives of Transition to Civilian Life and the Important Role of Identity," *Journal of Military, Veteran and Family Health* 4, no. 2 (2018): 28–36; Duncan M. Shields et al., "Mental Health and Well-Being of Military Veterans during Military to Civilian Transition: Review and Analysis of the Recent Literature," Canadian Institute for Military and Veteran Health Research, 2016.
[8] Cooper et al., "Transition from the Military into Civilian Life."

importance of understanding the enduring influence of military culture when an individual leaves the military and returns to a civilian environment that was once familiar but is no longer so. Military life is described as providing a sense of purpose, with military identity a "powerful and all-encompassing feature of life in service."[9] The suggestion here is that military life is more than simply a career choice. Rather, it offers a complete way of life for the duration of service, meaning that for the individual leaving the military a significant shift in identity is needed to separate the self from military culture. Furthermore, Engward et al. identify the military legacy as being significant specifically to the veteran adapting to living with limb loss.[10] The military legacy is an important identity factor to consider as part of the transition process and forms the backdrop to Tom's medical transition.

The Objectification of the Injured Body

Tom's military identity is central when Parker first introduces his protagonist to the reader. Tom is identified by his British Army number, BA5799, long before he is referred to by his name, which distances the reader from the character as an individual and instead reinforces BA5799's status as a product of the army and part of the military collective. When individuals enter the military for basic training, a process of separation from civilian society and civilian identities takes place, and identification with the military organization and culture is encouraged.[11] The new military identity is constructed in relation to the routine activities carried out as part of military service.[12]

BA5799 is introduced as a character of whom the reader receives no knowledge other than what is imparted through a military or medical lens. Parker's reader is introduced to BA5799 through objects described as being active participants in BA5799's care following his accident. The novel begins through the narration of the tourniquet, an unassuming object that stems the flow of blood from

---

[9] Forces in Mind Trust, "The Transition Mapping Study," 53–4.
[10] Hilary Engward, Kristina Fleuty, and Matt Fossey, *Caring and Coping: The Family Perspective on Living with Limb Loss* (London: Blesma, 2018), 29.
[11] Richard Godfrey, Simon Lilley, and Joanna Brewis, "Biceps, Bitches and Borgs: Reading Jarhead's Representation of the Construction of the (Masculine) Military Body," *Organization Studies* 33, no. 4 (April 1, 2012): 541–62; Duncan M. Shields et al., "Mental Health and Well-Being of Military Veterans during Military to Civilian Transition."
[12] Meredith Kleykamp and Crosby Hipes, "Coverage of Veterans of the Wars in Iraq and Afghanistan in the U.S. Media," *Sociological Forum* 30, no. 2 (2015): 348–68.

the body.¹³ This object is located in the pocket of BA5799's combat trousers; at the critical moment when BA5799 is injured, the tourniquet provides aid, asserting, "I was there when no one came and he was alone and couldn't move. I was still there as fear and pathetic hopelessness gripped BA5799."¹⁴ The tourniquet is a companion to BA5799, kept close to his body until needed. This narrative represents something, or rather someone, faithful and supportive, but also someone upon whom BA5799 is dependent for survival. The object acts as BA5799's comforting friend, creating the impression of a personal bond between the two as it recognizes BA5799's emotional state. This description of the tourniquet offers a sharp reminder that, in contrast to this seemingly close bond between the object and injured body, the character has been separated from human contact with both his military and civilian social groups. This temporary removal leaves BA5799 in a state of limbo, perpetuating an idea that undergoing medical procedures is solitary and isolates the body from everyday life, suspending the individual outside of shared experience.

Parker reinforces this idea further through his description of the intimate interaction between BA5799 and the breathing tube and catheter. The breathing tube takes responsibility for Tom's breathing and has awareness of his injuries, some of which are sensitive, such as to Tom's groin and testicles.¹⁵ Similarly, the catheter describes entering Tom's body: "I went into you too. I fed into your penis and up your urethra to your bladder."¹⁶ This clinical procedure goes beyond the usual boundaries of intimacy and suggests a fusing of the objects with the inner workings of Tom's body. The breathing tube and catheter have intimate knowledge of Tom's internal damage; for the reader, it may feel intrusive to be privy to these medical procedures. With the primacy of medical objects at the forefront of the narrative, Parker's reader is distracted from considering that the objects do not operate on their own; it is skilled military and civilian medical professionals who give these medical objects their agency. Centralizing objects, and the actions they take, reflects the unconscious body as being subject to the will of the medical process; the medical instruments appear more humanized than Tom, and he becomes literally objectified—a passive object upon which they work.

---

[13] This comparatively basic but crucial piece of equipment is the first step in providing medical intervention on the battlefield. For further discussion of the history of the tourniquet for military use, see R. L. Mabry, "Tourniquet Use on the Battlefield," *Military Medicine* 171, no. 5 (2006): 352–56.

[14] Harry Parker, *Anatomy of a Soldier* (London: Faber & Faber, 2016), 1.

[15] Ibid., 2, 23.

[16] Ibid., 125.

Transitioning from Able-Bodied to Amputee

Tom's transition is triggered by an unexpected and sudden event. Parker's protagonist becomes an amputee without time to prepare physically or psychologically for this life change. The physical suddenness of Tom's limb loss is significant to the process of transition that follows. Cooper et al. refer to this kind of "forced" transition from military to civilian as being abrupt, complicated, and traumatic. Engward et al. describe the trauma of sudden limb loss as including initial relief that the person injured is still alive, the realization that life has changed irrevocably, and the challenge of coping with and managing the unexpected life change.[17]

When Tom is released from hospital, he returns to a family home that has been adapted to improve accessibility for a wheelchair. Everyday domestic occurrences such as eating at a table, making a cup of tea, going to bed, and moving around the home are altered by limb loss, but these alterations are not always immediately perceived as being negative.[18] For example, in *Anatomy of a Soldier*, a makeshift bedroom is arranged for Tom in a dining room space that Tom associates with family Christmas celebrations, which initially sparks a positive association for Tom and he experiences a sense of relief at being back home.[19] However, later in the same chapter, Tom begins to realize how much his life has changed, and his frustrations grow at being unable to remain in control of all his care needs.[20] For Tom, there is thus irritation that he needs help from his parents, while for Tom's parents, the challenge is trying to work out how to help Tom, but not smother his independence. Parker's novel exemplifies the notion that limb loss affects not only Tom's life, as he is thrust into an existence of hospitals, health professionals, and physiotherapy. Tom's limb loss also affects his family, of which each member has to adjust to differing roles and care responsibilities for the limb loss and learn how to support, manage, and cope.[21] This family adjustment demonstrates the shared nature of transitioning into living with a life-altering injury, and the relationship of the individual to their home environment and family members as being significant to this transition.

---

[17] Research on the lived experience of being an amputee (Engward et al., 2018, 42) differentiates between two circumstances of limb loss: that which is expected and can be planned for, and that which is unexpected and happens with suddenness.
[18] For an exploration of the transition back into the family home following limb loss and consideration of how everyday domestic life is affected, see Engward et al. (2018).
[19] Parker, Anatomy of a Soldier, 200–201.
[20] Ibid., 203–5.
[21] For an exploration of the effect of limb loss on the family unit, see Engward et al. (2018).

Later in the chapter, Tom self-reflects and remarks, "I suppose being back here, at home, just made everything seem so stark. I've been a sick person in a bed, with no legs, broken in hospital. Now I'm getting stronger, I'm becoming a normal person with no legs."[22] There is an acceptance from Tom that while in hospital a person can be "broken" and fulfills the identity of a "sick" person, but once back at home, there comes pressure to return to domestic norms. Tom continues, "I'm back in the real world and I suddenly remember what I used to be able to do, what I might have achieved—and it feels like all that's been taken away."[23] Returning to a civilian environment with which Tom was familiar pre-limb loss, and within which Tom recognized himself as having perceived "normal" physical capabilities, emphasizes that Tom is trying to fit into an inadequate definition of what is "normal" within a civilian context for an amputee, and that he must therefore come to terms with a "new normal."

There is a further dynamic to Tom's reassessment of this "new normal," with regard to the military legacy, which Engward et al. recognize as being significant to the transition into being an amputee and veteran.[24] Woodward and Jenkins assert that military identity is grounded in military capability, and that military capability is measured through what the body is capable of.[25] This places Tom's body, and specifically his body's capability, as being important to his veteran identity and his reintegration into civilian society. As exemplified in the quotations above, Tom equates physical capability with life achievement and being able to exist successfully in the "real world." The way Tom chooses to frame his own limb loss and how he adjusts to accepting his limb loss as part of his "new normal" has a significant impact on Tom's self-identity as an amputee veteran.

Limb Loss and Prosthetic Gain

Beyond Tom's coming to terms with his physical capabilities post-limb loss, an overriding consideration for Tom is how others will perceive and judge him as an amputee veteran; this apprehension about the potential reactions of other people highlights an important aspect of transition from able-bodied to amputee

---

[22] Parker, *Anatomy of a Soldier*, 205.
[23] Ibid., 205.
[24] Engward et al., *Caring and Coping*, 48.
[25] Rachel Woodward and K. Neil Jenkings, "Military Identities in the Situated Accounts of British Military Personnel," *Sociology* 45, no. 2 (2011): 252–68.

for the individual as being the adjustment of their social identity. After Tom's amputation, Parker writes a chapter from the narrative perspective of a mirror, through which Tom looks at his body consciously for the first time following his amputation. Parker writes, "He knew I reflected what others saw, and it shocked him. He shook his head in disbelief. He was unnatural, created by violence and saved by soldiers and medics: he'd survived the unsurvivable and it showed. He felt disgusted."[26] The lens through which Tom sees himself is a projection of what he thinks others will see, which leads Tom to a negative assessment of his appearance post-limb loss. Tom's initial reaction is that others will perceive his body as "unnatural," and he is conscious of negative attitudes and judgments. At this early point in Tom's transition, his focus is on the social expectations of his post-limb loss body and how to return to the "norm" as Tom believes it to be socially defined, rather than the implications of the actual injury to his physicality and mobility, his recognition of which comes slightly later.

This transition is complicated further by Tom's accompanying veteran status and his preoccupation with what this signifies to civilian society. Part of Tom's self-disgust, as exemplified above, comes from the realization and guilt that he has survived an injury that until recently he likely would not have and, moreover, an injury many people still do not survive.[27] Parker's use of the phrase "created by violence" alerts the reader to this, as it is a reminder that Tom's body has been wounded and forever changed by the violence of combat. Aware that his body is a constant reminder of what happened to him, for both himself and wider society, Tom unwittingly becomes the embodied example of the damage war can cause to human life. Through the mirror Tom sees "the grotesque scars and folds of flesh and the pink skin grafts that covered his wounds. He saw the violence of the bomb. Who could love that, he thought."[28] Tom's self-judgment goes further than an association with war; he relates his wider social position back to his personal circumstances and thinks about how this may change people's feelings and opinions toward him.

Interactions with others outside of the family unit are also important for the amputee veteran's developing sense of self and acceptance of their limb loss.

---

[26] Parker, *Anatomy of a Soldier*, 192.
[27] Matt Fossey and Jamie Hacker Hughes, *Traumatic Limb Loss and the Needs of the Family* (London: Blesma, 2014). Fossey and Hacker Hughes (2014) acknowledge that for those in military service, due to improvements in body armor, front-line trauma techniques, and medical care, there has been a rise in people surviving IED explosions and associated blast injuries. Surviving this type of complex bodily trauma may mean individuals are left with limb loss or loss of limb function. It would thus become normalized for veterans with these complex injuries to have to negotiate decisions about a body that is damaged or limited in use.
[28] Parker, *Anatomy of a Soldier*, 193.

Engward et al. identify that for people who have lost limbs, talking to others who have been through similar circumstances is an important part of coping with the limb loss and adapting to life as an amputee.[29] Parker describes how talking to others who have been through similar experiences is a turning point for Tom, although Tom does not recognize the significance until later. For example, a man comes to visit while Tom is recuperating at home and talks to Tom about his own experience of limb loss. Tom recognizes the similarity in that the man "was broken but [he] found it hard to relate to him."[30] The man offers some friendly advice, "what [has] happened [will] make you appreciate life more," and says that Tom "probably didn't understand it yet, but one day [he] would."[31] At the time Tom is thankful for the visit but dismisses the advice. The significance of this conversation and the positive impact on Tom's sense of self are revealed later when Tom is prompted to say to his mother, "I wouldn't change it," in relation to his injury and what has happened to him; "It's hard to explain but it's already too much a part of who I am. Life's changed and it's been grim, but I'm experiencing so much."[32] This is evidence of Tom's developing recognition of his limb loss as part of his civilian identity as an amputee veteran. Cooper et al. assert that a shift in understanding of self-identity and resilience is important for a successful military and civilian transition and for renegotiating cultural norms in a civilian context.[33]

Tom's reframing of his experience into something that enriches his life and through which he "gains" greater self-understanding is a significant part of his gradual acceptance of himself as an amputee. Parker's exploration of this change in Tom's outlook is deepened through a description of Tom's interaction with his prosthetic limbs. When the reader meets Tom's first prosthetic leg, Parker writes that the leg addresses Tom directly and says, "You pressed your stump into me and we became one for the first time. A man was crouched in front of you and guided us together."[34] Here is a new object–body relationship, in which Tom's stump and his prosthesis work together to negotiate a sometimes physically painful relationship so Tom can learn to walk again. There is an intimate connection between Tom and an object implied once again in the assertion that "we became one for the first time,"

---

[29] Engward et al., *Caring and Coping*, 71.
[30] Parker, *Anatomy of a Soldier*, 207.
[31] Ibid.
[32] Ibid., 208.
[33] L. Cooper, N. Caddick, L. Godier, A. Cooper, M. Fossey, and H. Engward, "A Model of Military to Civilian Transition: Bourdieu in Action," *Journal of Military, Veteran and Family Health* 3, no. 2 (2017): 53–60.
[34] Ibid., 224.

which is reminiscent of the bond between Tom and the earlier medical objects. However, in the above quotation, there is evidence of less dependency and a more cooperative partnership. This is a significant step for Tom's reclaiming of his bodily identity. The prosthetic leg as narrator recognizes that in relation to Tom, "I adapt to you," which signifies that Tom is regaining authority and autonomy over his body during rehabilitation while being supported through the gaining of a prosthetic.[35]

The prosthetic aids Tom's mobility; and with its support, Tom experiences more physical freedom. When Tom receives his upgraded electric prosthetic leg, Parker writes, "You recognised my socket that only your odd-shaped stump, with its deep scarring, could fit," which indicates that the prosthetic is individual to Tom, with his unique stump "fingerprint."[36] De Preester suggests that true incorporation of limb prosthesis into the body involves a change in the feeling of body ownership over the prosthesis, which takes the object beyond simply being an extension of the body.[37] Tom's unique and individualized prosthetic limb thus becomes a way through which he reestablishes his individual bodily identity, rather than something that limits who he is and what he can achieve.

Using prosthetic limbs enables Tom to mobilize inside and outside of the home. Toward the end of the novel, Parker describes how Tom runs on a prosthetic limb that is adapted as a running leg. Messinger writes that in relation to the military past, sport and physical activity connect the veteran back to their past as service members, as a big part of the military experience is accomplishing a high level of physical activity.[38] Caddick and Smith also recognize that for the amputee, undertaking sport and exercise reflects "doing things" and taking responsibility for well-being[39]. Further, sport allows the individual to focus on achievement rather than their limitations and impairment.[40]

Tom's running is a significant marker of what could be perceived as "normal" mobility for someone physically fit and able-bodied, and it is important to explore Parker's inclusion of this particular activity for the transition experience of his character. Parker describes how Tom perseveres through the pain of adjusting to

---

[35] Ibid., 285.
[36] Ibid.
[37] Helena De Preester, "Technology and the Body: The (Im)Possibilities of Re-embodiment," *Foundations of Science* 16, no. 2 (2010): 119–37.
[38] Seth D. Messinger, "Getting Past the Accident: Explosive Devices, Limb Loss, and Refashioning a Life in a Military Medical Center," *Medical Anthropology Quarterly* 24, no. 3 (2010): 281–303.
[39] Nick Caddick et al., "Hierarchies of Wounding: Media Framings of 'Combat' and 'Non-Combat' Injury," *Media, War & Conflict* (January 13, 2020): 9.
[40] Nick Caddick and Brett Smith, "The Impact of Sport and Physical Activity on the Well-Being of Combat Veterans: A Systematic Review," *Psychology of Sport and Exercise* 15, no. 1 (January 1, 2014): 9–18.

running on a prosthetic and challenges himself to run faster and harder. Parker writes that Tom and the prosthetic work together to achieve this; "I compressed and sprang on below you and you puffed in and out above. We over-took another runner."[41] They are referred to as "we," a partnership in competition with another runner. Further, Parker writes, "It felt normal and light and fast and free—and you were running,"[42] but Tom falls over. This event is highly significant in what it indicates to Tom about his rehabilitation journey and with regard to what Parker tells the reader about what it is like to be an amputee. On falling over, Parker writes from the narrative viewpoint of the prosthetic limb:

> You looked at the deep red grooves down your palms and the black grit pushed under your skin. It stung and hardened into pain as you stared at them, but then you smiled and started to laugh at the pain and the blood that dripped from your hands. And tears came because you could, and it didn't matter anymore. It was normal. You replaced me with your other legs, shut the boot and drove to work.[43]

There are several significant aspects of this quotation to explore: first, the normalization of pain, in that Tom accepts pain as an inevitability of the process of adapting to his prosthesis and a "normal" part of being an amputee. Tom is also accepting of his emotional reaction to the pain, which the quotation implies is "normal" for Tom. Second, this prosthetic is recognized as one of many that Tom has to aid his mobility, shown through reference to "other legs," which gives a sense of the prosthetic, as the object narrator, having less of an identity than the character of Tom. This suggests that the emphasis moves away from the object as the dominant voice in the narrative and puts Tom in the position of authority over the decision of what prosthetic to select to aid his mobility best for his chosen activity.

Third, Tom's final act in the novel is to drive himself to work. This is a signifier of a "normal," everyday routine of working. Driving and being able to go to work are recognized as key markers of social independence for the amputee.[44] Engward et al. assert that being able to set goals related to pre-limb loss "normal" everyday activities such as employment is important for an individual and their family coping and living with limb loss.[45] The most significant aspect of the above quotation, though, may be the fall itself; falling as an amputee and accepting it as "normal" shows a self-acceptance of the injury and the ability to cope with it. In *Anatomy of a Soldier*, this demonstrates Tom's acceptance of his "new normal,"

---

[41] Parker, *Anatomy of a Soldier*, 311.
[42] Ibid.
[43] Ibid., 312.
[44] Engward et al., "The Family Perspective on Living with Limb Loss," 115.
[45] Ibid., 68.

in that falling over is a normal part of life as an amputee. However, falling over is something often more readily accepted by the amputee themselves than by those around them. Family members and onlookers can become understandably worried at seeing an amputee fall over, but for the amputee, the concern and attention from others at what has become a normal occurrence can be a source of frustration or self-consciousness.[46]

Falling over signifies that the body is in a state of unnatural movement. Turner writes that "social success depends on an ability to manage the self by the adoption of appropriate interpersonal skills and success hinges crucially on the presentation of an acceptable image," something the amputee may not always be able to achieve as they may face balancing issues.[47] Turner recognizes that body metaphors are important signals of social disruption; the balanced or imbalanced body is often used to speak about social order, and falling over signifies an imbalanced body and social disorder. For example, falling over in public can lead to the social judgment that the person in question is "drunk," which in turn is often associated negatively with being physically imbalanced and disorderly.[48] Tom's acceptance of falling over, and how he copes with his reaction to it, serves as a symbolic rejection of this rhetoric, in his reframing of the "normal" life of an amputee.

Renegotiating Sociocultural Norms and Social Identity as an Amputee Veteran

In the above discussion, there is a juxtaposition between Tom the amputee as a physically able runner, on the one hand, and as a social disrupter, on the other. In Parker's writing there is a sense that this medical transition is not linear. The amputee must cope with social stigma, multiple perspectives on limb loss, and conflicting attitudes toward what an amputee's social status is and should be, as well as their own preconceptions. In *Anatomy of a Soldier*, Tom confronts these attitudes directly when he ventures outside wearing his prosthetic leg. Parker writes from the view of the prosthesis:

> You saw them look and challenged them with a stare and they turned away embarrassed. You wished they wouldn't look at us; we weren't a freak show and you wanted to be ignored. But we were the strangest thing to walk down those

---

[46] Ibid., 62.
[47] Bryan S. Turner, "Body," *Theory, Culture & Society* 23, nos. 2–3 (2006): 223–9.
[48] Engward et al., "The Family Perspective on Living with Limb Loss," 62.

aisles all day. As soon as we were past and they knew you couldn't see them, they stopped picking tomatoes and stared at us walking away. They couldn't resist watching and they wondered how we did it. We were science fiction, you and I, and they didn't see the pain in your socket or the sweat collecting in your liners or the effort you expended to swing me down the bread aisle. All they saw was the magic of me and a young, upright man who had overcome the unsurvivable.[49]

This passage exemplifies the conflicting attitudes Tom confronts as a particularly visible amputee encountering strangers. It illustrates the judgment Tom faces, in being regarded as somehow "other," which therefore creates a social distance between Tom and other people. The quotation demonstrates the confusion and discomfort that such spectators face at simultaneously feeling embarrassed to stare at someone with these injuries, but also mesmerized by the impressive robotic sight of Tom; the confusion seems to come partly from a need of the public to comprehend whether Tom is more or less capable because of his injury. Brody explores the notion of living with disability and asserts that, apart from the physical disability itself, of equal importance is how others judge the disability and life with disability.[50] Brody contends that disability is a socially defined concept, and the quotation exemplifies the way in which attitudes toward those with physical differences are often polarized and experienced within the social sphere.

This dichotomy can be further examined through the hero–victim narrative, which Cree and Caddick recognize as a tension surrounding veterans.[51] Tom is seen as both limited and extraordinary, able to move in a seemingly "magic" way, but also a war-damaged victim. Tom's veteran identity is a significant aspect of many of his social interactions with others, both strangers and friends. Caddick asserts that experiences of war are "simultaneously narrative and embodied," as social human experience is enabled by the body but not reducible to it.[52] The embodied experience must be made sense of in relation to social experience suggesting that ultimately Tom's bodily identity will be predominantly socially defined and, therefore, Tom's sense of himself socially is an important part of his identity as an amputee veteran. Social connectedness and support within the civilian world are identified as being important for transition; Keeling asserts that veterans who are socially isolated experience the most difficult transitions.[53]

---

[49] Parker, *Anatomy of a Soldier*, 288.
[50] Howard Brody, *Stories of Sickness*, 2nd ed. (Oxford: Oxford University Press, 2003), 151.
[51] Alice Cree and Nick Caddick, "Unconquerable Heroes: Invictus, Redemption, and the Cultural Politics of Narrative," *Journal of War & Culture Studies* 13, no. 3 (2020): 258–78.
[52] Nick Caddick, "Life, Embodiment, and (Post-)War Stories: Studying Narrative in Critical Military Studies," *Critical Military Studies* 7, no. 2 (2021): 155–72.
[53] Keeling, "Stories of Transition."

Parker explores social connectedness further through a meeting between Tom and his friend in a pub post-limb loss. While they are talking, a member of the public approaches Tom and asks about his prosthetic leg, immediately associating it with a war injury. In conversation, the man uses the term "hero" in reference to Tom's injuries and remarks, "You lads are so brave."[54] Tom responds that he is not brave, "just trod on the wrong piece of ground," and says to his friend afterwards, "can't be too ungrateful—he meant well—but I hate that sort of thing."[55] It is clear from these exchanges that back in the civilian world, Tom's limb loss is regarded as defining his military service in the eyes of some people, but as a result of their lack of understanding of Tom's experience, and not because they want to socially exclude him.

These conflicting and polarized social attitudes toward veterans can be influenced by the media. Caddick et al. examine how the figure of the veteran has been portrayed by the British media. The authors identify, on the one hand, a portrayal of the injured veteran as heroic and, on the other, veterans as victims of warfare. Newspaper coverage of combat-related injury "present[s] a highly charged, sensationalized and emotive narrative rendering of combat injury."[56] This emphasis in the media coverage, Caddick et al. assert, encourages readers (and in turn the general public) to feel pride for the heroic soldier and their selfless actions, which are described in general as being honorable and worthy of respect. However, "wounded bodies confront societies with the damage of war. They make war real, visceral and concrete to publics who are often far removed from the violence itself."[57] War often takes place at a distance, "outside" of Western societies and out of view of the public, so the return of injured bodies is all the public sees as a representation of what happened.[58]

In a discussion on portrayals of veterans in US media, Kleykamp and Hipes assert that a dominant theme in media coverage is the victimization of veterans.[59] In Parker's narrative, immediately after the exchange with a member of the public, Tom's friend says, "Must be grim ... I'm not sure I could do it, mate. I'd probably have committed suicide if it happened to me."[60] The comment shows a subconscious adopting of this attitude of victimization; within the attempt at

---

[54] Parker, *Anatomy of a Soldier*, 268–9.
[55] Ibid., 269.
[56] Caddick et al., "Hierarchies of Wounding," 7.
[57] Ibid., 1.
[58] Alice Cree and Nick Caddick, "Unconquerable Heroes: Invictus, Redemption, and the Cultural Politics of Narrative," 258–78.
[59] Meredith Kleykamp and Crosby Hipes, "Coverage of Veterans of the Wars in Iraq and Afghanistan in the U.S. Media," 348–68.
[60] Parker, *Anatomy of a Soldier*, 269.

sympathy for limb loss is contained the attitude that life is not worth living with this form of disability, as socially defined in the context of the veteran narrative and which in turn isolates the amputee from their civilian peer group.

Conclusion

Harry Parker's novel *Anatomy of a Soldier* portrays two significant, related transitions: moving from able-bodied to amputee, and changing from soldier to veteran returning to civilian society. To describe the embodied experience of losing a limb and gaining a prosthetic, the novel is written from the narrative perspectives of the objects that assist Tom in his medical care, recovery, and rehabilitation. Imbuing medical instruments with a narrative voice humanizes medical and clinical procedures, which necessitates a suspension of the self for Tom and distances him from his social groups. Tom's bodily identity is reconstructed after his accident through the medical technologies used literally to put his physical body back together. This need for the reconstruction of the physical self-mirrors the need for a reconstruction of Tom's individual sense of self and civilian social identities. An individual's social identity is also influenced by social expectations and attitudes. For Tom this relates to attitudes toward disability, limb difference, and the mixed expectations of veterans. Parker's character is forced to define his new "normal" for his life as an amputee, and this is experienced against a backdrop of military-to-civilian transition, a process involving symbolic losses and gains in the individual's life. For Tom, these losses and gains are also experienced at a bodily level, in relation to his limb loss and gaining of a prosthetic. Beyond practical considerations, military-to-civilian transition is a personal, psychological, and emotional experience, and Tom's experience reflects the wider significance of individuals coming to terms with how "normal" life will change as a result of an accident, illness, or disease, and thus redefine what "normal" means to them, to cope with the long-term effects and changes. This chapter presents an alternative medical discourse to put a humanistic, rather than scientific, focus on the medical experience while showing how science and medicine are an integral part of "normal" life, and not something "other" to everyday experience.

Part 2

Practices

Introduction

This part investigates some of the humanities-informed practices that exist in medicine, including electronic recordkeeping of medical narratives, structural competence education and empathy training in the medical school curriculum, and the use of visual materials in the classification of patient pain. Writing from the disciplinary perspectives of emergency medicine, medical anthropology, and art history, authors Kamna S. Balhara, Joshua Franklin, and Gabi Schaffzin see such practices as cocreations of medicine and humanities that attempt to "humanize" medicine, but inadvertently result in perpetuating biomedical assumptions—not merely in their content but also in their forms and genres. The authors propose that such cocreations are evidence of medicine operating as a cultural practice that can shape aesthetic objects. Further, countering the inherent assumption that such "humanistic" practices might improve the medical encounter, the chapters also acknowledge the potential for dissatisfaction that can result from these practices from the perspective of the practitioner, the patient, or both.

Thinking through such dissatisfaction in an analytical way represents a commitment to the critical and ethical values that interweave these contributions and the volume as a whole. The chapters bridge their "medical humanities" orientation—their turn toward the realities of medical education and the clinical encounter—with a "health humanities" sensibility, questioning from an outside perspective the ways in which the humanities are brought to bear on medical contexts. The works identify how imported protocols from the humanities might not improve the delivery of care and instead produce new kinds of failures. The chapters' critical reflections on how cultural artifacts enter the clinic think about how these practices have become codified, and how careful attention can shape their future.

Chapter 4, by Balhara, approaches the electronic health record (EHR) as a historically bounded genre that can be critiqued as a "technoscientific object" through a philosophical lens. Following the media theories of Marshall McLuhan and Friedrich Kittler, Balhara finds that the EHR is a device that not only facilitates the communication between medical providers around the care of a patient but also transforms the doctor–patient relationship and the nature of illness. Concerns about the reshaped contours of the patient's narrative permeate physicians' own assessments of their adoption of the technoscientific form. Even as it fulfills the collection's emphasis on a critical value by illuminating medicine's own checkered assessment of the EHR and its implications, the chapter also performs ethical work by revealing the human consequences of adopting such technoscientific products in a medical space. Ultimately, the chapter proposes that the EHR might transform the style of medical communication itself, with both limitations and opportunities for the clinical encounter.

The challenge of narrativizing the medical encounter in the electronic medical record is taken up again in Chapter 5, by Franklin, which begins with a story of the author's recognition of his own limitations as a practitioner-in-training. Franklin offers the affordances of the genre of the electronic medical record as an invitation to reflect on the limitations of "structural competence education," a humanities-influenced curriculum taught in medical schools that aspires to compensate for the limitations of "cultural competency." Beyond literacy in and sensitivity to cultural differences, "structural competence" invites practitioners to use the tools of humanities disciplines (e.g., cultural history, anthropology, etc.) to consider the systemic and social determinants of health-shaping clinical encounters. Yet, Franklin finds that structural competence education is, practically speaking, an "umbrella term for social medicine pedagogy," and he argues that its limitations arise from unsolved dilemmas within anthropology, the discipline from which it was imported into medicine. He contends that, in turn, by solving the problems of structural competence education, the field of anthropology might also be transformed. In tracing such a two-way, mutually reinforcing relationship between the practices of the humanities and of medicine, the chapter fulfils the collection's ethical value of fortifying clinical research and scientific activity through the ways of knowing of the humanities while reconsidering how the humanities might be transformed by the knowledge practices of medicine.

Following the volume's emphasis on the critical value of medical humanities, Chapter 6, by Schaffzin, returns to the question of imported knowledge practices from the humanities into medicine, but from the vantage of art history and the history of science. Schaffzin traces the long history of the Visual Analogue Scale (VAS), a ubiquitous tool for the diagnosis of pain, to find that its roots lie in the evaluation metrics of early twentieth-century industrial management. From this surprising beginning, he argues, the quantification of pain in the patient has been commodified today as "a market that can be controlled and dominated." Through an analysis of the aesthetic design of the VAS as a "smooth line," Schaffzin finds that the tool is misleadingly suggestive of a kind of "freedom" for the "clinical subject," who experiences a "false sense of control" of their own self-definition while being caught in a hidden capitalist matrix underlying the health system. The deceptive design values of the VAS reveal the pain scale as a product imported from another context whose function within the medical establishment might prove to be ethically dubious. As with all the chapters in this part, Schaffzin's essay suggests that the interdisciplinary transplantation of knowledge practices from the humanities into medicine might not offer an unqualified solution to existing problems within medicine; rather, such importations might create further complications. Yet, as with Franklin's essay, the part as a whole presents the optimistic perspective that in responding to such challenges, medicine might be able to introduce solutions into the humanities as well.

On the Record: What Physician Texts Reveal about Physician Identities and the Electronic Health Record

Kamna S. Balhara

Introduction

The medical record has undergone numerous transitions in response to political, legal, bureaucratic, and technological forces.[1] Its most recent iteration, the electronic health record (EHR), has attracted significant conversation and controversy. First developed in the 1960s, the EHR received additional attention in the 1980s and 1990s after the Institute of Medicine identified it as a means of improving patient records. EHRs subsequently came into widespread use in the United States after President Obama's 2009 Health Information Technology for Economic and Clinical Health Act (HITECH), which set aside upwards of $19 billion to incentivize EHR use. Prior to HITECH, 17 percent of American physicians and 9 percent of hospitals were using EHRs.[2] By 2017, almost all hospitals and nearly 80 percent of office-based practices were using EHRs.[3]

While the definitive influence of EHRs on clinical care is not yet fully established, some studies point toward measurable positive impacts, including patient satisfaction with EHR use.[4] A 2011 review found that 92 percent of

---

[1] Richard F. Gillum, "From Papyrus to the Electronic Tablet: A Brief History of the Clinical Medical Record with Lessons for the Digital Age," *American Journal of Medicine* 126, no. 10 (October 1, 2013): 853–7, https://doi.org/10.1016/j.amjmed.2013.03.024.
[2] Jeanne Lambrew, "More than Half of Doctors Now Use Electronic Health Records Thanks to Administration Policies," White House President Barack Obama (blog), May 23, 2013.
[3] Vindell Washington et al., "The HITECH Era and the Path Forward," *New England Journal of Medicine* 377, no. 10 (September 7, 2017): 904–6, https://doi.org/10.1056/NEJMp1703370.
[4] Melinda Beeuwkes Buntin et al., "The Benefits of Health Information Technology: A Review of the Recent Literature Shows Predominantly Positive Results," *Health Affairs* 30, no. 3 (March 2011): 464–71; Jennifer King et al., "Clinical Benefits of Electronic Health Record Use: National Findings,"

published articles on health information technology recorded positive results in domains such as patient safety and clinical efficiency.[5] Despite this, ten years after its meteoric adoption across the United States, the EHR remains linked with physician dissatisfaction and burnout.[6] Common refrains populate physician complaints about the EHR, including erosion of the doctor–patient relationship, degradation of bedside skills, loss of autonomy, and encroachment into time away from work. This chapter will argue that the root of physician resistance to the EHR may also lie in the fundamental changes and perceived threats to physician identity wrought by the EHR. While some of these changes are emblematic of the larger commodification and corporatization of medicine, this chapter seeks to demonstrate that such changes are occurring from the "inside out," via the very structure and form of the medium of the EHR itself.

EHR as Technoscientific Object

The arrangements of power and knowledge intrinsic to EHR use have been previously described as a panopticon, an apparatus of power and surveillance that cultivates discipline among healthcare providers and enforces subordination to a bureaucratic authority.[7] Others have described how EHRs

---

Health Services Research 49, no. 1, pt. 2 (2014): 392–404, https://doi.org/10.1111/1475-6773.12135; Jihad S. Irani et al., "The Use of Electronic Health Records in the Exam Room and Patient Satisfaction: A Systematic Review," *Journal of the American Board of Family Medicine* 22, no. 5 (September 1, 2009): 553–62, https://doi.org/10.3122/jabfm.2009.05.080259; Jialin Liu et al., "Patient Satisfaction with Electronic Medical/Health Record: A Systematic Review," *Scandinavian Journal of Caring Sciences* 27, no. 4 (2013): 785–91, https://doi.org/10.1111/scs.12015.

[5] Buntin et al., "The Benefits of Health Information Technology."

[6] Mark W. Friedberg et al., "Factors Affecting Physician Professional Satisfaction and Their Implications for Patient Care, Health Systems, and Health Policy," *Rand Health Quarterly* 3, no. 4 (2013): 1; Greta B. Raglan et al., "Electronic Health Record Adoption among Obstetrician/Gynecologists in the United States: Physician Practices and Satisfaction," *Journal for Healthcare Quality* 39, no. 3 (2017): 144–52, https://doi.org/10.1111/jhq.12072; Chad D. Meyerhoefer et al., "Provider and Patient Satisfaction with the Integration of Ambulatory and Hospital EHR Systems," *Journal of the American Medical Informatics Association* 25, no. 8 (2018): 1054–63, https://doi.org/10.1093/jamia/ocy048; S. Emani et al., "Physician Beliefs about the Impact of Meaningful Use of the EHR," *Applied Clinical Informatics* 5, no. 3 (2014): 789–801, https://doi.org/10.4338/ACI-2014-05-RA-0050; Srinivas Emani et al., "Physician Beliefs about the Meaningful Use of the Electronic Health Record: A Follow-Up Study," *Applied Clinical Informatics* 8, no. 4 (2017): 1044–53, https://doi.org/10.4338/ACI-2017-05-RA-0079.

[7] Adam Reich, "Disciplined Doctors: The Electronic Medical Record and Physicians' Changing Relationship to Medical Knowledge," *Social Science & Medicine* 74, no. 7 (April 1, 2012): 1021–8, https://doi.org/10.1016/j.socscimed.2011.12.032; Jessica Dillard-Wright, "Electronic Health Record as a Panopticon: A Disciplinary Apparatus in Nursing Practice," *Nursing Philosophy* 20, no. 2 (2019), https://doi.org/10.1111/nup.12239.

lead to the electronic exile of the physical patient body to the virtual space.[8] Rather than viewing the EHR as a Foucauldian panopticon or heterotopia, however, this chapter will study the EHR as a technoscientific innovation that is reshaping physician practice, from the "inside out." Such innovations grow from the coalescence of science and technology. Technoscientization is a social phenomenon identified by Clarke and colleagues as a key apparatus of biomedicalization, which expands upon medicalization of human experience via advances in science and technology. Computerization and data-banking of medical knowledge are key technoscientific innovations in biomedicalization. Among the resultant processes of biomedicalization is not just the transformation of patient bodies via technoscientific advances but also the transformation of their identities. Examples include unexpectedly learning that one is a carrier of an inherited disease via genomic sequencing, or being able to transform from "infertile" to "mother" through fertility treatments.[9] Much of the emphasis on remodeled technoscientific identifies focuses on patients.[10] However, as operators, creators, and receivers of technoscientific innovations, physicians, too, are subject to a technoscientization of their identities. Exploration of the EHR as a technoscientific object in relation to physician identities is limited. Mishra applied an identity theory perspective to physician survey data to examine EHR assimilation.[11] Reich used sociological fieldwork to describe the EHR's impact as a disciplinary technology on physicians' professional relationships with medical knowledge and power. In a departure from previous work, this chapter will use texts written by physicians on the EHR as a primary source of data and apply a lens borrowed from German media theorist Friedrich Kittler to dissect how the EHR, as a technoscientific innovation, functions as a biomedical apparatus, fundamentally altering two core components of physician identity, that of a storyteller and of a diagnostician-detective.

---

[8] Marc Berg and Geoffrey Bowker, "The Multiple Bodies of the Medical Record: Toward a Sociology of an Artifact," *Sociological Quarterly* 38, no. 3 (1997): 513–37; Abraham Verghese, "Culture Shock—Patient as Icon, Icon as Patient," *New England Journal of Medicine* 359, no. 26 (December 25, 2008): 2748–51, https://doi.org/10.1056/NEJMp0807461.

[9] Adele E. Clarke et al., "Biomedicalization: Technoscientific Transformations of Health, Illness, and U.S. Biomedicine," *American Sociological Review* 68, no. 2 (2003): 161–94, https://doi.org/10.2307/1519765.

[10] Gayle A. Sulik, "Managing Biomedical Uncertainty: The Technoscientific Illness Identity," *Sociology of Health & Illness* 31, no. 7 (2009): 1059–76; Peter Wehling, "The 'Technoscientization' of Medicine and Its Limits: Technoscientific Identities, Biosocialities, and Rare Disease Patient Organizations," *Poiesis & Praxis* 8, no. 2 (2011): 67–82.

[11] Abhay Nath Mishra et al., "Electronic Health Records Assimilation and Physician Identity Evolution: An Identity Theory Perspective," *Information Systems Research* 23, no. 3 (2012): 738–60.

EHRs Determine Our Situation

Specifically, this chapter will treat the EHR as a technological medium that, via its production, reproduction, and storage of information, shapes and conditions its end-user, the physician. While Marshall McLuhan (1964) viewed media as an extension of the human body, Friedrich Kittler argued that "media are not pseudopods for extending the human body" and "they follow the logic of escalation that leaves us and written history behind it."[12] Media are not simply autonomous; they are exceedingly influential. "Media determine our situation,"[13] writes Kittler (1999) in the preface to *Gramophone, Film, Typewriter*, recognizing how media technologies shape their users and human affairs in turn.[14] Rather than viewing media as a way to dissect cultural and social movements, he views media as directly influencing those very movements. In Kittler's eyes, the development of the internet, for instance, "has more to do with human beings becoming a reflection of their technologies."[15] Rather than examining how external forces have shaped the EHR and physician practice, this chapter will adopt a Kittlerian approach in examining how the intrinsic structure and format of EHR technology has fundamentally altered certain key components of physician identity. Kittler further argued, "After all, it is we who adapt to the machine. The machine does not adapt to us."[16] Similarly, physician-author Abraham Verghese states that the EHR "was meant to serve [physicians], but at times the opposite seemed true."[17]

Kittler's book *Gramophone, Film, Typewriter* is a "story made up of … stories" that "collects, comments upon, and relays passages and texts that show … the novelty of technological media."[18] In order to study the adaptations and evolutions of culture in response to advances such as the gramophone, film, and typewriter, Kittler used poetry, literature, and essays contemporary to those innovations. Similarly, this chapter will use texts published by physicians about the EHR in widely read scientific journals as a primary source material to dissect the EHR's impact on physician self-perception, perceived loss of identities, and identities formed in response.

---

[12] Stuart Jeffries, *Grand Hotel Abyss: The Lives of the Frankfurt School* (London: Verso, 2016), 182.
[13] Friedrich A. Kittler, *Gramophone, Film, Typewriter*, trans. Geoffrey Winthrop-Young and Michael Wutz, Writing Science (Stanford, CA: Stanford University Press, 1999), xxxv.
[14] Ibid., xxxix.
[15] Stuart Jeffries, "Friedrich Kittler and the Rise of the Machine," *The Guardian*, 2011, sec. Opinion.
[16] Ibid.
[17] Verghese, "Culture Shock—Patient as Icon, Icon as Patient."
[18] Kittler, *Gramophone, Film, Typewriter*, xi.

Methods

The electronic archives of commentaries and essays in the *New England Journal of Medicine* (*NEJM*) and the *Journal of the American Medical Association* (*JAMA*) were searched from inception to May 2019 for articles including the words "electronic health record(s)" and "electronic medical record(s)." This search revealed 328 articles in *NEJM* and 599 in *JAMA*. After removal of duplicates, article titles or synopses were screened; articles that were clearly irrelevant; reviewed existing literature or commented on a research paper; focused solely on the financial, legal, bureaucratic, organizational, and logistical aspects of EHR implementation; or did not represent the point of view of a physician were excluded. First-person narratives on interactions with the EHR and articles describing the impact of and attitudes toward EHR implementation in key domains of clinical practice were included. In sum, twenty-five articles from *NEJM* and twenty-seven from *JAMA* were included for analysis. Themes of patient–physician communication, physician–physician teamwork, and written communication via narratives populated the majority of articles; questions of the meaning of physician work and rapport with diagnosis were common as well.

A Perceived Rupture in Identity

These texts reveal a perceived rupture and fundamental alteration in physician identity and sense of self. Toll describes one doctor, a "physician's physician" who delivers "humanity and competence," who is stunned to realize his "patients might be seeing him in a new way since the rollout of the [EHR]": no one is more surprised than him to see that a young patient's cartoon depicts him gazing at the computer with his back to her family.[19] Rosenbaum questions the enduring harm of the EHR via the "disruption of medicine which manifests as a disintegration, not just mental, but physical, causing physicians to come 'undone.'" The EHR leads one physician to be "distracted, losing his grip on the details of his patients' lives." The transition is so jarring as to manifest physically as illness; this physician "slumped around, shirt half-tucked, perpetually pulling a yellow handkerchief from his pocket to wipe his perspiring forehead. Everyone worried he was sick. His problem ... turned out to be the [EHR]."[20]

---

[19] Elizabeth Toll, "The Cost of Technology," *JAMA* 307, no. 23 (June 20, 2012): 2498.
[20] Lisa Rosenbaum, "Transitional Chaos or Enduring Harm? The EHR and the Disruption of Medicine," *New England Journal of Medicine* 373, no. 17 (2015): 1585.

Much is tinged with nostalgia: references to "past" or "bygone" eras, "old days," "traditional approaches," "time-honored" practices, and what "used to" happen abound in many physician articles on EHRs.[21] One physician looks to the archives of doctor/poet William Carlos Williams, as another explores patient notes kept by a great-grandfather.[22] As with all nostalgic references to the past, there is a tendency to overlook the failings of previous systems. However, a very real perception of loss persists. "It is easy to lose sight of yourself ... as you endure the countless hours spent ... entering data in [EHRs]," writes Safder.[23] Halamka and Tripathi, describing the rapid spread of the EHR, write that, "along the way ... we lost the hearts and minds of clinicians."[24] Rosenthal and Verghese question whether physicians have been led astray from their "original purpose" and question their ability to find meaning in a post-EHR world.

The Physician-Storyteller

The ability to listen to and transcribe patients' stories emerges as a defining characteristic of meaningful work for many physicians. The patient's "body is the text"; practicing medicine entails both "romance and passion"; and the keeping and telling of patient stories is described by many as an essential theme in clinical practice.[25] The EHR, however, throws that physician-storyteller identity into question by disrupting physicians' abilities to both gather and tell stories; "I suppose that my concern about [EHRs] and their templates is about losing the words that have connected me with generations of patients," writes Frey.[26]

---

[21] Pamela Hartzband and Jerome Groopman, "Off the Record—Avoiding the Pitfalls of Going Electronic," *New England Journal of Medicine* 358, no. 16 (April 17, 2008): 1656–8, http://dx.doi.org.ezproxy.cul.columbia.edu/10.1056/NEJMp0802221; Perri Klass, "Disconnected," *New England Journal of Medicine* 362, no. 15 (April 15, 2010): 1358–61. David I. Rosenthal and Abraham Verghese, "Meaning and the Nature of Physicians' Work," *New England Journal of Medicine* 375, no. 19 (2016): 1813–15; Ziad Obermeyer and Thomas H. Lee, "Lost in Thought: The Limits of the Human Mind and the Future of Medicine," *New England Journal of Medicine* 377, no. 13 (2017).

[22] John J. Frey, "At a Loss for Words," *JAMA* 297, no. 16 (April 25, 2007): 1751–2, https://doi.org/10.1001/jama.297.16.1751; Curtis G. Kommer, "Good Documentation," *JAMA* 320, no. 9 (September 4, 2018): 875–6.

[23] Taimur Safder, "The Name of the Dog," *New England Journal of Medicine* 379, no. 14 (October 4, 2018): 1301.

[24] John D. Halamka and Micky Tripathi, "The HITECH Era in Retrospect," *New England Journal of Medicine* 377, no. 10 (2017): 907.

[25] Verghese, "Culture Shock—Patient as Icon, Icon as Patient"; Rosenbaum, "Transitional Chaos or Enduring Harm?"; Allan H. Goroll, "Emerging from EHR Purgatory—Moving from Process to Outcomes," *New England Journal of Medicine* 376, no. 21 (May 25, 2017): 2004–6; Klass, "Disconnected"; Daniel R. Wolpaw and Dan Shapiro, "The Virtues of Irrelevance," *New England Journal of Medicine* 370, no. 14 (April 3, 2014): 2749.

[26] Frey, "At a Loss for Words," 1751.

The EHR was meant to facilitate transcription of patient encounters, but has in turn altered the nature of the encounter it was designed to record. What was once a conversation turns increasingly transactional. "Encounters have been restructured around the demands of the EHR: specific questions must be asked, and answer boxes filled in," write Hartzband and Groopman[27]; the very format of the EHR "directs [physicians] to ask restrictive questions rather than engaging in narrative-based open-ended dialogue."[28] Lifflander describes "particularly nefarious" EHR "hard stops," which mandate that a specific question be answered before moving to the next, literally disjointing the conversation.[29] Beyond the flow and content of verbal communication, the EHR also modifies the sharing of nonverbal cues; "the doctor focused on the screen rather than the patient has become a cultural cliché."[30] Indeed, studies of the gaze patterns of physicians corroborate this; 30 percent of physician gaze time is spent looking at the EHR.[31]

A common thread in these articles is not simply the loss of ability to truly hear the story, but the suppression of the physician's individual voice as a storyteller. This rupture in the physician-storyteller identity occurs via the devaluation of the handwritten word, the homogenization of physician expression via the use of prepopulated templates, and loss of meaning in storytelling.

Storytelling is inextricably linked to the act of writing, and handwriting is highly personal. Kittler describes how handwriting leaves behind "strangely unavoidable traces" of the body.[32] Mediums of storage and dissemination of the written word, however, diminish that highly personal connection. Kittler describes how the typewriter disrupted the intimate linkage of the eye, the hand, and the word, an interloper introducing an element of distance into the process of expression.[33] The introduction of the EHR operates a similar change. Edelman issues the death knell of handwritten physician narratives: "Electronic documentation ... has erased all vestiges of the hand-written word."[34] "Typing and clicking" has become the new writing, states Patel.[35] Not only has the sterile typed word taken the place of that which is handwritten, it has also assumed the

---

[27] Hartzband and Groopman, "Off the Record—Avoiding the Pitfalls of Going Electronic," 107.
[28] Ibid., 1657.
[29] Anne Lucy Lifflander, "Hard Times and Hard Stops," *JAMA* 321, no. 9 (March 5, 2019): 837.
[30] Rosenthal and Verghese, "Meaning and the Nature of Physicians' Work," 1814.
[31] Onur Asan, Paul D. Smith, and Enid Montague, "More Screen Time, Less Face Time—Implications for EHR Design," *Journal of Evaluation in Clinical Practice* 20, no. 6 (2014): 896–901.
[32] Kittler, *Gramophone, Film, Typewriter*, 8.
[33] Friedrich A. Kittler, *Discourse Networks 1800/1900*, trans. Michael Metteer and Chris Cullens (Stanford, CA: Stanford University Press, 1990), 195.
[34] Elazer R. Edelman and Brittany N. Weber, "Tenuous Tether," *New England Journal of Medicine* 373, no. 23 (2015): 2200.
[35] Jayshil J. Patel, "Writing the Wrong," *JAMA* 314, no. 7 (August 18, 2015): 671.

mantle of "the last word." "It might seem that the printed [or at least typed] word, which we are all conditioned to respect, would always be more definitive and have more impact than text written by hand," write Hartzband and Groopman.[36] Rosenbaum describes how lists of patients' conditions "pop up on the computer screen and, in their pristine, boldface type, somehow seem much more definitive than the words doctors used to scrawl in notoriously illegible handwriting."[37] Certainly, the assurance of universal legibility is an incontestable boon to patient safety; Patel, for one, describes looking forward to the EHR doing away with "shambolic handwriting" and "medical hieroglyphics."[38] But the fallibility of the handwritten word is also what makes it indelibly individual, and its replacement with standardized fonts and formatting displaces the individuality of the physician-storyteller and transforms fluid, evolving narratives into cold sterile edicts. Wu notes the emotionless and brutal efficiency of bad news delivered in a chart with a "blinking cursor."[39] Kommer, reflecting on his great-grandfather's "elegant handwriting" in personal patient anecdotes and his own "great pride in [his handwriting]" in the pre-EHR era, wonders whether his current "EHR-generated notes will shed any true insight to a future reader into how [he] cared for [his] patients."[40] The "loopy handwriting will be gone" along with "any trace of me," writes Frey.[41] Just as the typewriter is an "other," an intermediary that reduces the undulating flow of words from mind to hand to paper to staccato clicks and taps, the EHR, via the computer keyboard, takes away the visual signature of the storyteller.

Beyond erasing the physical appearance of the patient narrative recorded by an individual physician, the EHR effaces the storyteller's writing style. Concerns about "templated notes," "drop down menus, cut-and-paste text fields and lists," "answer boxes," and "boilerplate entries" populate many physician concerns about the EHR.[42] The patient narrative can often only be told through standardized click boxes. While free-text entry options exist, the use of pretemplated standardized

---

[36] Hartzband and Groopman, "Off the Record—Avoiding the Pitfalls of Going Electronic," 1657.
[37] Lisa Rosenbaum, "Living Unlabeled—Diagnosis and Disorder," *New England Journal of Medicine* 359, no. 16 (2008): 1652.
[38] Patel, "Writing the Wrong," 671.
[39] David Wu, "Virtual Grief," JAMA 308, no. 20 (November 28, 2012): 2095–6.
[40] Kommer, "Good Documentation," 375–6.
[41] Frey, "At a Loss for Words," 1752.
[42] Hartzband and Groopman, "Off the Record—Avoiding the Pitfalls of Going Electronic," 1657; Rosenthal and Verghese, "Meaning and the Nature of Physicians' Work," 1814; Pamela Hartzband and Jerome Groopman, "Medical Taylorism," *New England Journal of Medicine* 374, no. 2 (2016): 1; Goroll, "Emerging from EHR Purgatory—Moving from Process to Outcomes," 2005; Gordon D. Schiff and David W. Bates, "Can Electronic Clinical Documentation Help Prevent Diagnostic Errors?," *New England Journal of Medicine* 362, no. 12 (March 25, 2010): 1066.

language is encouraged for the facilitation of billing. "The things in the margins are the most important, if not to the patient, then to me," writes Frey, but in the restrictive confines of the EHR's narrative spaces, there is no room for personal annotations.[43] In defining what physicians should write, the EHR also defines what parts of the narrative the physician should value; Patel notes that while mired in the computer's "numbers ... and the notes," he no longer writes down much, and what he fails to write down are perhaps the things that matter most to his patient.[44] The EHR does not provide space for clinicians to express their "thought processes, intuitions, and recommendations."[45] The result is the loss of independent, personal expression. The standardized language of the EHR homogenizes physicians' voices, which are supplanted by electronic anonymity in the form of the toneless, unvarying voice of the EHR. In an effort to reduce time spent typing, physicians have also started to employ voice recognition systems. Once anchored to the EHR by the keyboard, the physician is also now tethered by a microphone; via the use of such voice recognition software, not only does the EHR coopt the physician's written word, it also encroaches upon the domain of the spoken word, as physicians train themselves to adapt speech, modify pronunciation, and modulate volume to assure seamless dictation.

The physician's written expression is made uniform; the content, too, becomes the same. There is a perception that the only story produced is the same story repeatedly. Rosenbaum describes a physician whose "notes have been rendered uselessly homogenous by the tyranny of clicks and auto-populated fields."[46] While he once used his notes to distinguish one patient from the next, he now feels that he "never saw them before" and "can't even picture their faces." Flows of information have become "meaningless,"[47] and notes "signifying nothing" litter the EHR.[48] Searching for meaning in "novella-length EHR notes" is "a tiring and cynical hunt."[49] Automatically inserted phrases generate "awkward," often incomprehensible syntax.[50] Kittler describes "optical fiber networks [turning] formerly distinct data flows into a standardized series of digitized numbers"[51]; similarly, the data entry constraints and copy-forward functionality of the EHR

[43] Frey, "At a Loss for Words," 1751.
[44] Ibid.
[45] Kommer, "Good Documentation."
[46] Rosenbaum, "Transitional Chaos or Enduring Harm?," 1587.
[47] Rosenthal and Verghese, "Meaning and the Nature of Physicians' Work," 1814.
[48] Lisa Rosenbaum, "The Not-My-Problem Problem," *New England Journal of Medicine* 380, no. 9 (February 28, 2019): 881.
[49] Kommer, "Good Documentation."
[50] Robert E. Hirschtick, "Copy-and-Paste," JAMA 295, no. 20 (2006): 2335.
[51] Kittler, *Gramophone, Film, Typewriter*, 1–2.

turn formerly distinct patient narratives into a standardized series of increasingly repetitive and granular lists, labels, and checklists. Fanestil questions whether "clicking on a box" means anything for the patient's health in real life, "as if health care happens on the monitor or the silicon chip in my laptop."[52] When transcribing the patient, the physician, in sole command of neither hand, speech, or voice, no longer controls content. Patients must be labeled via predetermined problem lists and menus. These menus offer diagnosis codes from the *ICD-10 Clinical Modification (International Statistical Classification of Diseases and Related Health Problems)*. There are over 69,000 diagnosis codes to choose from, compared to 14,000 in the most recent iteration. Yet, real patients "seldom conform neatly to the language and numbers" of such systems.[53] The labels offered by the EHR grow increasingly specific and, in their specificity, lose their ability to parlay a meaningful bigger picture. Notes are "no longer constructed to be read," writes Hirschtick.[54] Words are written with the purpose of satisfying financial and regulatory requirements; in altering their purpose, they are robbed of meaning. As such, the power of the storyteller in meaning-making is challenged. Beyond meaning, there is also a fear of loss of authenticity. The time-consuming nature of the EHR leads to a reliance on shortcuts, including copy/paste, insertion of preset text, automated importation of data, and authorship takeover of a preexisting note. Physicians describe how notes are now populated with "misleading inaccuracies or fraud" or "chart lore"; "disease labels," for instance, are "immortalized by being cut and pasted."[55] The "compulsion to leave no box unchecked often creates a neat construct of a patient that can be a meta-fiction."[56] What's more, one describes how "the practice of making up answers to bypass a hard stop" is not uncommon, and "the EHR can offer no guarantees that [one] performed the examination that is so thoroughly documented."[57]

How are physicians adapting to this change in their identity? "The blanks on our screens can be filled with words, but the process of understanding cannot be auto-populated," writes Rosenbaum.[58] Given the devolution of the physician-storyteller identity as it pertains to the transcribed patient history, how do physicians reestablish that process of understanding? Just as Kittler

---

[52] Bradley D. Fanestil, "The Tyranny of the Measuring Cup," *JAMA* 301, no. 15 (April 15, 2009): 1515.
[53] Elizabeth Toll, "278.00 Obesity, Not Otherwise Specified," *JAMA* 309, no. 11 (March 20, 2013): 1123.
[54] Robert E. Hirschtick, "John Lennon's Elbow," *JAMA* 308, no. 5 (August 1, 2012): 463.
[55] Rosenthal and Verghese, "Meaning and the Nature of Physicians' Work"; Jeffrey Chi and Abraham Verghese, "Clinical Education and the Electronic Health Record: The Flipped Patient," *JAMA* 312, no. 22 (December 10, 2014): 2331–2; Verghese, "Culture Shock—Patient as Icon, Icon as Patient," 2749.
[56] Chi and Verghese, "Clinical Education and the Electronic Health Record: The Flipped Patient," 2231.
[57] Lifflander, "Hard Times and Hard Stops," 838; Kommer, "Good Documentation," 876.
[58] Rosenbaum, "Transitional Chaos or Enduring Harm?," 1587.

notes that it is we who adapt to the changes wrought by technology, physicians are adapting in response to the EHR in order to maintain their intimate rapport with narrative. As an antidote to the "countless hours spent ... entering data in [EHRs]," Safder suggests we must "make sure to get the name of the dog," encouraging physicians to continue to seek humanizing details of patients' stories even when there is no official space for them in the EHR.[59] Wolpaw and Shapiro extol the "virtues of irrelevance" as antidotes to the facelessness of the EHR, emboldening physicians to ask questions about the details of patient lives that may seem irrelevant in an era hyperfocused on what can be measured.[60] Perhaps it is no coincidence that the coming of age of narrative medicine in the early 2000s paralleled the rise of the EHR. Counter, and perhaps in response, to the EHR's devaluation of story, narrative medicine reinvigorates the role of the narrative. Increasingly, physicians are seeking "extracurricular" training in close reading and reflective writing to reestablish a "medicine infused with respect for the narrative dimensions of illness and caregiving."[61] Stepping beyond the bounds of the EHR, physicians are finding new spaces in which to listen to and tell stories in their own voices, in workshops, medical humanities journals, afterhours reading groups, and even online, in group chats on social media platforms. Cognizant perhaps of the new limits constricting the physician-storyteller identity within the EHR, physicians are also taking on new identities as cocreators or facilitators of the patient narrative. Kahn advocates for patients to be able to view their charts, citing the "enormous benefit arising from patients' opportunity to factcheck their own histories."[62] Others highlight the possibilities for using the EHR as a "relational tool" to foster greater patient engagement and activation in "positioning the screen as a bridge rather than a divider."[63] Czernik describes the restorative possibilities for patients and physicians alike, describing how sharing a screen was helping a resident build "more than just an acquaintance with her patient."[64] Increasingly, physicians are realizing that they should equip patients with greater agency over their health narratives.[65]

[59] Safder, "The Name of the Dog," 1301.
[60] Wolpaw and Shapiro, "The Virtues of Irrelevance," 1283.
[61] Rita Charon, "Narrative Medicine: A Model for Empathy, Reflection, Profession, and Trust," *JAMA* 286, no. 15 (October 17, 2001): 1901.
[62] Michael W. Kahn et al., "Let's Show Patients Their Mental Health Records," *JAMA* 311, no. 13 (April 2, 2014): 1292.
[63] Amina White and Marion Danis, "Enhancing Patient-Centered Communication and Collaboration by Using the Electronic Health Record in the Examination Room," *JAMA* 309, no. 22 (June 12, 2013): 2327.
[64] Zuzanna Czernik and C. T. Lin, "Time at the Bedside (Computing)," *JAMA* 315, no. 22 (June 14, 2016): 2400.
[65] Katherine A. Mikk, Harry A. Sleeper, and Eric J. Topol, "The Pathway to Patient Data Ownership and Better Health," *JAMA* 318, no. 15 (October 17, 2017): 1434.

Wang suggests that "medical documentation should be synced to the vernacular, not ... scholarly jargon" so that patients can more easily access their health information.[66] "Wouldn't we be closer to our patients' experience if we got into the habit of thinking about them in language they would find meaningful and useful?" writes Kahn, citing a colleague's email.[67] In creating new programs such as OpenNotes, physicians are now permitting patients to actively participate in the creation of their EHR narrative by giving them access to read and provide feedback on clinicians' electronic notes. Goroll encourages clinicians to go one step further by integrating patient-generated reports into the EHR; Oldfield and Duvall encourage a "coauthored narrative," while Feldman invites her patients directly to the computer to type in their thoughts.[68] Schiff and Bates further advocate for EHRs to serve "as a place where clinicians, together with patients, document succinct evaluations" while "together on the same side of the screen."[69] A new initiative called OurNotes does exactly that, proposing that patients coproduce electronic notes with physicians. Ownership of narrative is further placed in patient's hands via programs such as the Veterans' Affairs' My Life My Story program, developed by two psychiatrists, wherein patients share their stories with volunteers who transcribe this patient-powered narrative and embed it back into the EHR for clinicians to access. Adopting these new identities permits physicians to circumvent the checkboxes and templates of the EHR to generate narratives within and without its bounds.

Physician as Detective

Detection, diagnosis, and problem-solving also lie at the core of physician identities. This core tenet of physician self-definition, as physician-sleuth or doctor-as-detective, appears under siege in these texts: the EHR appears to dissolve the mystery associated with the patient encounter, dull the critical thinking that defines the diagnostician, alter identity formation for physicians-in-training, and change the faces and places of the process of detection.

---

[66] C. Jason Wang, "Medical Documentation in the Electronic Era," *JAMA* 308, no. 20 (November 28, 2012): 2092.
[67] Kahn et al., "Let's Show Patients Their Mental Health Records," 1292.
[68] Ellen Feldman, "The Day the Computer Tried to Eat My Alligator," *JAMA* 304, no. 24 (2010): 2362.
[69] Schiff and Bates, "Can Electronic Clinical Documentation Help Prevent Diagnostic Errors?," 1067–8.

The EHR offers easy access to previous results; physicians "meet a fully formed iPatient long before seeing the real patient."[70] Litvin describes how, thanks to the EHR, she knows most of the patient's story before meeting him. Perhaps there is an inevitable sense of a loss of mystery; the patient's story comes to a sudden, anticlimactic denouement when the once-longitudinal process of discovery is telescoped into a brief moment of data review. The enigmatic, undifferentiated patient is rarely encountered; the EHR houses not only diagnostic data but also the diagnostic impressions of previous physicians who have seen the patient. A common vein in these articles is the necessity of grappling with a glut of data, which transforms the thrill of sailing an uncharted territory into the mundanity of wading through a swamp of information. EHRs produce a "new electronic sea of results" and "mountains of noise"; an "exponential accumulation of data" leads to "note bloat," making every patient a "big data challenge."[71] The physician-detective struggles to identify what is relevant: "voluminous" notes distract from "key cognitive work," leading to a "vain search" through "meaningless repetition in multiple notes for the single [change representing] a new development."[72]

Ironically, however, the EHR may make the process of diagnosis artificially easy, altering how physicians seek and process information. Automated data importation allows results to populate charts at the click of a button, reducing the need for selectivity. Macros allow paragraphs of predetermined language, including pre-populated differential diagnosis lists applicable to a chief complaint, to appear in a patient's EHR chart with a single click, eclipsing the narrative and cognitive fieldwork that typically goes into crafting an assessment. What results, then, is the "product of a word processor, not of physicians' thoughtful review and analysis."[73] The theme of the presence of the EHR leading to an absence of thinking pervades multiple articles: the EHR "strains our collective ability to think," could hinder physicians in "synthesizing, analyzing, thinking critically," goes against "creative clinical thinking [with] automaticity," and "dilutes independent assessment."[74] Multiple physicians argue that the immediate availability of information encourages an overreliance on electronic

---

[70] Verghese, "Culture Shock—Patient as Icon, Icon as Patient," 2749.
[71] Hartzband and Groopman, "Off the Record—Avoiding the Pitfalls of Going Electronic," 1657; Rosenthal and Verghese, "Meaning and the Nature of Physicians' Work," 1814; Obermeyer and Lee, "Lost in Thought," 1209; James J. Cimino, "Improving the Electronic Health Record—Are Clinicians Getting What They Wished For?," *JAMA* 309, no. 10 (March 13, 2013): 991.
[72] Hartzband and Groopman, "Off the Record—Avoiding the Pitfalls of Going Electronic," 1656–7.
[73] Ibid., 1657.
[74] Obermeyer and Lee, "Lost in Thought," 1209; Rosenbaum, "Transitional Chaos or Enduring Harm?," 1588; Hartzband and Groopman, "Off the Record—Avoiding the Pitfalls of Going Electronic," 1658; Rosenthal and Verghese, "Meaning and the Nature of Physicians' Work," 1814.

data, with a corresponding erosion in the key detective skills of history-taking and physical examination.[75] Zulman suggests that physicians overly invested in the computer may miss highly individual "phenotypic observations" that would shed light on a diagnosis, while Lifflander notes that engaging with the EHR prevents physicians from drawing out the history that is needed for a diagnosis.[76] What's more, hidden in these masses of information may be nuggets of disinformation and "noisy data," leading to "cognitive bias in decision-making."[77] Labels that persist in the chart, such as electronic flags for frequently presenting patients whose social and medical vulnerabilities make them reliant on emergency departments as safety nets, unwittingly propagate implicit biases and threaten accurate diagnosis.[78]

Edelman (2015) warns against "letting the collation of data characterize us as physicians."[79] Not only has the EHR forced mutations in established identities, it is fundamentally altering identity formation for physicians-in-training. Physicians who practiced in the era of pen and paper note a silent, subconscious evolution in the professional identity formation of new physicians as they adapt to the EHR. Hartzband and Groopman describe how EHRs make it easy for trainees to avoid taking their own histories or developing their own thought processes. Rosenthal and Verghese note that the "skills learned early by today's medical students and house staff—because they are critical to getting the work done—are not those needed to perform a good physical exam or take a history, but rather the arts of efficient 'chart biopsy,' … in the electronic age."[80] The EHR has redefined what the physician's "work" is and, in doing so, has insidiously altered medical curriculum. Verghese further notes that this "expedient way" of approaching patients "is not formally taught, and yet residents seem to have learned it no matter where in the United States they trained."[81] What's more, trainees have not only learned this approach, they have also learned to value it, for what defines a "good" trainee appears to have changed. "Students quickly

---

[75] Edelman and Weber, "Tenuous Tether"; Verghese, "Culture Shock—Patient as Icon, Icon as Patient"; Rosenthal and Verghese, "Meaning and the Nature of Physicians' Work"; Chi and Verghese, "Clinical Education and the Electronic Health Record: The Flipped Patient"; Wang, "Medical Documentation in the Electronic Era."
[76] Donna M. Zulman, Nigam H. Shah, and Abraham Verghese, "Evolutionary Pressures on the Electronic Health Record: Caring for Complexity," JAMA 316, no. 9 (September 6, 2016): 924; Lifflander, "Hard Times and Hard Stops."
[77] Patel, "Writing the Wrong," 672.
[78] Michelle Joy, Timothy Clement, and Dominic Sisti, "The Ethics of Behavioral Health Information Technology: Frequent Flyer Icons and Implicit Bias," JAMA 316, no. 15 (October 18, 2016): 1539–40; Jayshil J. Patel, "The Things We Say," JAMA 319, no. 4 (2018): 341–2.
[79] Edelman and Weber, "Tenuous Tether," 2201.
[80] Rosenthal and Verghese, "Meaning and the Nature of Physicians' Work," 1813.
[81] Verghese, "Culture Shock—Patient as Icon, Icon as Patient," 2749.

realize that their clinical performance indirectly draws on their skills to use the EHR ... mastering [it] can often pass for familiarity with the actual patient," writes Chi.[82] It becomes difficult to tell whether a student "has independently formed an assessment or has just mastered how to extract information from the computer," he continues.[83] Future generations of physicians may know no other way of working up a patient, and, in this manner, the change operated by the EHR on the physician's diagnostic identity is complete.

These texts reveal not only a perceived cognitive torpor in the process of detection in the EHR era but also a perception of alteration in the spaces and faces that define detection. Rather than hunting for clues at the material patient body, physicians interrogate the virtual recesses of the EHR. The physical space of detection is no longer "the bedside"; Wolpaw writes that the very "geography" of medicine has changed.[84] "The majority of what we define as 'work' takes place away from the patient," write Rosenthal and Verghese.[85] "It is ironic and emblematic that we sit down in front of our computers, getting comfortable for our chart encounter, whereas with our patients, the reason we're here, we generally position ourselves for a quick exit," continues Wolpaw.[86] Despite the physical proximity to patients, there is a cognitive distance; we form "intimate relationships" with the EHR and "remotely [monitor] patients who may lie only feet from the computer."[87] Not only is there perceived isolation from patients, there is a perception that detection now occurs in isolation from colleagues. Prior to the EHR, "medicine was a fraternal order" and "clinicians thought in groups ... [working] together on problems too difficult for any single mind to solve."[88] Now, however, "increasing reliance on EHRs as a means of communication distances team members from one another," write Singh and Graber; "very few meetings ... occur face to face," add Rosenthal and Verghese.[89] The EHR dissolves the collegial companionship of diagnosis: "Days go by without seeing a referring physician in the reading room," writes Hise about

---

[82] Chi and Verghese, "Clinical Education and the Electronic Health Record: The Flipped Patient," 2331–2.
[83] Ibid., 2332.
[84] Daniel R. Wolpaw, "Seeing Eye to Eye," *New England Journal of Medicine* 365, no. 22 (December 1, 2011): 2052.
[85] Rosenthal and Verghese, "Meaning and the Nature of Physicians' Work," 1814.
[86] Wolpaw, "Seeing Eye to Eye," 2053.
[87] Ibid., 2052; Edelman and Weber, "Tenuous Tether," 2200.
[88] Rosenthal and Verghese, "Meaning and the Nature of Physicians' Work," 1813; Obermeyer and Lee, "Lost in Thought," 1209.
[89] Hardeep Singh and Mark L. Graber, "Improving Diagnosis in Health Care—The Next Imperative for Patient Safety," *New England Journal of Medicine* 373, no. 26 (December 24, 2015): 2495; Rosenthal and Verghese, "Meaning and the Nature of Physicians' Work," 1813.

what used to be the favorite part of his day.[90] The EHR also renders obsolete the physical spaces of collaboration: Rosenthal and Verghese describe the dissolution of the doctors' lounge, those "central locations where community internists, specialists and surgeons ate together, socialized, and 'curb-sided' each other for patient consultations."[91] A sense of physical exile permeates many articles: thinking occurs "alone, bathed in the blue light of computer screens," with "countless hours" spent in "windowless rooms" and "snug bunkers."[92] The EHR-era physician-diagnostician is thus socially and physically isolated.

However, just as physician identities have adapted to changes in the storyteller role by finding other spaces and partners for the production of narratives, the identity of the physician-diagnostician is also evolving in response to the EHR. Rather than allowing the EHR to supplant the internal process of critical thinking, physicians are externalizing the diagnostic process by using the EHR as an exterior brain. Benjamin welcomes the durability of the EHR as a storage medium, so that physicians do not have to rely on memory or recollection alone for important patient details.[93] Physicians not only accept the EHR as a repository of data but also seek to take advantage of its abilities to process that data. The EHR's capacity for storing immense amounts of data can allow it to serve as a virtual collation of physician experience; Frankovich and colleagues and Zulman and colleagues describe how real-time clinical decisions can be made based upon amassed patient information in an EHR when individual experience is insufficient to make a diagnosis.[94] Others highlight the EHR's potential in machine learning–based decision-making algorithms and relevant "just-in-time" access to online resources.[95] In an article that charts the evolution of the "master diagnostician," Dhaliwal and Detsky describe "the diagnostician of the future" as one who is expert at using EHRs to measure diagnostic error rates by following up on patients, to employ diagnostic checklists, and to reach for computer-based diagnostic support tools.[96] Pageler, Friedman, and Longhurst, too, suggest that

---

[90] Joseph Henry Hise, "And Then Came the PACS," *JAMA* 318, no. 4 (July 25, 2017): 331.
[91] Rosenthal and Verghese, "Meaning and the Nature of Physicians' Work," 1813.
[92] Obermeyer and Lee, "Lost in Thought," 1209; Safder, "The Name of the Dog," 1301; Verghese, "Culture Shock—Patient as Icon, Icon as Patient," 2748.
[93] Regina Benjamin, "Finding My Way to Electronic Health Records," *New England Journal of Medicine* 363, no. 6 (August 5, 2010): 505–6.
[94] Jennifer Frankovich, Christopher A. Longhurst, and Scott M. Sutherland, "Evidence-Based Medicine in the EMR Era," *New England Journal of Medicine* 365, no. 19 (November 10, 2011): 1758–9; Zulman et al., "Evolutionary Pressures on the Electronic Health Record: Caring for Complexity."
[95] Obermeyer and Lee, "Lost in Thought"; Cimino, "Improving the Electronic Health Record—Are Clinicians Getting What They Wished For?"
[96] Gurpreet Dhaliwal and Allan S. Detsky, "The Evolution of the Master Diagnostician," *JAMA* 310, no. 6 (August 14, 2013): 579–80.

the negative impacts of the EHR on future physicians are due to the maladaptive responses of the current generation, and that a formal integration of the EHR into medical education can actually be positively formative for trainees. Schiff and Bates exhort clinicians to "take back ownership of the medical record," and Hartzband and Groopman write that "[physicians] need to make this technology work for [them], rather than allowing [themselves] to work for it."[97] To do so, physicians must acquire new identities. The physician-diagnostician has many faces: observant examiner of the body, astute and empathetic history-taker, and critically thinking clinician. But in the era of the EHR, the physician-diagnostician must acquire a new face. This face, write Obermeyer and Lee, is that of a physician "trained in statistics and computer science, who can contribute meaningfully to algorithm development and evaluation."[98] The collegial team convening in the doctor's lounge may have gone by the wayside, but physicians are also adapting their conceptions of partnership. Recognizing that much of clinical communication occurs electronically, Khanna, Wachter, and Blum suggest making the EHR a partner privy to real-time conversations: physicians will need to recognize that the EHR "is as much as a member of the team as any physician, nurse, or member of the support staff" since it is a "valued resource" that may one day be able to positively "participate in those conversations."[99] Obermeyer and Lee describe the importance of viewing algorithms as "thinking partners" in a "team sport."[100] Teams of diagnosticians should include not only physicians but also new partners as well, including software designers, healthcare information technology innovators, engineers, and psychologists.[101] Schiff and Bates further note that the EHR could guide the process of "thoughtful assessment" if physicians adopt yet another partner in their practice, the patients themselves: EHRs can "foster thoughtful assessment," they write, if clinicians "craft thoughtful differential diagnoses and note unanswered questions together with their patients."[102] Shared decision-making can occur when physicians and patients are sharing screens.[103]

---

[97] Schiff and Bates, "Can Electronic Clinical Documentation Help Prevent Diagnostic Errors?," 1068; Hartzband and Groopman, "Off the Record—Avoiding the Pitfalls of Going Electronic," 1658.
[98] Obermeyer and Lee, "Lost in Thought," 1211.
[99] Raman R. Khanna, Robert M. Wachter, and Michael Blum, "Reimagining Electronic Clinical Communication in the Post-Pager, Smartphone Era," JAMA 315, no. 1 (January 5, 2016): 21–2.
[100] Obermeyer and Lee, "Lost in Thought," 1211.
[101] Robert S. Rudin, David W. Bates, and Calum MacRae, "Accelerating Innovation in Health IT," New England Journal of Medicine 375, no. 9 (September 1, 2016): 815–17; C. Jason Wang and Andrew T. Huang, "Integrating Technology into Health Care: What Will It Take?," JAMA 307, no. 6 (February 8, 2012): 569–70.
[102] Schiff and Bates, "Can Electronic Clinical Documentation Help Prevent Diagnostic Errors?," 1067.
[103] Czernik and Lin, "Time at the Bedside (Computing)."

Conclusion

These texts, sourced from essays written by physicians in two well-known scientific journals, provide a rich vein of data on how physician identities are evolving in response to the structure and function of the medium of the EHR. Other observers of the evolution of medicine have previously described how commercial and market interests have rendered doctors subordinate, while some have pronounced dead the "golden age of doctoring" due to "pervasive macrostructural influences."[104] This chapter demonstrates, however, that the technological microcosm of the EHR is also capable of operating a large-scale change from the inside out; with its mandated checkboxes, limits on narrative, cognitive shortcuts, and diagnostic possibilities, the EHR, as a technoscientific innovation, is rendering physicians into reflections of technologies, with a subsequent dissolution of previously established identities. While a sense of loss is pervasive in many of these texts, there is also a sense of progress, evolution, and adaptation in response to the EHR. Though the disappearance of these identities gives rise to dissatisfaction, there is a faintly optimistic acquiescence to the influence, promise, and possibility of the EHR. Physicians insist that they are not "Luddites," "technophobes," or "anachronistic curmudgeons."[105] Just as patients are gaining new illness identities and biosocial communities via technoscientific advances, physicians, too, are replacing previous identities and communities with new ones. While physicians of the era of medicalization may have relied upon the roles of storyteller and diagnostician as a means to concentrate their primacy, the EHR propels physicians into the era of biomedicalization by forcing them to adopt new technoscientific identities, those of a cocreator and facilitator of narratives, and of a participant within (rather than the sole proprietor of) the process of detection. The EHR does, indeed, "determine our situation."[106] Rather than heralding the end of a golden age, however, the EHR perhaps serves as both a symbol and usher of a new age of heightened symbiosis between physician, patient, and technology.

---

[104] Ibid.
[105] Hartzband and Groopman, "Off the Record—Avoiding the Pitfalls of Going Electronic," 1658; Wu, "Virtual Grief," 2095.
[106] Kittler, *Gramophone, Film, Typewriter*, xxxix.

5

Mixed Feedback: The Promise of Structural Competency Education

Joshua Franklin

During my second year of medical school, a few months before I was to start my clinical rotations, I spent an afternoon visiting the pediatric gender clinic where I was conducting anthropological fieldwork. I followed the physician as she saw a patient, a transgender boy who was starting to take oral contraceptives to change his menstrual cycle. After we left the room, the physician suggested that I try writing a progress note about the encounter; she would review it, and it would be good practice for the next stage of my medical training. I froze, staring at the blank Epic electronic health record interface. Later that evening, tucked in my notebook between some quotations from Robert Desjarlais's *Shelter Blues* and a few key points from a late-night renal review session about the BUN/Cr ratio, I wrote down my reflections on what had happened: "I felt unprepared, acutely aware of my medical novice status."

Why did I struggle so much to write the progress note? Certainly, it was due, in part, to my lack of knowledge as a medical student. But while I would have felt similarly unprepared after any patient encounter, there was something about the collision of my medical training with the world of my anthropological work. I was anxious—I was worried about my own efficacy, but also about the future of this transgender boy and about an unfulfilled need for certainty in relation to the practices of both medical diagnosis and anthropological critique. I thought of what many critical trans and feminist scholars have documented about the complicated relationship that medical professionals have with gender diversity, often playing an instrumental role in sustaining oppressive discourses of normative gender.[1] In the hands of physicians and other healthcare workers,

---

[1] Julian Gill-Peterson, *Histories of the Transgender Child* (Minneapolis: University of Minnesota Press, 2018); Sahar Sadjadi, "The Endocrinologist's Office—Puberty Suppression: Saving Children

nonnormative gender identities often become pathologies or problems to be managed. I was worried that fixing this boy's life in an electronic file represented the problematization of his experience, his gender identity, and his desires, and I was frozen by my sense that anything I wrote might implicate me in this practice of wielding knowledge as power.

Wanting to preserve the idiosyncrasy and richness of one family's experience, I reached for an anthropological counternarrative; I was left with a vague anxiety about uncertainty and complexity. Does being an anthropologist commit me to being a failing medical student? And if all of my immersion in critical scholarship about transgender medicine did not prepare me to answer these questions, I wondered, how do we make use of medical anthropology and knowledge of related disciplines in medicine?

Anthropology in Medical Education

In their classic essay about medical education, anthropologists Byron Good and Mary-Jo DelVecchio Good dispel the illusion of the medical humanities—anthropology in particular—as the savior of medicine. "Anthropology in medical schools," they wrote, "thus occupies an ambiguous position; critic of the role of the natural sciences and the individualized and mechanistic forms of reasoning about disease and its treatment, critic of the social organization of medicine, and critic of the nostalgic view of the human sciences as the producers of caring."[2] Medical anthropologist Nancy Scheper-Hughes is more pointed: "Clinical medical anthropology has become a new 'commodity,' carefully sanitized, nicely packaged, pleasant tasting (no bitter aftertaste)—the very latest and very possibly the most bourgeois product introduced into the medical education curriculum."[3] Several decades have passed since these articles were written, and yet, as an anthropologist in medical training, I still wonder exactly how to offer something anthropological to my clinical community.

---

from a Natural Disaster?", *Journal of Medical Humanities* 34, no. 2 (June 2013): 255–60, https://doi.org/10.1007/s10912-013-9228-6; Dean Spade, "Resisting Medicine, Re/Modeling Gender," *Berkeley Journal of Gender, Law & Justice* 18, no. 1 (2003): 15–37, https://doi.org/10.15779/z38nk3645g.

[2] Byron J. Good and Mary-Jo DelVecchio Good, "'Learning Medicine': The Constructing of Medical Knowledge at Harvard Medical School," in *Knowledge, Power, and Practice: The Anthropology of Medicine and Everyday Life*, ed. Shirley Lindenbaum and Margaret Lock, Comparative Studies of Health Systems and Medical Care (Berkeley: University of California Press, 1993), 103.

[3] N. Scheper-Hughes, "Three Propositions for a Critically Applied Medical Anthropology," *Social Science & Medicine (1982)* 30, no. 2 (1990): 191, https://doi.org/10.1016/0277-9536(90)90079-8.

Medical education is a prominent site where social scientists have attempted to make good on critiques of medicine and intervene in medical practice. While this work has a long history, the past several years have witnessed the development of a structural competency framework in medical education. Structural competency attempts to remedy some of the shortcomings of cultural competency, an earlier paradigm of social science pedagogy in medical training, which often ignored structural racism and economic inequality in favor of, at times, stereotypical cultural explanations. Writing from the vantages of sociology, anthropology, and medicine, Jonathan Metzl and Helena Hansen note, while cultural competency pedagogies "enhance clinical dialogue in vital ways, they do little to address the complex relationships between clinical symptoms and social, political, and economic systems."[4] Metzl and Hansen proposed a structural competency that would consist of five core competencies: recognizing the structures that shape clinical interactions, developing an extraclinical language of structure, rearticulating "cultural" presentations in structural terms, observing and imagining structural intervention, and developing structural humility. But structural competency has eclipsed this concrete definition and now represents an umbrella term for social medicine pedagogy.

Some of the same problems that beset cultural competency and mobilized a critique of it now haunt its successor: structural competency is what cultural competency lacks, and so structural competency is defined less in terms of what it *is*, than what cultural competency could not be. Many of these persistent challenges are variations on a central problem of expertise. How can we simultaneously explore the vast work of anthropologists and others on these topics without claiming this knowledge as a form of mastery, as Scheper-Hughes cautioned? Metzl and Hansen (2014) caution about the limits of the structural competency paradigm: "The final component of structural competency is the trained ability to recognize the limitations of structural competency. Here, students demonstrate a critical awareness of medical education's realistic goals and endpoints."[5] Yet, how can we ensure that our efforts do not simply reinscribe precisely the forms of medical hegemony that social and humanistic critique seeks to hold up for scrutiny?

Despite this expanding body of scholarly literature arguing for the inclusion of social and humanistic knowledge in medical curricula, these topics are often

---

[4] Jonathan M. Metzl and Helena Hansen, "Structural Competency: Theorizing a New Medical Engagement with Stigma and Inequality," *Social Science & Medicine, Structural Stigma and Population Health*, 103 (February 1, 2014): 128, https://doi.org/10.1016/j.socscimed.2013.06.032.
[5] Ibid., 131.

marginalized within medical curricula even when they are formally included. And many in medicine outrightly reject the premise of their importance. One such person is Stanley Goldfarb, a physician and former administrator at my institution, who pitted the social and biological against each other in a polemic for the *Wall Street Journal*: "These educators focus on eliminating health disparities and ensuring that the next generation of physicians is well equipped to deal with cultural diversity, which are worthwhile goals. But teaching these issues is coming at the expense of rigorous training in medical science."[6] In the face of such skepticism and political opposition, medical anthropologists and other social scientists and humanists have made a strong case for the ethical and practical necessity of social medicine education.[7]

I am likewise committed to the importance of structural competency. However, I attempt in this essay to elucidate through practical experience what is still lacking from these pedagogies, particularly with respect to the way that learners are interpellated in the discourse and practice of structural competency. I draw on the work of theorists Lauren Berlant and Robyn Wiegman to theorize the disciplinary formation of structural competency, finding a neglect of trainee subjectivity in the conceptualization of social medicine pedagogy. I argue that medical social sciences and humanities are places where we are able to displace our anxieties and concerns about the unfinished ethical work of medicine and sustain our hope for their resolution. In other words, understanding the *purpose* of social medicine training does not mean fully grasping its *promise*. This is not a critique of structural competency per se; rather, I argue that the problems of structural competency reflect a central problem of anthropology's disciplinary vision that becomes starkly apparent when anthropological thinking is injected into spaces of medical education.

The Promise of Social Medicine Pedagogy

In *Cruel Optimism*, in her discussion of the satisfactions of consumption, Lauren Berlant writes about "the thing within any object to which one passes one's

---

[6] Stanley Goldfarb, "Take Two Aspirin and Call Me by My Pronouns," *Wall Street Journal* (September 12, 2019), sec. Opinion, https://www.wsj.com/articles/take-two-aspirin-and-call-me-by-my-pronouns-11568325291.

[7] Scott D. Stonington et al., "Case Studies in Social Medicine—Attending to Structural Forces in Clinical Practice," *New England Journal of Medicine* 379, no. 20 (November 15, 2018): 1958–61, https://doi.org/10.1056/NEJMms1814262.

fantasy of sovereignty for safekeeping."[8] I want to suggest that anthropological and humanistic interventions in medical training may become precisely such a place of safety. As Berlant puts it, "Any object of optimism promises to guarantee the endurance of something, the survival of something, the flourishing of something, and above all the protection of the desire that made this object or scene powerful enough to have magnetized an attachment to it."[9] As I have discussed, structural competency frameworks are different in various ways from older models of cultural competency. Yet, these new frameworks are still able to sustain very much the same sort of promise. This is in part because student and faculty engagement with the curriculum materializes medical education in a particular way, reflecting also how students see themselves in relation to medicine and its institutions, as well as something about how anthropology constructs its own objects. In order to see how this is the case, we first must ask: What does humanistic and social medical education promise to medical students?

My entrance into this work was as a student course director for a course at my institution required for all first-year medical students, called "Introduction to Medicine and Society" or, more informally, "Doctoring." This course was revised through a student initiative, and top-down teaching methods ("information delivery paradigms") were replaced with what the course designers called a pedagogy of critical consciousness, which is defined as "a state of understanding how power and difference shape social structure and interaction ('reading the world'), coupled with an orientation toward pragmatic action."[10] Taught through a combination of lectures, small group discussions, and individual reflective writing, the aim of the class is to explore social issues through the lens of personal experience, critical scholarship, and social theory. The course occurs over twelve sessions during the first semester of medical school and is divided into three parts— "Foundations," "Stratification, Privilege, and Disparity," and "Medical Culture and the Physician's Role"—and is organized around the recurrent theme of the physician's relationships with patients, peers, and communities.[11]

---

[8] Lauren Gail Berlant, *Cruel Optimism* (Durham, NC: Duke University Press, 2011), 43.
[9] Ibid., 48.
[10] Diane K. Dao et al., "Integrating Theory, Content, and Method to Foster Critical Consciousness in Medical Students: A Comprehensive Model for Cultural Competence Training," *Academic Medicine* 92, no. 3 (March 2017): 335–44, https://doi.org/10.1097/ACM.0000000000001390.
[11] The "Introduction to Medicine and Society" course is also referred to as "Doctoring" 1A and is the first in a five-semester-long series of "Doctoring" courses. "Doctoring" IB and IC take place during later preclinical semesters. "Doctoring" II takes place monthly during students' clerkship year, when they are immersed in clinical rotations. Students stay with the same fourteen-person group throughout this time, often with the same faculty facilitators. Over the course of this sequence, the

Although the course did not use the language of structural competency when it was developed in 2013, it was based on similar concepts, and when it was revised in 2015, the term "structural competency" became a central one, with the first two class sessions devoted to it. There are some meaningful differences between the way the course's architects characterize their objectives and the strategies laid out in the structural competency framework. In particular, the "Doctoring" course involves a significant number of reflective activities drawn from what might be termed a narrative medicine framework, and it also includes an emphasis on communication skills. Nevertheless, the course's creators explicitly aimed to foster a "process of learning that transcends both list-based and open-mindedness approaches," and they rely on the language of social structure that characterizes the structural competency framework to do so. As such, the course fits within a broad movement in contemporary social medicine education that seeks to center questions of power and society in response to a perceived overemphasis on culture and individual values, synecdochally termed structural competency.

Another unique and important feature of the course is that it is designed to be constantly revised through a process of feedback from students. In part, this derives from the larger structures of medical education at the institution, which have regular avenues for feedback, as is common in postsecondary and graduate education. But these feedback mechanisms are even more central to "Doctoring"; this is, in part, a recognition of the unique nature of the course content, as well as a reflection of the understanding that students may know more than faculty in many ways. In addition to the regular course and instructor feedback that the medical school solicits for every course, "Doctoring" incorporates student feedback by having students work alongside faculty. Second-year students work over the summer to revise lesson plans; fourth-year students serve as course facilitators; and the course has a student codirector (this was the position I held). This extensive student involvement makes the course exceptionally open to feedback.

In the feedback process, I observed that some themes appeared again and again. When bringing in participant experiences, such as in activities designed to elicit all group members' experiences of a certain aspect of identity or reactions to a particular text, students often objected to what they perceived to be tokenization, or a disproportionate burden placed on marginalized students

---

content focus of the sessions shifts to be more narrowly focused on the techniques of doctoring, rather than the wide view of health and illness in the context of society that is taken by "Doctoring."

to teach those with privilege about their communities. Students bemoaned the many topics that were omitted, on a macro level (e.g., not having a session devoted to obesity) or within broad themes (e.g., not addressing intimate partner violence within a session on gender). At the same time, students sometimes felt that some topics or themes were superfluous (e.g., watching an ethnographic film portraying homeless drug users was felt to be voyeuristic and stereotyping). Students often reacted strongly to activities that were designed to foster empathy, but may risk a flattening of experiences (e.g., an activity that asks students to imagine different moments of bodily failure in their own lives is seen to draw false equivalences between temporary athletic injury and serious disability). At times, some students were troubled by a lack of "hard" (i.e., quantitative) evidence. At others, the problem seemed to be a lack of narrative or experiential evidence.

As is evident from this partial list, much of the feedback from students is contradictory. What does this disagreement signify? The answer depends on how student feedback itself is conceptualized. The usual way is that these student voices are understood as commentary about the curriculum, the content of the course, and its format and organization. As in other educational settings, this kind of feedback may essentially figure students as *consumers* of educational content. Faculty and administrators are beholden to this student feedback insofar as their success is measured in terms of positive course ratings. It is worth spelling out the essentially consumer logic of this practice, as it reifies the division between student and teacher that this critical pedagogy was established in part to complicate. By focusing the course on the social context of medicine, the creators envisioned that students would contribute insights that their teachers did not have—for instance, around gender, race, or disability—borne of personal experience or academic training. The potential for student contribution, in turn, would offer an opportunity to depart, even if only briefly, from training hierarchies that mainly recapitulate structural forms of power and inequality. And yet when students see themselves as consumers to be listened to, it undermines this project of imagining an alternative relationship that challenges the racialized and gendered hierarchies that overdetermine medical training.

But it could also be seen as an enactment of precisely the kind of reflection that a critical consciousness pedagogy seeks to foster. The course aims to provoke students to reflect on their experiences through the lens of social theory as a way of coming to terms with the social and structural context of health and illness. Reading feedback in this way, student critiques of various aspects of the course do not index the course's failures, but rather its successes. Feedback becomes an unrecognized object for the practice of the very skills in which the course purports to train students. In this sense, this feedback is a reflection of students who are concerned not with a bounded collection of literature or a core set of clinical competencies but with a broader set of questions about the meaning of being a physician and practicing medicine. As a student once asked incredulously during a feedback session while I was working on revising the curriculum, "What kind of doctors do you want us to become?"

In other words, these feedback activities reflect what it is that social medicine pedagogy promises—to institutions, to teachers, and to students. Conflict over course content, then, represents a kind of displacement, transforming deep uncertainty about what it means to be a physician into a sharp concern with medical curricula. That is, in addition to the mobilization of social science knowledge to address health inequities and improve healthcare, these curricula speak to the complex moral questions that such issues provoke. In their own critique of cultural competency, Arthur Kleinman and Peter Benson wrote, "There is something more basic and more crucial than cultural competency in understanding the life of the patient, and this is the moral meaning of suffering—what is at stake for the patient; what the patient, at a deep level, stands to gain or lose."[12] I would suggest that it is precisely this moral meaning that the cruel optimism of structural competency is meant to safeguard, as students' feedback seems to reflect the perception of what still escapes social medicine pedagogies.

As Seth Holmes and Maya Ponte argue, one of the central tasks in medical education is becoming a certain kind of subject.[13] As they show, medical students in their clinical year are not only learning how to frame patient narratives using specialized jargon; they are learning to frame their own experiences and identities. What is at stake in student critiques of readings, activities, or lecturers is not a disciplinary debate about conflicting sociomedical theories. Rather, what matters is the values that students see represented in these different discourses of culture and meaning and, in particular, how they understand their own identities in relation to these curricular elements.

[12] Arthur Kleinman and Peter Benson, "Anthropology in the Clinic: The Problem of Cultural Competency and How to Fix It," *PLoS Medicine* 3, no. 10 (October 24, 2006): 1675, https://doi.org/10.1371/journal.pmed.0030294.

[13] Seth M. Holmes and Maya Ponte, "En-Case-Ing the Patient: Disciplining Uncertainty in Medical Student Patient Presentations," *Culture, Medicine, and Psychiatry* 35, no. 2 (June 2011): 163–82, https://doi.org/10.1007/s11013-011-9213-3.

The divergence between the purpose of social medicine pedagogy and its promise only becomes apparent when we attend to these questions of trainee subjectivity. If we figure medical students only as consumers of educational content, we can only understand such practices in terms of the knowledge and skills they contain and communicate. But if we take a question such as "what kind of doctors do you want us to become?" seriously, we can recognize that the promise of structural competency and other contemporary curricula is a moral one, too.

Desiring Social Medicine

In thinking about what an academic discipline promises to a morally charged practice such as medicine, I am drawing from the work of theorist Robyn Wiegman who examines how identity knowledges are shaped by an underlying political desire. Wiegman astutely asks, "What has enabled or emboldened, allowed or encouraged scholars to believe that justice can be achieved through the study of identity? How have identity objects of study been imbued with political value, and what does 'the political' mean in those academic domains that take critical practice as the means and measure for pursuing justice?"[14] She argues that practices of critique in the fields she refers to as "identity knowledges" are rooted in a political desire that must be constantly renewed through a series of acts of renaming and reframing. She traces shifts in the terms that define fields such as gender studies and critical race theory and finds a series of substitutions that are intended to preserve an optimistic investment in these disciplines. We see very much this kind of substitution and refinement in the efforts to reform social medicine education. Even as educators in medicine critique older paradigms and conjure new conceptual scaffolds for teaching the social in medical schools, they are sustaining a kind of political desire, the moral promise of structural competency education.

In the context of commodified medical education seen through the kinds of formalized feedback structures I have discussed here, such interventions advance a vision of "doing justice in the classroom": that is, the hope that transforming what happens in education spaces is connected to the broader struggle for equity in healthcare. Education certainly is a space of possibility for social change and social justice. However, doing justice in the classroom in

---

[14] Robyn Wiegman, *Object Lessons*, Next Wave (Durham, NC: Duke University Press, 2012), 4–5.

the context of a neoliberal society might simply stop at the classroom door. The risk is that the transformational energy of students rightly concerned with the stark injustice of the US healthcare system might be redirected and ultimately absorbed by radical curricula. This is the core problem that Wiegman identifies as the tacit assumption of identity knowledges—and here we can include medical anthropology—which is the unquestioned belief that critique within the discipline will produce certain political effects or satisfy certain political desires. It is the precarity of the political desire that necessitates continual revision, in the form of feedback I have described here, as well as the larger-scale shifts in educational paradigms in medical education.

Recognizing the continuity of this desire allows us to appreciate that if structural competency seems to present anew many of the challenges of cultural competency, it is not because the creators of the new paradigm misunderstood the lessons of the old one. Rather, I would suggest that the problems of structural competency reflect a central problem of what anthropologists, and other social scientists and humanists, believe about their own disciplines. This is what Wiegman refers to as a "field imaginary," citing Donald E. Pease: "That domain of critical interpellation through which practitioners learn to pursue particular objects, protocols, methods of study, and interpretive vocabularies as the means for expressing and inhabiting their belonging to the field."[15]

It is natural to think about the intersection of medicine and anthropology in the spaces of medical education in terms of a promise to medical students rather than a promise to the humanities, because part of medical anthropology field's imaginary is the expectation that anthropological critique will transform medical practice, and not the other way around. Such a distinction between theory and practice generates critical energy, but also, I think, forecloses the most interesting possibilities for collaborative engagement between social science and medicine.

I began this essay with a moment of uncertainty that I experienced in the clinic that was my field site at the beginning of my medical training. This moment framed an important question about the practical usefulness of scholarship in medical anthropology. But it also suggests that these encounters at the interstices of medicine and anthropology might yield interventions into the field of anthropology, rather than simply produce applications in medicine. This does not constitute a grand plan for teaching anthropology in medicine or the practice of medical anthropology. But I argue that we should attend to

---

[15] Ibid., 14.

the *desires* of social medicine pedagogy—its promises and attachments—and not merely its content. This would allow us to see clearly that the turmoil of curricular change conceals an enduring wish, which is that anthropology might deliver an answer to the question of, in the words of my student, what kind of doctors we wish to become.

6

The Perceived Freedom of the Visual Analogue Scale

Gabi Schaffzin

This chapter traces the history of the Visual Analogue Scale (VAS), used today as a graphic measurement tool in over half of all pain trials. In what follows, I am primarily concerned with how the design of a seemingly benign information-gathering object—a two-dimensional, monochromatic line—has a direct effect on the information gathered. I begin with a breakdown of what this simple, line-based scale, with roots in the experimental psychology of Wilhelm Wundt, looked like in its early forms, making the case for why its visual properties are critical to a history of graphic pain studies, and asking how its key features propelled the VAS through industrial and psychological studies in the first part of the twentieth century. Later, the chapter draws upon a variety of works, including N. Katherine Hayles's account of the rise of cybernetics and posthumanism, and Elizabeth Wilson's history of computation and affect, to consider the rise of pain management through a specifically graphic and quantitative system. Touching upon a mid-century shift in how pain is conceptualized, measured, and reported on, I will be showing how a well-capitalized pharmaceutical industry today utilizes the VAS, a tool that, as I will demonstrate, has been designed for the organization and management of populations, to reify the patient in pain as a market that can be controlled and dominated. Throughout, my primary concern is to consider the design of the tool—that is, the smooth line, and its implementation in a process that is associated with the offer of a sense of freedom to the clinical subject, a sense that, I will finally propose, is false.

The Graphic Rating Scale

The use of a horizontal line as a basis for indicating units of time or some other entity is a relatively modern innovation, going back only about 250 years.[1] In 1921, however, the line as a graphic scale for quantitative evaluation was assigned a particular role with respect to interpretation and power in the field of psychology. That year, the American Psychological Association published an abstract in its *Psychological Bulletin* in which the authors Mary Hayes and Donald Paterson make a rather momentous declaration about the line. "The Graphic Rating Method," they state, "is a new method for securing the judgment of superiors on subordinates."[2] Thus, the ubiquitous use of the simple line and its associated design parameters were elevated to a system for securing judgment and power within psychology. The authors emphasized a pair of primary benefits to clinicians using the scale: its lack of direct quantitative terms and its flexibility with respect to incrementation. These benefits would eventually prove critical to the graphic rating method's proliferation throughout the medical field in both the clinical and laboratory settings—first as the Graphic Rating Scale (GRS) and eventually as the VAS. Understanding its widespread popularity requires delving into two historical contexts. First, in this section, we must unpack the design decisions made in the name of the tool's typographical reproduction in order to pinpoint what elements of its design proved most valuable to its innovators and users. Second, in the following section, I will highlight the GRS's deep roots in an industrial psychology that understood both the scale's user and the subject (sometimes the same person) as impulsive in service of—not as opposed to—that actor's volition. This view, as I will demonstrate, was an inherent assumption of the then burgeoning field of industrial psychology, wherein a human subject operated in a manner akin to a cog in the larger corporate machine.

The GRS, as introduced by the Scott Company Engineers and Consultants in Industrial Personnel of Philadelphia in 1921, is a straight horizontal solid line of indeterminate length. Four or five "short descriptive adjectives" sit directly below the line providing a rater guidance on the various degrees against which he evaluates his subject. In the rating form published by Paterson

---

[1] Daniel Rosenberg and Anthony Grafton, *Cartographies of Time*, 1st ed (New York: Princeton Architectural Press, 2010), 19.
[2] Mary H. S. Hayes and Donald G. Paterson, "Experimental Development of the Graphic Rating Method," ed. Shepherd I. Frantz and Samuel W. Fernberger, *Psychological Bulletin* 18 (1921): 98.

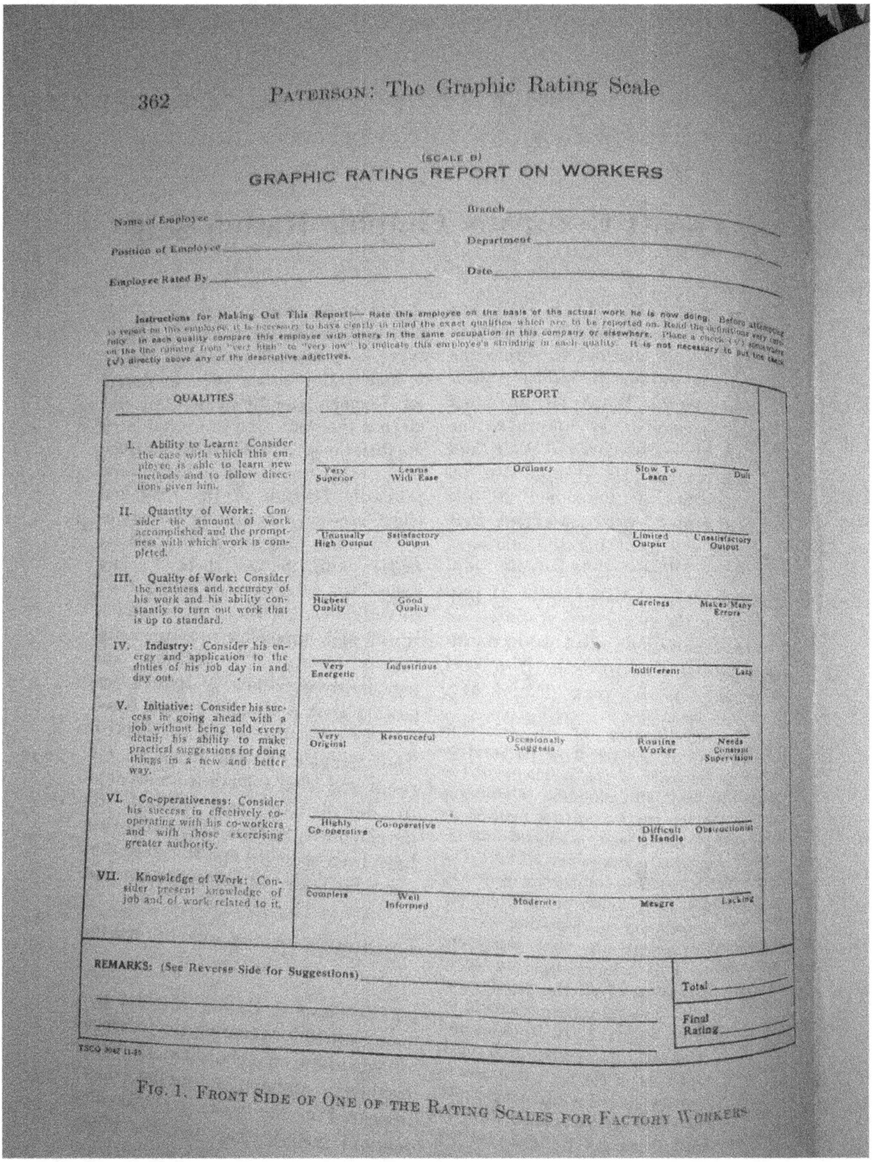

Figure 6.1 Graphic rating report on workers (Paterson, 1923).

in a subsequent article from 1923 (Figure 6.1), for instance, the first quality, "Ability to Learn," is accompanied by a GRS with "Ordinary" centered directly below the midpoint of the line in small type (perhaps 8 pt to the line's 1 pt height). To the left of "Ordinary," "Very Superior" hugs the edge, and "Learns with Ease" sits about 30 percent of the way in from the end. "Dull" and "Slow to Learn" are similarly spaced from the right edge. The text of each block is centered within.³

The next six qualities on the "Graphic Rating Report on Workers" reproduced by Paterson are similarly arranged, some of which include a midpoint label (see "V. Initiative"), while others do not (see "II. Quantity of Work"). The report includes a space at the top of the page for information about the rater and the subject, as well as the location and date of evaluation. Underneath the seven qualities, a space for remarks is designated by an outline and three blank lines, as well as a reminder that a rater may "See Reverse Side for Suggestions." To the right of the remarks area, a short line is labeled "Total," below which another is labeled "Final Rating." Each rule (a typesetter's term for a line) on the page is solid on this particular example. Later on in the paper, however, Paterson includes a version of the report featuring a "Rating Scale for Executives" (Figure 6.2).⁴ This version of the report includes all dotted lines for any rule outside of the actual GRS, indicating the critical nature of the style of lines on the GRS. That is, why should the typesetter be burdened with differentiating between the styles used for each rule if the style change is not critical to the form's use?

As Paterson describes it, an evaluator "may make as fine a discrimination of merit as he chooses," thanks primarily to the lack of preset delineations on each GRS rule.⁵ Further, because the labels are purely qualitative in nature, per Paterson, "the person who is making the judgment is freed from direct *quantitative* terms in making his decision of merit in any quality."⁶ "These two facts," he goes on, "eliminate the restrictions on natural judgments which other rating methods impose."⁷ Thus, using dotted rules for the form's metadata acts to—deliberately or not—emphasize the continuous and nondiscrete nature of the GRS lines in contrast.

Notably, Freyd's 1923 review of the GRS—a paper published in the *Journal of Educational Psychology* and oft-cited by both GRS- and VAS-utilizing studies from within a wide variety of fields, even as recently as 2019 and 2022⁸—reproduces

---

³ Donald G. Paterson, "The Scott Company Graphic Rating Scale," *Journal of Personnel Research: Official Publication of Personnel Research Federation* 1, nos. 8–9 (1923): 362.
⁴ Ibid., 364.
⁵ Ibid., 363.
⁶ Ibid., original emphasis.
⁷ Ibid.
⁸ Lu Feng Yao et al., "Minimally Invasive Treatment of Calcaneal Fractures via the Sinus Tarsi Approach Based on a 3D Printing Technique," *Mathematical Biosciences and Engineering* 16, no. 3 (February 26, 2019): 1597–610, https://doi.org/10.3934/mbe.2019076. See also Michael Giummarra, Loretta Vocale, and Matthew King, "Efficacy of Non-surgical Management and Functional Outcomes of

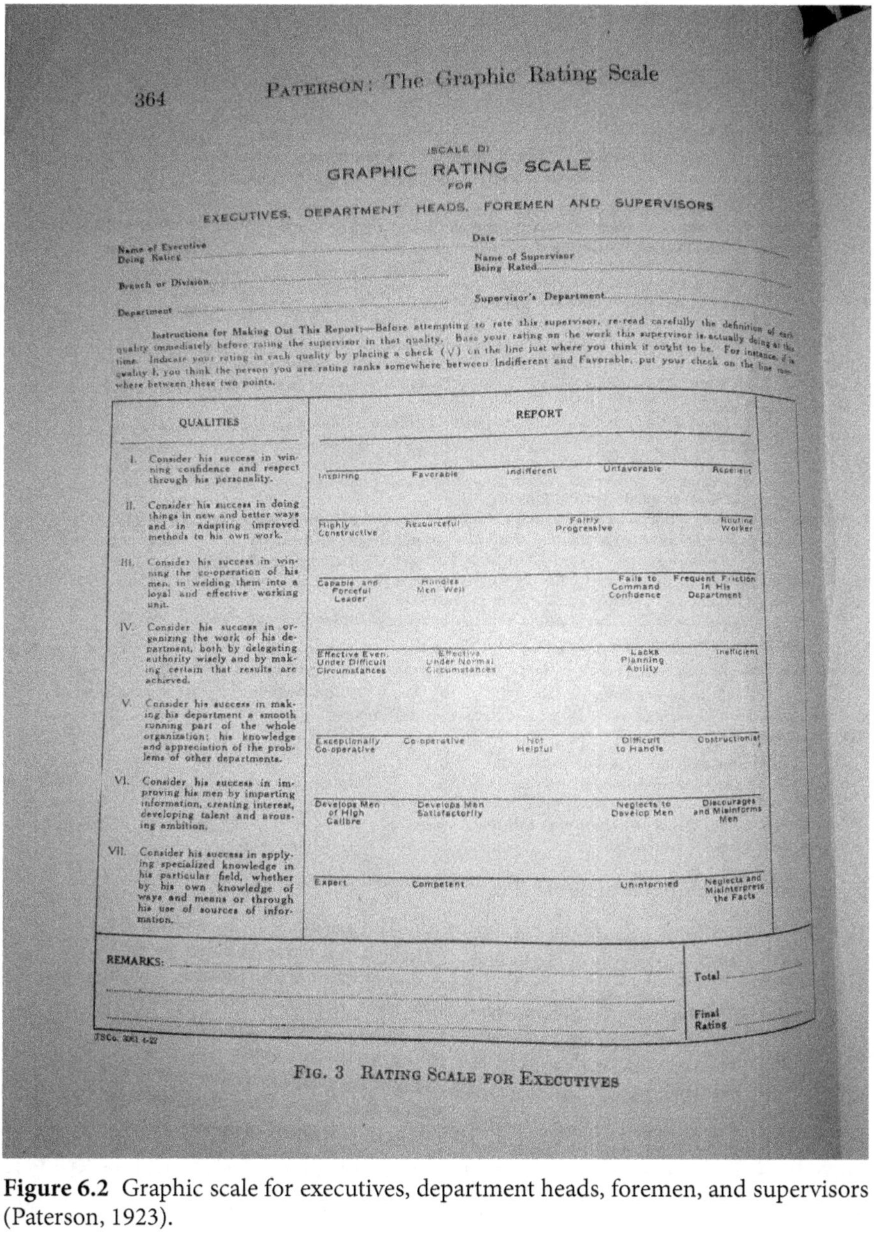

Figure 6.2 Graphic scale for executives, department heads, foremen, and supervisors (Paterson, 1923).

```
GRAPHIC RATING OF...  .....  ...        ......................  ...  .....  . ....
              Instructions for Using the Rating Scale
```
1. Let these ratings represent your own judgments. Please do not consult anyone in making them.
2. In rating this person on a particular trait, disregard every other trait but that one. Many ratings are rendered valueless because the rater allows himself to be influenced by a general favorable or unfavorable impression which he has formed of the person.
3 When you have satisfied yourself on the standing of this person in the trait on which you are rating him, place a check at the appropriate point on the horizontal line. You do not have to place your check directly above a descriptive phrase. You may place your check at any point on the line.

3. Does he appear neat or slovenly in his dress?

| Extremely neat and clean. Almost a dude. | Appropriately and neatly dressed | Inconspicuous in dress | Somewhat careless in his dress | Very slovenly and unkempt |

9. How does he impress people by his physique and bearing?

| Looked down on | Unimpressive physique and bearing | | Noticeable for good physique and bearing | | Excites admiration. Very impressive |

13. How flexible is he?

| Hidebound. Runs in a rut | Slow to take up new ideas | Progressive tendencies | Quick to pick up new ways and habits | Is always adapting himself and taking up new ideas |

18. Is he quiet or talkative?

| Talks seldom. When questioned answers briefly | Does not uphold his end of the conversation | Moderately talkative | More than upholds his end of the conversation | Great talker. Always going |

Figure 6.3 Graphic Rating Scale (Freyd, 1923).

a report with dotted rules (Figure 6.3).[9] The paper also includes graphs[10] and a table with solid lines,[11] indicating that printing solid lines was not an impossibility for the publisher. This raises the question: would the GRS work as a delineated line, as opposed to Paterson's continuous rule? To answer this, we need to both consider the publication date and perform an inspection of the typographic properties of the rest of the paper. The majority of the article was most likely compiled on a Linotype machine, a mechanism not equipped to produce solid

---

Partial ACL Tears: A Systematic Review of Randomized Trials," BMC Musculoskeletal Disorders 23, no. 332 (April 8, 2022), https://doi.org/10.1186/s12891-022-05278-w.
[9] Max Freyd, "The Graphic Rating Scale," Journal of Educational Psychology 14, no. 2 (1923): 92, https://doi.org/10.1037/h0074329.
[10] Ibid., 95–6.
[11] Ibid., 98.

TABLE I.—INTERCORRELATIONS OF AVERAGE RATINGS (84 CASES)
Decimal Points are Omitted

Trait	1	2	3	4	5	6	7	8	9	10	11	12	13	14	15	16	17	18	19	20
1. Present-mindedness		43	40	-03	16	34	40	22	25	06	00	-13	45	45	-06	23	19	16	13	51
2. Good-nature	43		19	03	-22	25	25	16	34	00	51	34	29	51	06	29	13	16	25	16
3. Neatness in dress	40	19		-19	-25	00	29	-13	25	03	51	16	34	25	34	19	-06	19	16	19
4. Cool-headedness	-03	03	-19		19	37	22	54	37	-13	19	16	-19	13	-19	19	-16	-25	37	-19
5. Self-assertion	16	-22	-25	19		19	25	16	03	16	06	-13	16	22	-16	16	40	22	-03	37
6. Accuracy in work	34	25	00	37	19		06	45	06	13	-03	00	-19	19	03	13	06	03	22	34
7. Freedom from self-consciousness	40	25	29	22	25	06		25	51	03	25	06	25	25	-03	59	00	25	16	-03
8. Cautiousness	22	16	-13	54	16	45	25		13	-16	00	40	-06	00	-22	06	-03	-28	03	00
9. Good bearing	25	34	25	37	03	22	51	13		34	34	-06	25	03	-03	13	06	25	37	40
10. Self-esteem	06	00	03	-13	16	13	03	-16	34		48	-40	16	00	06	06	-03	43	19	37
11. Even-temper	00	51	51	19	06	-03	25	00	34	48		34	06	00	-16	06	03	-16	25	06
12. Appreciation of others	-13	34	16	16	-13	00	06	40	-06	-40	34		-03	-03	-34	-13	06	-54	16	-19
13. Flexibility	45	29	34	-19	16	-19	25	-06	25	16	06	-03		43	16	22	13	37	-34	66
14. Sociability	45	51	25	13	22	19	25	00	03	00	00	-03	43		31	56	03	51	03	31
15. Open-heartedness	-06	06	34	-19	-16	03	-03	-22	-03	06	-16	-34	16	31		22	-19	51	-19	-00
16. Sociability with other sex	23	29	19	19	16	13	59	06	13	06	06	-13	22	56	22		-03	51	13	06
17. "Nerve"	19	13	-06	-16	40	06	00	-03	06	-03	03	06	13	03	-19	-03		-13	37	19
18. Talkativeness	16	16	19	-25	22	03	25	-28	25	43	-16	-54	37	51	51	-13			-19	37
19. Artistic taste	13	25	16	37	-03	22	16	03	37	19	25	16	-34	03	-19	13	37	-12		03
20. Quickness in work	51	16	19	-19	37	34	-03	06	40	37	06	-19	66	31	-06	06	19	37	03	

Figure 6.4 Intercorrelations of average ratings (Freyd, 1923).

rules quickly. Instead, typing a series of periods in succession would help produce the dotted lines for an in-paper exhibit. Any solid lines on the subsequent graphs in the publication appear to be hand-drawn or traced, indicating that those figures were compiled using a combination of Linotype plates, as well as copper etchings (or, perhaps, flexographic plates—sections of chemically engraved rubber).[12] The table[13] (Figure 6.4) would have been "locked up" in a press individually, as it sits on a page by itself, allowing the typesetter to use both lead rules (for solid lines) and lining figures for the numerals without worrying about accommodating large blocks of type around it.[14] The discontinuous nature of the Freyd GRS lines, then, were not meant to represent that the scale should be delineated, but were instead done in the name of a more efficient printing process.

In 1924, Freyd published another version of the same form. Whereas in his 1923 publication he included eighty-seven dots per GRS rule, this time he included ninety dots. The discrepancy between dot counts in the 1923 and 1924 papers further supports my assertion that his graduated lines were based on printing decisions and not one related to the quantitative properties or specific design of the GRS itself (especially as he did not seem to be paying

---

[12] Per Clive Message, art logistics manager at the Lancet Journals, hot metal type was used in conjunction with copper engraving through the 1970s. A brief review of industry norms throughout the early to middle part of the century indicates a relative lack of change in typesetting, compositing, and printing technologies for publications such as the journals in question. See Philip B. Meggs and Alston W. Purvis, *Meggs' History of Graphic Design*, 5th ed. (Hoboken, NJ: Wiley, 2012).

[13] Max Freyd, "The Graphic Rating Scale," *Journal of Educational Psychology* 14, no. 2 (1923): 98, https://doi.org/10.1037/h0074329.

[14] Numerals aligned in a table require a different set of characters than those in line with text. These are called lining, or tabular, figures.

much attention to how many delineations existed along his lines). However, while Freyd still argues in both 1923 and 1924 that an evaluator is freed from directly delineated lines when presented with a GRS, certainly anyone using his lines would be enticed to mark on or between a specific dot, effectively negating that freedom. He never directly addresses this inconsistency. Rigg provides no reasoning for their use of dots in their study on "Propaganda in the Enjoyment of Music," though the large typewritten X indicates that the choice is similarly based on a typesetting problem, especially as the X is not on the same baseline as the periods—something that would be difficult to accomplish within one line of Linotype output, or "slug."[15]

In addition to using dotted lines for typographic purposes, there have also been a number of efforts over the history of the GRS to adjust the line style and arrangement, resulting in the publication of both graduated lines (horizontal or vertical lines with small perpendicular tick marks along the way) and broken lines. One of the earliest examples of the former comes from a psychology study by Moffie in 1942: the instructions on the form read, "Make a straight, vertical mark on the line … it need not necessarily be under a descriptive phrase."[16] Moffie never goes on to explain why the graduation marks are present, but in 1953, Dreger readily admits that their graduated scale to evaluate college-level courses "violates several principles considered best for rating scales, in particular, using definite marks along the rating line."[17] The author continues: "It was thought, possibly unjustifiably, that the use of marked points would encourage use of any part of the scale rather than just the white space in the middle."[18] The design of the GRS, then, is specifically attuned to the ways that a user will interact with it. This feature is something we can trace to its original founder, Walter Dill Scott, and his research into instinct and impulse.

Scott's Wundtian Lineage

In his 1923 article introducing the GRS, Paterson credits Beardsly Ruml with "originating the graphic rating method as well as supervising its experimental

---

[15] Melvin G. Rigg, "Favorable versus Unfavorable Propaganda in the Enjoyment of Music," *Journal of Experimental Psychology* 38, no. 1 (1948): 78–81, https://doi.org/10.1037/h0056077.
[16] D. J. Moffie, "The Validity of Self-Estimated Interests," *Journal of Applied Psychology* 26, no. 5 (1942): 609, https://doi.org/10.1037/h0056402.
[17] Ralph Mason Dreger, "A Simple Course Evaluation Scale," *Journal of Experimental Education* 22, no. 2 (1953): 145.
[18] Ibid.

development."[19] Ruml, who was instrumental in the establishment and growth of the Social Sciences Department of the University of Chicago,[20] cofounded the Scott Company Engineers and Consultants in Industrial Personnel with Walter Dill Scott. At the time of Paterson's publication, Scott was president of Northwestern University and president of the American Psychological Association. He had formerly been founding director of the Bureau of Salesmanship at the Carnegie Institution of Technology and the 1917 recipient of the Distinguished Service Medal as a colonel in the US Army for his work establishing a rating method for officers.[21] Scott was one of the first people in the United States to combine industrial management with the emerging field of applied psychology.

Scott's background in psychology was rooted in his doctoral work with Wilhelm Wundt at the University of Leipzig at the turn of the century. Wundt, who is best known as the founder of experimental psychology, opened the first "laboratory" for psychological studies in 1879. Under Wundt, Scott wrote a dissertation that, through an historical exploration of human impulses (*triebe*) from 1755 to 1900, argues that a Wundtian definition of instinct "better than any other, summarizes the various historical treatments of the subject, while at the same time harmonizing with the modern psychological views."[22]

As Scott explains it, Wundt's approach to human impulse is "of a reflex-mechanical nature,"[23] which is worth unpacking further if we are to understand the implications of Scott's training in the development of the GRS. Scott goes on to quote Wundt: "These (innate impulses), however, are, as we say, states of a particular striving or reluctance, in which an existing feeling of pleasure or pain causes bodily movements, the effect of which is directed to the intensification of the feeling of pleasure or to the elimination of the feeling of lack."[24] Scott

---

[19] Donald G. Paterson, "The Scott Company Graphic Rating Scale," *Journal of Personnel Research: Official Publication of Personnel Research Federation* 1, nos. 8–9 (1923): 361.

[20] William H. McNeill, *Hutchins' University: A Memoir of the University of Chicago, 1929–1950*, illustrated ed. (Chicago: University of Chicago Press, 2007), 12.

[21] "Walter Dill Scott, Northwestern University Archives," The Presidents of Northwestern, 2009, http://exhibits.library.northwestern.edu/archives/exhibits/presidents/scott.html.

[22] "welche besser als irgend eine andere die verschiedenen historischen Behandlungen des Gegenstandes zusammenfasst und gleichzeitig mit den modernen psychologischen Ansichten harmoniert." Walter Dill Scott, *Die psychologie der triebe historisch-kritisch betrachtet* (Leipzig, 1900), 52, http://hdl.handle.net/2027/njp.32101061248017. Many thanks to Teresa Fankhänel of Technische Universität München for help with translation.

[23] Ibid., 43.

[24] "Diese (angeborenen Triebe) sind aber, wie wir sagen, Zu stände eines bestimmten Strebens oder Widerstrebens, bei denen ein vorhandenes Lustoder Unlustgefühl Körperbewegungen her beifürt, deren Effekt auf die Verstärkung des Lustgefühls oder auf die Beseitigung des Unlustgefühls gerichtet ist." Wilhelm Max Wundt, *Grundzüge der physiologischen Psychologie* (Leipzig: W. Engelmann, 1893), 593, quoted in Scott, *Die psychologie der triebe historisch-kritisch betrachtet*, 43.

uses Wundt here to tie impulsive bodily movements to psychological, not physiological, systems. Critically, Wundt suggests that instinctual movement is not the same as a physical reflex because the former is an act of volition. Scott goes so far as to describe instinctual movements as dignified by their being influenced by will, especially in opposition to reflexes. For Scott's understanding of Wundt—an understanding that he would bring back to the United States with him soon after completing his doctorate—an impulsive bodily movement is indicative not only of the "unconscious" but also of *what a subject wants*: "the first stage in the development of the will."[25]

The GRS (and, eventually, the VAS) is an attempt by a researcher to trigger an impulse—it asks an evaluator to make a mark based on a feeling or observation. In his book *The Theory of Advertising* (1903), Scott spends an entire chapter explaining the power of suggestion and how advertisers take advantage of it to encourage or inspire a consumer to spend money. If, as Scott suggests, humans are easily inspired to act by simple advertising copy,[26] then it follows that when seeking an impulsive—and, as such, volitional—response from an evaluator, then there must be as little suggestion as possible. In the same work, Scott offers his "Law of Suggestion": "Every idea of a function tends to call that function into activity, and will do so, unless hindered by a competing idea or physical impediment."[27] Ideas such as breaks in lines and graduation, then, must be eliminated from the scales in order to remove any suggestions. Enter the VAS—a descendant of the GRS stripped even more bare than those lines put forth by Paterson and his contemporaries.

The Visual Analogue Scale

In a letter to the editor of the June 24, 1961, issue of the *British Medical Journal*, three researchers from the RAF Institute of Aviation argued that the statistical analysis for an article published previously in the same journal was done using faulty data. Specifically, the study in question—centered around respiratory diseases among workers—offered binary choices ("yes" and "no") for questions that, the letter's authors argued, should in fact be more continuous in nature:

---

[25] "das erste Stadium in der Entwickelung des Willens." Scott, *Die psychologie der triebe historisch-kritisch betrachtet*, 52.
[26] Walter Dill Scott, *The Theory of Advertising: A Simple Exposition of the Principles of Psychology in Their Relation to Successful Advertising* (Boston: Small, Maynard, 1903), 60.
[27] Ibid., 47.

It would seem that the use of such a technique for subjective assessment fails to extract the maximum information, by not providing any quantitative measure of degree, and may even have produced false information by having forced a biased answer from those in doubt. Clarification by further questions or elucidation by an interview may provide more information, but still does not achieve the maximum.[28]

The writers offer instead what they call "a continuous scale" and include a visual example: a single thin horizontal line with two thin vertical marks at each end. Cantered under the left mark is the word "Never" and under the right, "Every day."[29] They suggest that the line be 10 cm long and that a quantitative score might be gathered from a subjective answer by measuring the distance in millimeters from the left end to the mark placed on the line by the subject. Eight years later, one of the authors of the letter would publish a paper and give this new scale the name by which we recognize it today: the VAS, effectively a GRS without the intermediate labels. The term analogue was used because the line represents a spectrum of values, not a pre-delineated scale.[30]

Prior to the 1961 letter, only Dreger (1953)—whose scale is referenced above in my discussion of graduated GRSs (i.e., scales that did not adhere to the Scott Company's original guidelines)—argued for a bipolar line. After defending the use of tickmarks along their scale, Dreger adds, "Since the scale is meant for a quick expression of feeling ... the fewest descriptive phrases consonant with clarity had to be included."[31] Here, we can once again make a connection from a Wundtian emphasis on impulse to the "quick expression of feeling," one that minimizes an evaluator's time to consider an answer before marking the line.

Per Tousignant (2011), the middle of the twentieth century saw the anesthesiologist Henry Beecher publish field-shifting arguments regarding the subjective nature of pain, requiring that pain studies be designed around large numbers of subjects (three subjects had been the previous minimum).[32]

---

[28] J. L. Gedye, R. C. B. Aitken, and Helen M. Ferres, "Subjective Assessment in Clinical Research," *British Medical Journal* 1, no. 5242 (June 24, 1961): 1828.
[29] Ibid.
[30] R. C. Aitken, "Measurement of Feelings Using Visual Analogue Scales," *Proceedings of the Royal Society of Medicine* 62, no. 10 (October 1969): 989–93.
[31] Dreger, "A Simple Course Evaluation Scale," 145, 147.
[32] Noémi Tousignant, "The Rise and Fall of the Dolorimeter: Pain, Analgesics, and the Management of Subjectivity in Mid-Twentieth-Century United States," *Journal of the History of Medicine and Allied Sciences* 66, no. 2 (2011): 145–79.

Pain studies were being redesigned to accommodate the newly required scale of "n-values," and there needed to be tools that could quickly and reliably record pain data that can then be crunched by statisticians. For Beecher et al., the VAS may have been a perfect tool to address many of the considerations raised by the researchers relating to how best to record the intensity of felt pain in the patient during subjective clinical studies. In *Measurement of Subjective Responses*, Beecher notes that "Keele recognized ... the difficulty of verbalizing descriptions of pain."[33] Certainly, when Beecher used the term "verbalizing," he was referring to the subject's ability to come up with the right word to describe pain. There is also the scenario, however, when a patient in pain literally cannot speak, either due to incapacitation or the severity of the pain. With a VAS, a subject need not speak. They may just leave a mark on or point to a line. The nonverbal nature of the VAS also helped mitigate those situations when the physician, researcher, or technician does not speak the same language as the patient.[34]

It is no coincidence, then, that the 1960s saw the emergence of VAS usage in pain studies specifically. This began with a collaboration between psychiatrist Issy Pilowsky and physician Michael Bond at the University of Sheffield. Colleagues of theirs had been using a graphic scale (Clarke and Spear, 1964) around that time, and so the pair recorded subjects' pain by asking each one to pencil-mark on a blank ten-centimeter line.[35] On one side of the line, "I have no pain at all" was written, and on the other side, "My pain is as bad as it could possibly be."[36] The 1966 paper is often cited as the first implementation of a GRS-like scale in a pain-related study. Bond, during a conference on "Innovation in Pain Management," noted that he "asked patients to estimate their pain levels, and incidentally the analogue scale for measurement of pain first appeared in Sheffield at about that time."[37] The line had thus arrived at pain research.

---

[33] Henry K. Beecher, *Measurement of Subjective Responses: Quantitative Effects of Drugs* (New York: Oxford University Press, 1959), 63.
[34] G. B. Langley and H. Sheppeard, "The Visual Analogue Scale: Its Use in Pain Measurement," *Rheumatology International* 5, no. 4 (July 1, 1985): 145–8, https://doi.org/10.1007/BF00541514.
[35] Unfortunately, Clarke and Spear's 1964 paper was only published as an abstract, and it is unclear if their line had the GRS's intermediate or the VAS's bipolar labels.
[36] M. R. Bond and I. Pilowsky, "Subjective Assessment of Pain and Its Relationship to the Administration of Analgesics in Patients with Advanced Cancer," *Journal of Psychosomatic Research* 10, no. 2 (1966): 203, https://doi.org/10.1016/0022-3999(66)90064-X.
[37] L. A. Reynolds and E. M. Tansey, eds., *Innovation in Pain Management* (London: QMUL History C20Medicine, 2004), 21.

Decision-Making

A simple line promising at once freedom and reliability, the VAS mediates what N. Katherine Hayles calls "the disembodiment of information."[38] In *How We Became Posthuman*, she writes that "decisions are important not because they produce material goods but because they produce information."[39] The story of the VAS is one of decisions. One year before Freyd wrote about the graphic scale, he published "A Method for the Study of Vocational Interests" (1923), an essay on the best methods for placing students in the right jobs. He writes, "One of the goals ... of the worker in the field of Applied Psychology, is to harmonize the individual with his vocational environment."[40] Nearly one hundred years later, the VAS is used to inform decisions on a plethora of levels: whether or not to believe,[41] to diagnose,[42] to treat,[43] or to go to market.[44] And each of these decisions embodies its own labyrinth of judgments and recommendations. As Annemarie Jutel writes, "Diagnosis ... serves an administrative purpose as it enables access to the services and status, from insurance reimbursement to restricted-access medication, sick leave and support group membership."[45]

When Bond and Pilowsky decided to use the VAS for their study on felt pain, they were doing so with the understanding that the scale was not only an appropriate tool for the measurement and tracking of the subjective experience but also an efficient and reliable one. It was not until Beecher, however, that the idea that reliable pain measurement required efficiency and volume proliferated. In light of this, as well as the VAS's lineage (via the GRS) as a tool for the likes of Walter Scott and Company, we must consider the VAS to be used as a decision mechanism. Just like the machines in the factories studied by the Scott Company,

---

[38] Katherine Hayles, *How We Became Posthuman: Virtual Bodies in Cybernetics, Literature, and Informatics* (Chicago, IL: University of Chicago Press, [1999] 2010), 21.
[39] Ibid., 22.
[40] M. Freyd, "A Method for the Study of Vocational Interests," *Journal of Applied Psychology* 6, no. 3 (1922): 243, https://doi.org/10.1037/h0072563.
[41] Akihiko Masuda et al., "A Parametric Study of Cognitive Defusion and the Believability and Discomfort of Negative Self-Relevant Thoughts," *Behavior Modification* 33, no. 2 (March 1, 2009): 250–62, https://doi.org/10.1177/0145445508326259.
[42] James S. Factor and Harald Azuma, "Visual Analog Scale and Method of Use for the Diagnosis and/or Treatment of Physical Pain," United States US6258042B1, filed September 17, 1999, and issued July 10, 2001, https://patents.google.com/patent/US6258042B1/en.
[43] Langley and Sheppeard, "The Visual Analogue Scale."
[44] Martin S. Angst, William G. Brose, and John B. Dyck, "The Relationship between the Visual Analog Pain Intensity and Pain Relief Scale Changes during Analgesic Drug Studies in Chronic Pain Patients," *Anesthesiology* 91, no. 1 (July 1, 1999): 34–41, https://doi.org/10.1097/00000542-199907000-00009.
[45] Annemarie Jutel, "Sociology of Diagnosis: A Preliminary Review," *Sociology of Health & Illness* 31, no. 2 (March 1, 2009): 278, https://doi.org/10.1111/j.1467-9566.2008.01152.x.

the VAS brings in raw material in the form of pencil marks and processes it to become "useful" to the physician, nurse, researcher, and so on.

Returning to Jutel, the author begins her essay by declaring that "diagnoses are the classification tools of medicine."[46] How might we understand the implications of a classificatory tool, especially in the context of design decisions that led to its form? Geoffrey Bowker and Susan Leigh Star's 2000 work, *Sorting Things Out*, offers a thorough and valuable look at the ways which tools of classification have been designed and implemented in a postwar West and how scholars might best study them going forward. In their penultimate chapter, the pair seeks to reconcile the ethnographies and histories of classificatory tools and the theoretical underpinnings informing their investigation. Bowker and Star write:

> Information is only information when there are multiple interpretations. One person's noise may be another's signal or two people may agree to attend to something, but it is the tension between contexts that actually creates representation. What becomes problematic under these circumstances is the relationships among people and things, or objects, the relationships that create representations, not just noise.[47]

Critical for this discussion here, then, is to consider what the relationship might be between the scale and the subject, and the scale and the individual using its data (or, as Hayes and Paterson might refer to the latter, the judge). To the subject in pain, the VAS is a smooth line with only two poles. The possibilities for selection are, literally, endless, as there are no rules requiring a decision to be snapped to any specific location on the line. To the judge, the line is delineated— most likely one hundred times, if dividing a 10 cm length by millimeters. While the judge is privy to the view of the VAS as both a single smooth surface and a graduated line, the subject is not. The diagnosis is made, medication given or taken away, pharmaceuticals approved and brought to market, and the individual being surveyed has, based on the graphic in front of them, no idea what sort of influence the mark they made has on that decision.

Consider the use of the term "analogue": opening his 1969 paper in support of the use of VAS in psychological studies, Aitken notes of rating scales unlike the graphic method: "A digital system is imposed on the observer, when the freedom of an analogue system would be welcome."[48] It is logical that the term "Visual

---

[46] Ibid.
[47] Geoffrey C. Bowker and Susan Leigh Star, *Sorting Things Out: Classification and Its Consequences*, first paperback ed., Inside Technology (Cambridge, MA: MIT Press, 2000), 291.
[48] Aitken, "Measurement of Feelings Using Visual Analogue Scales," 989.

Analogue Scale" emerges in the latter half of the century, at exactly the same time that computers and computing culture were proliferating into research laboratories (among other venues)—a time when the term "digital," per the researchers at the *Oxford English Dictionary*, "underwent an explosion in usage and in meaning."[49] Analogue scales are, on their surfaces, in direct opposition to the digital, the binary, the discrete. But once the placement of the mark on the VAS is measured, the data is no longer analogue, but in discrete units.

Affect and the Subject

This transformation and the power it exercises might best be understood by first taking a sidebar through psychologist and science studies scholar Elizabeth Wilson's book *Affect and Artificial Intelligence* (2010). Wilson's argument is multifaceted. She makes the case for a reconceptualization of AI away from the stereotypical view of it as a "cool," emotionless field for unfeeling mathematicians and computer scientists, and toward a significantly warmer, more emotional domain in which these professionals engage in emotion-rich activities. She also suggests that the proliferation and improvement of AI technologies will increase when all parties involved agree on the aforementioned reframing. She uses biographies of both humans (chess master Gary Kasparov, computer science pioneer Alan Turing, logician Walter Pitts, etc.) and machines (IBM's Watson, virtual psychoanalyst ELIZA, its descendant PARRY, and MIT robot Kismet), alongside theories taken from the social sciences, culture of technology, and psychoanalysis to weave an argument that challenges many assumptions that society holds about computers and computing.

Wilson's work is important to my own study primarily when she begins to probe our relationship to what she terms "calculating machines"—she "advocates greater emotional attachment" to them, appealing to users: "yes, please, feel them."[50] She amplifies those who argue for a more complicated, emotional relationship between the user and the device; quoting Clifford Nass and Byron Reeves: "We have found that individuals' interactions with computers, television,

---

[49] Richard Holden, "Digital," *Oxford English Dictionary* (blog), August 16, 2012, https://public.oed.com/blog/word-stories-digital/.
[50] Elizabeth A. Wilson, *Affect and Artificial Intelligence (In Vivo: The Cultural Mediations of Biomedical Science)* (Seattle: University of Washington Press, 2010), xii, http://www.columbia.edu/cgi-bin/cul/resolve?clio14020718.

and new media are fundamentally social and natural."[51] Of particular interest here is Joseph Weizenbaum's psychoanalytic artificial intelligence program ELIZA and the ways that the MIT researcher sought to reveal the program's inner workings in an effort to "detach users from their peculiar affection for it."[52] "Once a particular program is unmasked," Weizenbaum writes, "once its inner workings are explained in language sufficiently plain to induce understanding, its magic crumbles away; it stands revealed as a mere collection of procedures."[53] Wilson uses ELIZA and Weizenbaum to open a pathway to the work of Sylvan Tomkins, whose *Affect Imagery Consciousness* (four volumes published over thirty years, starting in 1962) is a sweeping work on the way that affects and cognitive processing work together in the human psyche to help us process and utilize information.[54] Critically, Wilson explains that "affects … are analogic events: being ashamed or afraid or interested is a highly variegated experience. Accurate measurement of the affects typically requires continuous rather than discrete calibration."[55]

Pain, Tomkins would argue, is already a highly analogic event and, as such, one that would garner much affect. Returning, then, to the VAS, we might consider the relationship between the subject and the smooth analogue scale—upon which a seemingly endless possibility of choices is present—to be one infused with great affect as well. Wilson argues that "when relatedness … between digital and analog … is obstructed, there is a high price to pay."[56] That is, artificial barriers between these two seemingly opposite concepts put us at risk of missing the ways that the construction of human experiences through the layering of the analogue and the digital is at the foundation of these experiences in the late twentieth and early twenty-first centuries. The history of VAS is littered with words like "freedom,"[57] "interesting,"[58] and "sensitivity,"[59] but also

---

[51] Byron Reeves and Clifford Ivar Nass, *The Media Equation: How People Treat Computers, Televisions, and New Media as Real People and Places*, CSLI Lecture Notes, no. 63 (Stanford, CA: Cambridge University Press, 1996), 5.
[52] Wilson, *Affect and Artificial Intelligence*, 92.
[53] Joseph Weizenbaum, "ELIZA—A Computer Program for the Study of Natural Language Communication between Man and Machine," *Communications of the ACM* 9, no. 1 (January 1, 1966): 36, https://doi.org/10.1145/365153.365168.
[54] Silvan S. Tomkins, *Affect, Imagery, Consciousness*, ed. Bertram P. Karon, 4 vols. (New York: Springer, 1962).
[55] Wilson, *Affect and Artificial Intelligence*, 116–17.
[56] Ibid., 108.
[57] Aitken, "Measurement of Feelings Using Visual Analogue Scales."
[58] Freyd, "The Graphic Rating Scale."
[59] Bond and Pilowsky, "Subjective Assessment of Pain and Its Relationship to the Administration of Analgesics in Patients with Advanced Cancer."

"validity,"[60] "reliability,"[61] and "objective."[62] To the outside observer of the system and to the judge, the layering of analogue and digital is clear; to the patient—the subject, the pained—it is hidden.

Return again to Paterson and his written instructions: "Rate this employee on the basis of the actual work he is now doing."[63] Imagine, then, a factory in 1920s America: machines on the floor churning out widgets; workers manning their stations; foremen patrolling the catwalks above them, clipboards in hand, rapidly marking the 10 cm lines in front of them. In this scenario, the judges are hidden, but the fate of each employee rests on those clipboards. To be sure, the situations involving the factory worker and the subject in pain are not perfectly analogous. For the latter, they see the line being marked, while the former does not. However, for both, what is being measured is not inherently quantifiable; the data taken may be used in an individualized or aggregated manner; and both are submitting data that will eventually influence their futures. And within the use of this designed tool, meant to disembody information and take advantage of the subject's affect, are layers of power relationships that must be unpacked.

Power and the Judge

In the biopolitical realm, knowledge of the human—at once global, quantitative (i.e., concerning the population), and analytical (i.e., concerning the individual)— is exploited by the loci of power to divide, categorize, and act "upon populations in order to securitize the nation."[64] As the nineteenth century came to a close, the negative effects of laissez-faire policies turned the tide toward a more active liberal state, one that enabled citizens to maximize their liberties. Picking up at the beginning of the twentieth century, it takes no stretch of the imagination to understand how technologies like the rating scales of the Scott Company might have been welcomed into a society seeking to solidify who is normal and who is not. Beecher's work was strongly inspired by his work on the battlefield, the ultimate space for (what Foucault would refer to as) the securitization of

---

[60] Aitken, "Measurement of Feelings Using Visual Analogue Scales."
[61] Mary H. S. Hayes and Donald G. Paterson, "Experimental Development of the Graphic Rating Method," ed. Shepherd I. Frantz and Samuel W. Fernberger, *Psychological Bulletin* 18 (1921): 98–9.
[62] Freyd, "The Graphic Rating Scale."
[63] Paterson, "The Scott Company Graphic Rating Scale," 362.
[64] Majia Holmer Nadesan, *Governmentality, Biopower, and Everyday Life*, Routledge Studies in Social and Political Thought 57 (New York: Routledge, [2008] 2011), 25.

the population.⁶⁵ When the physician returned from war, he published and implemented what he had learned so that a newly empowered pharmaceutical industry might move toward an effective analgesic testing. The ultimate goal was the widespread availability of pain killers. As Nadesan notes, "By stressing 'self-care,' the neoliberal state divulges paternalistic responsibility for its subjects but simultaneously holds its subjects responsible for self-government."⁶⁶

The overwhelming justification for the use of a line-based scale is one of empowerment—the "freedom" discussed in the previous section—and distancing the subject from the direct mechanisms of quantification. And yet, this tool is meant to measure the intensity of pain. As it moves from the individual as a mark on a line to the collective as a numerical value representing distance, that mark is effectively erased. Does a patient in great pain press hard with their pencil on the piece of paper? Do they place a lighter mark because the pain has sapped their strength? Do they just point, as getting their eyes to focus on the line might be too difficult given the headache they are battling? In all of these instances, the VAS sanitizes the affect of the subject as soon as a value is noted by the physician, recorded by the technician, and smoothed by the data scientist.

Above, I referenced N. Katherine Hayles: "Decisions are important not because they produce material goods but because they produce information." The next line of that passage is: "Control information, and power follows."⁶⁷ The VAS's early proliferation as a rating tool and its surface-level simplicity make it a perfect case study in the control of information through the design of an information-gathering tool. It is just a single line drawn on a piece of paper; how can it possibly affect the shape of information being gathered? In fact, its unassuming form ensures that the information gathered is as unaffected as possible. Without preset steps, the subject should feel free to move about the line as they wish. Without suggested vocabulary (save for the phrases at each pole), they need not find their own words to describe their pain.

But to understand the history of VAS means to understand the measurement system and vocabulary that was used to build and adapt it over the past one hundred years. We give our pain ratings like we are grading a student or evaluating an employee. We seek to manage our pain like we might an assembly-line

---

⁶⁵ Michel Foucault, *Security, Territory, Population: Lectures at the Collège de France, 1977–78*, ed. Michel Senellart, François Ewald, and Alessandro Fontana, trans. Graham Burchell (Basingstoke: Palgrave Macmillan, 2007), 11.
⁶⁶ Nadesan, *Governmentality, Biopower, and Everyday Life*, 33.
⁶⁷ Hayles, *How We Became Posthuman*, 52.

worker. Our individual, subjective experience is in one moment recorded and considered and, in another, grouped and calculated. When we talk about pain with our doctors, insurance agents, or pharmacists, we are using a language that can be tied back to the way people were measured and controlled. On the surface—literally—we are empowered to declare our pain using a mark we make ourselves. That power is fleeting, however, and without a proper understanding of the ways that it works, we risk a false sense of control.

Part 3

Contingencies

Introduction

The chapters in this part illustrate how aspects of lived, bodily experience pose challenges for traditional biomedical knowledge frameworks. From the points of view of disability studies and critical theory, history, and literary studies, Travis Chi Wing Lau, John A. Carranza, and Benjamin Gagnon Chainey raise questions about how biomedicine offers an incomplete understanding of illness and embodiment. Their attention to bodily realities, such as disability, terminal illness, and death, reveals epistemological shortcomings. As these chapters highlight, humanistic tools, including critical thinking, attention to historical context, and rhetorical analysis, can help account for bodily ambiguity and uncertainty. These chapters assert the need for the ethical, critical, and stylistic values that are interwoven throughout the collection, illustrating that their combination can expand our sense and definition of human life.

This part provides innovative models for addressing ambiguities not by trying to pin them down but by showing the wealth of their potential to open up new discussions and better account for lived experiences. While the challenges of disability, terminal illness, and end of life might seem to call the authority of biomedical regimes into question, these chapters also nod to the potential changes that could be made to medical institutions by listening more closely to bodily realities.

Using disability studies as the critical framework, Chapter 7, by Lau, evaluates the state of the field of medical and health humanities through a discussion of the historical challenges of intersecting disability studies with medical forms of knowledge. A "crip turn" is necessary, he argues, in order for medical care—and medical humanities itself—to account properly for the notions of disability that have too often been placed at the margins of discourse. "Crip time," in particular, can offer not just medicine but also medical humanities a more capacious framework for challenging "curative violence," since the teleology of cure is itself antithetical to the lived experience of disability. For Lau, infusing a hospitalist-oriented medical humanities with crip theory is both a political and an "ethical investment" that prompts a rethinking of the field's (sometimes unscrutinized) aim to improve the delivery of care.

Building on this examination of how and why teleologies that defy a notion of "cure" are left out of medical humanities discourse, Chapter 8, by Carranza, an historian, takes an unusual disciplinary approach by treating a series of literary texts—Armistead Maupin's *Tales of the City*—as a series of historical documents that chart the HIV/AIDS epidemic in Los Angeles. For Carranza, whose essay begins with a personal account of the discovery of an annotated copy of *Tales of the City*, the methods of historical analysis can be applied with unexpected payoffs to works of literature in which the author explicitly takes on the role of a narrative eyewitness to a community event. In contrast to approaches in medical humanities that attend to the author's body or to medical professionals' responses to illness, Carranza's analysis finds that *Tales of the City* offers historical evidence of a terminal illness experience, as recorded by a surviving community. In this account, the AIDS crisis registered in Maupin's novels is not only a "snapshot ... of [a] specific moment ... in history" but also a model for how an unconventional application of disciplinary strategies (here, the historical analysis of fiction) might make space for new forms of ambiguity in understanding illness—an ethical intervention in conceiving of illness as both narratively embodied and historically bounded.

Chapter 9, by Gagnon Chainey, returns to the AIDS crisis and its representation in literature from a different angle, with a particular focus on the ethical merit of reconsidering the medicalized experience of dying through a literary frame. Turning from his central example of the French novelist Hervé Guibert, who wrote about his own experience of AIDS at the end of his life, Gagnon Chainey considers whether a good death might be a form of (self-)care—and if so, how it can be learned, taught, and practiced. The question becomes pressing, the author argues, in light of new legislation such as the Medical Assistance in Dying (MAID), a law allowing for assisted death enacted federally in Canada in 2016. Through a sophisticated analysis of the tension between univocality and polyphony between patient and caregiver that is legally required in making a claim for a medically assisted death, Gagnon Chainey argues for the essential role of literature, such as Guibert's, in providing a kind of training in the empathetic articulation that care providers at the end of life require in order to make sense of their experience of supporting the dying individual. "Literature is never a still life," Gagnon Chainey writes, "it is a moving and a dying life." Attentive to both the nuances of literary form and to the dangers of an unexamined importation of "empathy" into end-of-life caregiving, Gagnon Chainey asks readers to make space for ambiguity in expression and to become newly aware of the gulf between medical knowledge and embodied reality. Taken together, the chapters in this part advocate for a more nuanced interrogation of bodily states that defy the curative aims and trajectories of biomedicine.

7

Toward a Crip Medical Humanities

Travis Chi Wing Lau

The recent semantic shift from "medical humanities" to "health humanities" has brought with it a much-needed transformation in research and pedagogy that decenters physicians and the medical establishment in favor of recognizing the marginalized, "multiple stakeholders in healthcare settings, including nonphysician healthcare professionals, patients," caregivers, and global populations impacted by public health and medical interventions.[1] While this emergence of the health humanities as an interdisciplinary field has been generally received as "a radical and welcome move"[2] and continues to gain momentum globally, the medical humanities still dominates in many academic and healthcare settings. Since the 1970s, medical humanities programs, certificates, and elective coursework have gained traction among medical schools and STEM departments as a means of cultivating more empathetic, "well-rounded" future clinicians capable of practicing patient-centered medicine. Yet, as critics of the medical humanities have long pointed out, this emphasis on "feeling rather than methods of knowing" reduces the medical humanities to "feel-good narratives" that are still, by and large, "constructed, defined, and used within a medical frame of reference."[3] Even as medical humanists such as Rita Charon (2016) have argued for narrative medicine *as medical practice*, the medical humanities are still often framed in service of medicine, especially as these programs are so often housed, funded, and

---

[1] Lisa M. DeTora and Stephanie M. Hilger, "Introduction: Bodies and Transitions in the Health Humanities," in *Bodies in Transition in the Health Humanities: Representations of Corporeality* (Abingdon: Routledge, 2019), 3.

[2] Paul Crawford, "Introduction: Global Health Humanities and the Rise of Creative Public Health," in *The Routledge Companion to Health Humanities*, ed. Andrea Charise, B. J. Brown, and Paul Crawford, Routledge Companions to Literature Series (Abingdon: Routledge, 2020), 3.

[3] Sari Altschuler, *The Medical Imagination: Literature and Health in the Early United States* (Philadelphia: University of Pennsylvania Press, 2018), 198.

practiced in medical schools and STEM-focused research centers.⁴ As a result, the disparate approaches that make up the medical humanities, particularly those more critical of medicine as an institution and industry, are seldom positioned to do so, or can only do so superficially. To put this in Otniel Dror's words, the very "integration of the humanities into the 'medical humanities' has implicitly medicalized the humanities, thereby suppressing those dimensions of the humanities that can significantly contribute to medicine," such as analytical frameworks for systemic inequalities in healthcare, or critical histories of biomedicine that trace its enduring imbrication with society and culture.⁵

In response to such critiques of the limits of medical humanities, many scholars have articulated the urgent need for self-reflexivity about how the medical humanities can intervene beyond simply the refinement of medical practice. William Viney, Felicity Callard, and Angela Woods (2015) advocate for a "critical medical humanities" that embraces the field's multidisciplinary heterodoxy toward greater collaborations and risk-taking among practitioners who are working in vastly different institutional spaces and interpretive frameworks. In this light, the medical humanities are generative because it does not conform to a singular field identity or set of methodological parameters that might otherwise limit forms of inquiry. Yet, in their qualification of what makes their "*critical* stance" critical, they insist that a "critical medical humanities" is "not in the service of a particular political agenda or particular epistemological priorities, or indeed in favour of a precise programme of reform."⁶ While this qualification suggests an openness to dissent and to ongoing interrogations of the fields' norms, it also risks reproducing the already limited capacity for humanistic critiques of *medicine as political* by gesturing broadly toward disciplinary plurality rather than identifying precise agendas for reform. Furthermore, their reductive characterizations of the two major camps of medical humanities—either "servile" or "hostile, dogged, sceptical, and separable from the medical practices it seeks to target"—reinforce a trivializing vision of the medical humanities as being ineffectual if the approach commits too intensely either to accommodating medicine or to critiquing it. The description of the latter camp echoes familiar indictments of minority fields like critical race studies, queer

---

⁴ Rita Charon, Sayantani DasGupta, Nellie Hermann, Craig Irvine, Eric R. Marcus, Edgar Rivera Colón, Danielle Spencer, and Maura Spiegel, *The Principles and Practice of Narrative Medicine* (New York: Oxford University Press, 2016).
⁵ Otniel E. Dror, "De-Medicalizing the Medical Humanities," *European Legacy* 16, no. 3 (2011): 317.
⁶ William Viney, Felicity Callard, and Angela Woods, "Critical Medical Humanities: Embracing Entanglement, Taking Risks," *Medical Humanities* 41, no. 1 (2015): 3.

studies, and disability studies whose "hostilities" have, in fact, advanced the medical humanities by providing conceptual vocabularies and methodologies.[7] It is the latter of these fields that I take up in this essay as a key example of how a "critical medical humanities" simply cannot be both critical *and* apolitical. If, as Alan Bleakley notes, "it seems hard for medicine to admit that science is not only political (knowledge is power), but also intrinsically aesthetic" in that the "aesthetic (*what* and *how* we appreciate and value, and how we educate for sensibility) is deeply tied to the political," disability studies is a field uniquely positioned to insist on the ethical necessity and critical purchase of such an admission as the medical and health humanities continue to define themselves as fields.[8]

Irreconcilable Differences?

What is at stake in putting disability studies in dialogue with medical humanities? Over fifteen years ago, Diane Price Herndl (2005) reflected on her experience as a scholar trying to navigate both of these burgeoning academic fields. Herndl observed an ongoing disciplinary divide between them, which she argued stems primarily from their disparate historical formations as institutionalized fields of study and the resulting opposition of their critical objectives:

> Disability studies originated from the activism of people with disabilities ... the medical humanities began in the institution of the medical school and for the most part has relied on institutional funding or at least the benevolence and interest of physicians; the support for such programs is often tenuous as they are seen as supplemental, at best. Were the medical humanities to take on changing the profession as a charge, with the implicit criticism of medicine that such a move implies, funding would almost certainly disappear. Medical humanists (at least those who work in medical schools) therefore find that to be heard at all, their message cannot alienate physicians. Thus, while disability studies takes as its primary goal changing policies, environments, and minds, medical humanities seeks to improve the status quo.[9]

---

[7] Ibid., 4.
[8] Alan Bleakley, *Medical Humanities and Medical Education: How the Medical Humanities Can Shape Better Doctors*, Routledge Advances in the Medical Humanities (Abingdon: Routledge, 2015), 2.
[9] Diane Price Herndl, "Disease versus Disability: The Medical Humanities and Disability Studies," *PMLA* 120, no. 2 (2005): 595.

In Herndl's assessment, the medical humanities' material dependencies and obligations to medical schools and the physicians who run them render the field less likely to be critical of the very institutions that sustain it. Rather than bite the hand that feeds it, the medical humanities as a field has little incentive to agitate for change when it must inevitably capitulate to its primary audience that also happens to be its patron. Disability studies, in contrast, emerged out of rights-based activism that was always already in tension with the medical model, which locates impairment in individual bodyminds and diagnoses them as the pathological objects of curative intervention. To jettison the medical model in the medical humanities would risk making its work inaccessible and be much more threatening to physicians and medical students already trained to be skeptical of the humanities' value to their profession.

In the related field of history, a similar debate about the relationship between medical and disability history usefully contextualizes why their integration remains so vexed. Beth Linker (2013), in response to the growing numbers of special journal issues and monographs in disability history, asks "if disease and disability have been interconnected throughout history, why has the literature in the history of medicine almost wholly been dominated by the former?"[10] Charting the trajectory of medical history as it became housed in the US university medical school system after Henry Sigerist, Owsei Temkin, and Erwin Ackerknecht arrived at Johns Hopkins, Linker fleshes out the institutional reasons why medical history became invested in disease narratives "with an ever-increasing emphasis on curative medicine" branded as more "scientific."[11] Even when disability is the object of inquiry, medical historians still tended to subordinate it to "biomedical disease etiology and control" because such a move "remained a fairly safe mode of inquiry, both professionally and financially."[12] As a disability historian herself, Linker critiques historians of medicine for their tendency "to see disability as a different ontological and phenomenological category than disease," which pushes disability into the "margins of medical history," instead of doing the more difficult work of putting it "front and center to be fully theorized and systematically studied" on its own labile terms.[13]

---

[10] Beth Linker, "On the Borderland of Medical and Disability History: A Survey of the Fields," *Bulletin of the History of Medicine* 87, no. 4 (2013): 506.
[11] Ibid., 509, 512.
[12] Ibid., 510, 512.
[13] Ibid., 502.

Although Linker takes medical historians to task for their refusal to be in dialogue with disability scholars, she also suggests that disability demands a different kind of historiography:

> Something inherent to the very categories of disease and disability makes the latter more challenging to write about, more resistant to a linear narrative. Under the biomedical model of disease—a model that emerged in tandem with the professionalization of medical history as a discipline of study—disease is a fairly well-defined ontological category that offers a kind of stability in meaning with definitional parameters. Disability, on the other hand, is often unstable in its meaning and not an easily recognizable category. Disease as a theoretical and historical topic offers a "certain coherence, neatly bridging issues of causation, experience, and response," whereas disability does not.[14]

Histories of disability insist on disability's contingency as an experience, identity, and conceptual category that shifts meaning over time and in different cultural contexts. Such an approach departs substantially from the tidy, transhistorical accounts of disease etiologies and medical innovation. Linker underscores that disability very often accompanies or originates from disease and that the history of disabled people is also the history of their encounters with healthcare institutions and the medical establishment. To that end, the historically coconstitutive nature of disability and disease suggests that "medical historians have been doing disability history all along," and to deny their relationship or insist on their bifurcation is ahistorical.[15] Medical history and disability history are neither "rival siblings" nor "conjoined twins," Linker concludes, but actually bear "family resemblances" and even share a "common family heritage": similar objects of study and the same founding generation of scholars who collaborated in the same intellectual circles.[16]

Disability scholars Catherine Kudlick and Julie Livingston, in their responses to Linker's provocations, similarly parse the fundamental difference between these fields as one of politics, which animate scholarly "work that might provoke discomfort because it openly confronts the problem of disability within the context of institutional discrimination, social prejudice, inhospitable environments, and other misconceptions past and present in analyses that invariably implicate us."[17] Echoing Herndl's point about medical

---

[14] Ibid., 515–16.
[15] Ibid., 502.
[16] Ibid., 500, 535.
[17] Catherine Kudlick, "Comment: On the Borderland of Medical and Disability History," *Bulletin of the History of Medicine* 87, no. 4 (2013): 541.

humanities' tendency toward maintaining the status quo, Kudlick provides an affective reason for why medical historians would avoid engaging with disability: it disrupts the dominant narrative of medical triumphalism by implicating medicine in having "played an active, if often unintended part in promoting prejudice, social isolation, and systemic discrimination against disabled people."[18] This implication is revelatory in that it holds medicine accountable for its

> tremendous institutional and cultural authority to define, adjudicate, to pathologize, an authority that was often conjoined to the power of the state ... [and] reminds us that medicine held the trump cards for those caught up in its web, even if those historical subjects did not understand themselves to be diseased or in need of repair.[19]

From a disability studies standpoint, diagnosis and cure are hardly value-free nor benign in their "devastating consequence," especially for those historically marginalized communities whose discrimination was justified by both medicine and the state framing them as disabled.[20] Throughout their exchange, Linker, Kudlick, and Livingston each emphasize how disability studies pursues politically "discomforting" critiques of medicine to rectify this historical power imbalance that continues to impact the lived experience of sick and disabled people. This defining characteristic of the field emerges directly out of disability studies' origins in social justice activism and advocacy that made possible groundbreaking civil rights legislation like the Americans with Disabilities Act of 1990. If the medical humanities (critical or otherwise) wants to claim disability studies as part of its larger scholarly collective, even drawing on its progressive imaginary, it cannot do so selectively by shying away from the disability studies' more trenchant interventions, which make it a useful "critical modality ... with which to investigate the mechanism by which scientific [and medical] language, masquerading as technology, encodes and transmits a social agenda."[21] Exposing and revising medicine's social agendas is precisely what is crip about disability studies and why the medical humanities urgently needs a crip turn.

---

[18] Ibid., 544.
[19] Ibid., 563.
[20] Paul Baynton C., "Disability and the Justification of Inequality in American History," in *The New Disability History: American Perspectives*, ed. Paul K. Longmore and Lauri Umansky, The History of Disability Series (New York: New York University Press, 2001), 33–57.
[21] James C. Wilson, "Making Disability Visible: How Disability Studies Might Transform the Medical and Science Writing Classroom," *Technical Communication Quarterly* 9, no. 2 (March 1, 2000): 159–60.

Crip Lives, Crip Theory

In efforts to historicize and unpack medicine's social agendas, scholars of disability have drawn attention to how "the prevailing metaphors of medical education continue to be heavily mechanistic (the body is a machine), linear (find the cause, create an effect), and hierarchical (doctor as expert), while its dominant narrative tends to be a story of restitution (patient becomes ill; patient is cured by physician expert; patient is restored to pre[-]illness state)."[22] Aside from underscoring how medicine is constituted by and operates through metaphor, disability studies resists each of these metaphors: that bodily health is defined by a set of normative functions that can become impaired or disordered, that illness and disability must necessarily follow a progress narrative toward curative resolution, and that physicians hold the expertise and authority in adjudicating how such bodies must be managed. These metaphors underpin what disability studies has called in Western contexts the "medical model," which

> frames atypical bodies and minds as deviant, pathological, and defective, best understood and addressed in medical terms. In this framework, the proper approach to disability is to "treat" the condition and the person with the condition rather than "treating" the social processes and policies that constrict disabled people's lives.[23]

By individualizing disability as inherent to a body or mind and casting that disability as a problem to be ameliorated or eliminated by medicine, the medical model stigmatizes the disabled by contributing to the belief that disability can only be undesirable. Furthermore, this belief places the onus on disabled people to "fix" or "overcome" their disability or at least be committed to the improvement of their conditions toward a hopeful return to normative health. To counter this essentializing of disability, activists in 1970s and 1980s adopted the "social model," which emphasized how environments, ideologies, and institutions produce disability through social oppression and exclusion.[24] The locating of disability not in individual defects but in social barriers, such as inaccessible buildings or discriminatory legislation, provided the disability rights movement a concrete platform on which to advocate for social change. Less visible yet no

---

[22] Johanna Shapiro et al., "Medical Humanities and Their Discontents: Definitions, Critiques, and Implications," *Academic Medicine* 84, no. 2 (February 2009): 194.
[23] Alison Kafer, *Feminist, Queer, Crip* (Bloomington: Indiana University Press, 2013), 5.
[24] Tom Shakespeare, "The Social Model of Disability," in *The Disability Studies Reader*, ed Lennard J. Davis, 4th ed. (New York: Routledge, 2013), 217.

less disabling is what Tobin Siebers has called the "ideology of ability," or the cultural preference for able-bodiedness that, "at its most radical ... defines the baseline by which humanness is determined, setting the measure of body and mind that gives or denies human status to individual persons."[25] Such ideology becomes so pervasive that it becomes compulsory through cultural and medical enforcement.[26] Biomedical discourse thus contributes to this cultural encoding of disabled bodies as lesser or lacking by insisting on naturalized standards for embodiment to which all bodies are compared. Disability Studies in turn denaturalizes such standards by tracing their historical formations within the ideologically laden discourses of physiognomy, statistics, and eugenics.[27]

Yet, while the social model continues to provide the foundations for disability activism and scholarly praxis, some scholars have returned to the medical model in the process of understanding the limits of the social model beyond its political practicality. Because the social model differentiates between individual impairment and socially constructed disability, this approach has been critiqued for its neglect of the everyday phenomenological experience of disabled people. By consigning disability to the realm of the social, the social model tends to sideline the real pain and suffering that accompanies disability while also faulting disabled people for seeking medical assistance or curative intervention. Instead of aligning with either the social or medical model or abandoning both models, Alison Kafer has proposed a political/relational model of disability, which

> neither opposes nor valorizes medical intervention; rather than simply take such intervention for granted, it recognizes instead that medical representations, diagnoses, and treatments of bodily variation are imbued with ideological biases about what constitutes normalcy and deviance. In so doing, it recognizes the possibility of simultaneously desiring to be cured of chronic pain and to be identified and allied with disabled people. ... I am arguing for increased recognition of the political nature of a medical framing of disability.[28]

The model is both *political*, in that it refuses to accept the medicalization of disability as unquestionable or empirically objective, and *relational*, in that it addresses how ableism affects everyone regardless of whether they identify as disabled. This expansion of disability as a category enables a more coalitional

---

[25] Tobin Siebers, *Disability Theory* (Ann Arbor: University of Michigan Press, 2008), 8.
[26] Robert McRuer, *Crip Theory: Cultural Signs of Queerness and Disability*, Cultural Front (New York: New York University Press, 2006).
[27] Lennard J. Davis, "Introduction: Normality, Power, and Culture," in *The Disability Studies Reader*, ed. Lennard J. Davis (New York: Routledge, 2013), 1–16.
[28] Kafer, *Feminist, Queer, Crip*, 6.

politics that unites disabled people whose disabilities take different forms and disabled people with their friends, families, and caregivers. The political/relational model does not seek to alienate medicine as a static monolith: it recognizes moments of solidarity in which medicine can better the lives of disabled people but not without difficult negotiations and conversations with physicians and caregivers, many of whom still see disability as a personal tragedy or moral failure. For Kafer, "seeing disability as political, and therefore contested and contestable," also means imagining different futures for disabled people beyond stigma, medicalization, incarceration, and genocide.[29]

Joining other disability theorists like Margaret Price, Ellen Samuels, and Jay Dolmage thinking about accommodations in higher education, Kafer considers how disability actually "reorients" time: "Crip time is flex time not just expanded but exploded: it requires reimagining our notions of what can and should happen in time, or recognizing how expectations of 'how long things take' are based on very particular minds and bodies."[30] Having developed out of earlier theorizations of time by queer scholars as deviations from heteronormative expectations of reproductive futurity and development, crip time puts into question the expectations that disabled people should always be on the therapeutic path that returns them to health. In opposition to crip time, then, is what Kafer calls "curative time," which Beth Linker described earlier as medicine's fixation on a linear timeline of diagnosis, prognosis, treatment, and cure. Curative time is the temporal dimension of the medical model's "curative imaginary," a worldview and "understanding of disability that not only *expects* and *assumes* intervention but also cannot imagine or comprehend anything other than intervention."[31] Within this teleological framework, "the only appropriate disabled mind/body is one cured or moving toward cure," so those with chronic or uncurable conditions are inevitably "cast ... out of time, or as obstacles to the arc of progress."[32] The "unhealthy disabled," to use Susan Wendell's (2001) formulation, are further stigmatized because they come to embody medicine's failures as costly lost causes—a harmful stereotype only exacerbated by the insurance industry's narrow views of who and what is worthy of care.[33]

Building upon Kafer's concept of the coercive curative imaginary, Eunjung Kim identifies the violent effects of cure in the sense of both "denying a place for

---

[29] Ibid., 10.
[30] Ibid., 27.
[31] Ibid, original emphasis.
[32] Ibid., 28.
[33] Susan Wendell, "Unhealthy Disabled: Treating Chronic Illnesses as Disabilities," *Hypatia* 16, no. 4 (2001): 17–33.

disability and illness as different ways of living" and "the physical and material violence against people with disabilities that are justified in the name of cure."[34] Kim counterintuitively challenges cure as purely salutary by attending to what she terms "curative violence," a phenomenon that "occurs when cure is what actually frames the presence of disability as a problem and ends up destroying the subject in the curative process."[35] The valorization of cure dismisses the potential for unforeseen harms that may accompany curative techniques, including other forms of disability and debility, and also detracts from developing other forms of support for those who cannot access cure or those who cannot benefit from it (i.e., palliative care). Though the medical humanities have better attended to the subjective experiences of those undergoing therapeutic care, the field must move beyond compassion and witnessing, both of which can passively enable the curative violences that pervade healthcare by bypassing any confrontations with how medicine can actually "make life with disability difficult and unlivable."[36] Such violences are evident in everything from chemotherapy to mastectomies. When medical humanists uncritically advocate for "doing better medicine," this well-meaning point can often mean a harmful complicity with curative imperatives when disability is left out of the conversation. This complicity is also one of the uncomfortable implications that Kudlick identifies as an obstacle to disability's fuller presence in medical history and, as I argue, in medical humanities contexts.

A Field's Crip Future

If the medical humanities is to claim crip, it must begin to ask what forms of knowledge are being valued and who is producing that knowledge. I draw here on Rosemarie Garland-Thomson's call in bioethics for "conserving disability," where she proposes a revaluation of disability as a resource—epistemological, ethical, and narrative—worthy of "preserving intact, keeping alive, and even encouraging to flourish" in the face of ableism that would deny its worth.[37] Calling out the dangerous eugenic logic underpinning medical practices like neonatal testing and gene editing technologies like CRISPR, which frequently

---

[34] Eunjung Kim, *Curative Violence: Rehabilitating Disability, Gender, and Sexuality in Modern Korea* (Durham, NC: Duke University Press, 2017), 14.
[35] Ibid.
[36] Ibid., 10.
[37] Rosemarie Garland-Thomson, "The Case for Conserving Disability," *Journal of Bioethical Inquiry* 9, no. 3 (September 1, 2012): 341.

imagine a perfected future purged of disability, Garland-Thomson insists on disability's inherent value as part of human biodiversity, but also in the radically temporal ways Kafer identifies of crip time:

> So disability's contribution, its work, is to sever the present from the future. More precisely, disability can be a narrative resource that does not trade the present in on the future ... [it] contributes a narrative of a genuinely open future, one not controlled by the objectives, expectations, and understandings of the present.[38]

Disabled lived experience should be valued because of how it generates crip knowledges that can challenge the prescribed narratives of our present and imagine more inclusive futures not yet realized. To quote the disability activist slogan, "nothing about us without us," a crip medical humanities should ask (1) which bodyminds are being prioritized as the field's leaders, (2) how these leaders shape the field's primary scholarly conversations, and (3) which bodyminds are only worthy of being the objects of inquiry rather than the subjects pursuing that inquiry. *Are we speaking for or over sick and disabled people, or are we not really speaking about them at all?* Given how many physicians and medical professionals have since taken up the field, a reflexivity not just of method but of positionality seems most urgent, especially as medicine is "where theory meets practice, where thinking about human variation is powerfully brought to bear on bodies and minds at risk."[39]

What would the field look like if disabled scholars or disabled medical professionals were at its center? This question is meant to echo recent discussions in disability studies about "cripistemologies" or the ways of knowing and understanding grounded in disability lived experience. By "structurally placing crip(s) at the beginning or center of the production of knowledge,"[40] a cripistemological approach validates disabled people as knowledge makers and "demonstrates that theorizing is and always should be multi-directional (and multitudinous), that it is not brought from on high to a movement in order to fuel and direct it: disability movements, queer movements, crip movements, and others are always and have always been excessively and pleasurably generating new theories."[41]

---

[38] Ibid., 352.
[39] G. Thomas Couser, "What Disability Studies Has to Offer Medical Education," *Journal of Medical Humanities* 32, no. 1 (March 1, 2011): 29.
[40] Merri Lisa Johnson and Robert McRuer, "Cripistemologies: Introduction," *Journal of Literary & Cultural Disability Studies* 8, no. 2 (2014): 158.
[41] Ibid., 145.

Whose knowledges get to matter remains a persistent concern for me as a scholar, like Herndl, trying to find a place in the intersections of disability studies and medical humanities. As I sit in medical and health humanities conferences and symposia, I still find discussions of disability often seem like afterthoughts or conceptual abstractions entirely separated from disabled lives. If, as Martha Holmes has suggested, that "another layer in the divide between medical humanities and disability studies may be anxiety about identifying as disabled, either in a narrative or as a scholar," more publicly disabled scholars shaping medical humanities discourse seems that much more necessary.[42]

I want to be clear that to crip the medical humanities is not simply to rebrand the field to make it more relevant[43] or to make it more marketable for institutions that have already tended to exploit the field as proof of their commitment to interdisciplinarity or somehow bridging the gap between the "two cultures" of the humanities and the sciences. Whether it be "critical medical humanities" or "health humanities," to crip the field is to *politicize* it or, more specifically, to emphasize that the field has always been political. Forged from activist reclamations of "crippled" as a slur, crip designates a politicized community identity and a contestatory position vis-à-vis medicalization and cure.[44] When medical humanists say they want to "include" disability and disability studies, this cannot take the form of tokenizing inclusions in the name of disciplinary "diversity," because disability "is not just another 'Other': it reveals and constructs notions of citizenship, human difference, social values, sexuality, and the complex relationship between the biological and social worlds."[45] I take seriously Alison Kafer's reminder that to claim crip is also an affective investment and an ethical investment in different futures for those in medicine, those cared for by medicine, and ultimately our fields of study.

---

[42] Martha Stoddard Holmes, "Embodied Storytellers: Disability Studies and Medical Humanities," *Hastings Center Report* 45, no. 2 (2015): 13.
[43] Craig M. Klugman, "How Health Humanities Will Save the Life of the Humanities," *Journal of Medical Humanities* 38, no. 4 (2017): 13.
[44] Kafer, *Feminist, Queer, Crip*, 16.
[45] Kudlick, "Comment," 793.

8

Tales of the City as Historical Document: HIV/AIDS, Serialization, Urban Landscapes, and Sexuality

John A. Carranza

Introduction

I first learned of the *Tales of the City* series from sex advice columnist and podcast host Dan Savage. One of his callers had just come out of the closet as a gay man and needed guidance about what to expect in his new identity. Savage recommended the novel to the caller, and since I had never heard of the book, I decided to purchase a copy as well. Armistead Maupin's characters were captivating and endearing. San Francisco, as the backdrop of the story, buzzed with an aura of excitement and romance. Mirroring the soap opera format, each of the chapters in the early novels ended with cliff-hangers that compelled me onward. The first *Tales of the City* novel is now a book I frequently gift, and on one occasion, after visiting a local used bookstore, I found one copy that was in better shape than the others on the shelf and was pleased to find the following inscription in it:

> Dear Trinity,
>
> It was so nice seeing you and Jesse and Leo in San Francisco ... The "Tales of the City" is a fabulous drama that I stumbled across 14 years ago. They made it into a miniseries ... I watched one show within the series and was hooked. I then read all the books. I hope these books bring you as much pleasure and enjoyment as they did me.

I shared the same sentiment as this anonymous stranger after reading the series. One might question whether the recipient shared these same feelings, either about the person giving the book or the story itself, since the copy had ended up in the used bookstore. Nevertheless, I kept the used copy for myself and gave away a brand-new copy I had bought previously.

Over the next few months, I read through the remaining five books in the series, which ended with *Sure of You* (1989). I put off the continuation of the series, which began again with *Michael Tolliver Lives* (2007), and chose to consider the type of historical documentation that relied on Maupin's first-person point of view. As an historian, I was amused by the way in which Maupin managed to work Jim Jones and Jonestown and Queen Elizabeth II's visit to San Francisco into whimsical storylines. I grew with the characters as they aged, and their problems became more rooted in the immediate reality around them, especially once the AIDS epidemic began. *Tales of the City* began as a serial in the *San Francisco Chronicle* in 1976 and was written in bursts that eventually came to a temporary end in 1978, but reappeared in 1981 and 1983. In the interim periods between publishing the serial, Maupin revised the entries to better fit the format of a novel.[1] Maupin's observations and first-hand experiences were central to developing multidimensional characters and a sketch of San Francisco that was captivating to audiences. The resultant novels straddle the line between fiction and reality because of Maupin's experiences, which provide a partial representation of the past.

The first six novels of the *Tales* series function as useful artifacts that illuminate the recent past for readers today. Maupin was highly observant of the people and events that shaped the world around him; much of what he experienced informed the characters and the events that shaped their lives. Maupin's introspection was reflected in the characters he created and helped to inform his activism and outspokenness during the AIDS crisis. In the context of the medical humanities, literature read as a piece of history has the power to reveal how illness and health were constructed based on the knowledge available in the past, what it looks like in the present, and to imagine what it might look like in the future. Steven F. Kruger's analysis of AIDS narratives elucidates these points when he states that "cultural narratives of AIDS play a crucial role in attempts to understand the past, present, and future of the epidemic, providing a stabilizing framework within which to place unpredictable, disturbing, world-threatening events so that these seem to make sense as part of a coherent story." These narratives, according to Kruger, have the ability "to determine treatment protocols, research agendas, education and political priorities."[2] This bears

---

[1] J. Kaliss, "Two Writers' Wry Views of Romance," *Noe Valley Voice* (July 1986): 12.
[2] Steven F. Kruger, *AIDS Narratives: Gender and Sexuality, Fiction and Science* (New York: Routledge, [1996] 2011), 80–1.

itself out as he outlines the importance of the individual narrative, which is characterized by a person's journey with HIV from infection to AIDS and the decline in health. Additionally, the population narrative traces the history of the epidemic from the beginning, to the present, and to a possible future. Both narratives are not absolute and can be disrupted by any number of factors that could slow down the spread of disease.[3] *Tales of the City* is but one example that complicated the individual and population narratives by drawing together the author's personal experiences of an epidemic and fixing them on Maupin's widely read characters.

Historians and Historical Method

Historians are tasked with relating events or people of the past to an audience living in the present. History and fiction share narratives as the primary means for conveying stories, but they ultimately diverge in how a narrative is used. Hayden White has written about the significance of "historical imagination," which was at its peak from 1800 to 1850, and emphasized the importance of "man's responsibility for his own fate."[4] The task at hand for historians was to remind readers of the past so that they might "effect an ethically responsible transition from the present to future."[5] Historians reach their audiences by composing histories informed by theoretical concepts and narratives. In doing so, the historian is at once deciding what their analysis will center on and how they will explain that analysis using existing frameworks.[6] The historian approaches their craft through the use of emplotment, formal argument, and ideological implication that each has four modes used for explanation.[7] White demonstrates the importance of formality in creating a narrative of the past, but incorporates little of how literature can be used to inform those narratives.

David Carr maintains that narratives in fiction convey a sense of credibility but have been contentious within the discipline of history. This contention lies within historians' desire to remain objective in how they relay the past to readers in the present, and became evident throughout the 1980s as historians sought

---

[3] Ibid., 73, 75–7.
[4] Hayden V. White, "The Burden of History," *History and Theory* 5, no. 2 (1966): 132, https://doi.org/10.2307/2504510.
[5] Ibid.
[6] Hayden V. White, *Metahistory: The Historical Imagination in Nineteenth-Century Europe* (Baltimore, MD: Johns Hopkins University Press, 1973), 30–1.
[7] Ibid., 29.

to quantify the past to align more with the social sciences.[8] Carr explained that fiction should not be equated with falsehoods, because in fiction there is never a real claim to represent reality—which never gives the opportunity to question falsity. To avoid any question about falsehoods, an author simply labels their work a "novel." Yet, to assert that historians' work includes elements of fiction is not to claim that histories include inherent falsehoods, but rather that they display the machinations of the historian's imagination at work.[9] The imagination does not simply create new ideas or characters, but enables the writer to see beyond present sense reactions.[10] Finally, Carr emphasizes that humans typically inhabit a world that makes a mess of the "beginning, middle, and end" sequence that characterizes fiction, and he maintains that the best fiction is like reality in that there are unintended consequences for the characters. The reality of a narrative is not ordered reality. Historical narrative is part of the human experience in which the present is always in conversation with the past and the future.[11]

Carr's philosophy demonstrates that while one might view fiction and history as distinct entities united by narrative, there is little discussion as to how fiction might be used to help construct a historical narrative fiction. How does the imagination and the lived reality of an author, such as Armistead Maupin, contribute to a robust and continuously expanding body of knowledge about the 1970s and 1980s in the United States? What do such works convey to the reader about the place of health, sexuality, and the city in the past? How does literature and the experience of the author effectively bring the reader into their way of seeing the world around them?

Tales of the City addresses these questions by acting as an archive of the author's experiences as well as an artifact from the 1970s and 1980s of the queer community in San Francisco. The series began with an article Armistead Maupin intended to write for the *Pacific Sun* about men and women cruising for dates at a Safeway grocery store. Maupin quickly learned that these men and women were reticent about discussing their intentions with a reporter, but the scene became the inspiration for what Maupin originally called "The Serial." Shortly thereafter, the story moved to the *San Francisco Chronicle* and was branded "Tales of the City."[12] The events and situations that the characters found themselves entangled in were frequently informed by Maupin's personal experiences living in

---

[8] David Carr, *Experience and History: Phenomenological Perspectives on the Historical World* (New York: Oxford University Press, 2014), 201–2.
[9] Ibid., 205–6.
[10] Ibid., 206–7.
[11] Ibid., 207–9.
[12] Armistead Maupin, *Logical Family: A Memoir* (New York: Harper Collins, 2017), 180–3, 187.

San Francisco.¹³ These experiences, partially veiled behind the veneer of fiction, give *Tales* in its serial and novel forms the aura of historical artifact. The artifact is any object that remains with us from the past, which includes, but is not limited to, government records, diaries, newspapers, and photographs. The artifact is in fact a trace of the past that exists whether a historian uses it or not and, only upon the historian using it to support an argument, becomes evidence.[14] Historian John Tosh's useful introduction to the history profession, *The Pursuit of History*, maintains that literature opens up the possibility to inform the present of what people in the past were engaged in socially and intellectually, and that fiction can even describe the physical world as it was.[15] Carolyn Steedman's analysis of George Eliot's *Middlemarch* confirms Tosh's observation and proposes that the novel as a historical artifact can be used for reading the social and cultural environments of Eliot's past.[16] *Tales of the City* is all the more significant because of how it describes San Francisco and incorporates elements of the 1970s and 1980s into its storylines.

Finally, if the novels function as an artifact of the past, there is the possibility that they may function as an archive that yields perspective on the AIDS epidemic for present readers. Steedman's analysis of *Middlemarch* points to how, in the absence of an archive, Eliot read backfiles of newspapers to better understand the political circumstances that led to the British Parliament's First Reform Bill and the popular reaction to it.[17] Ann Cvetkovich presents what she calls the archive of feelings that are "both material and immaterial … incorporating objects that might not ordinarily be considered archival, and at the same time, resisting documentation because sex and feelings are too personal or ephemeral to leave records."[18] Cvetkovich sees documentary as an archive that reaches well beyond what one believes the traditional archive to look like and that brings together an assemblage of archival materials that are widely accessible and capable of creating an archive of emotion that documents trauma.[19] While the visual nature of documentary certainly adds depth to what we might consider an archive, Maupin's novels could also be read as an archive of emotion that

---

[13] Ibid., 167.
[14] Keith Jenkins, *Re-thinking History* (London: Routledge, 1991), 59–60.
[15] John Tosh, *The Pursuit of History: Aims, Methods and New Directions in the Study of Modern History*, 5th ed. (Harlow: Longman, [1984] 2010), 99.
[16] Carolyn Steedman, "To Middlemarch: Without Benefit of Archive," in Dust: The Archive and Cultural History, Encounters (New Brunswick, NJ: Rutgers University Press, 2002), 103–7.
[17] Ibid., 99–102.
[18] Ann Cvetkovich, *An Archive of Feelings: Trauma, Sexuality, and Lesbian Public Cultures* (Durham, NC: Duke University Press, 2003), 244.
[19] Ibid., 244.

accounts for comedy and trauma in the lives of the characters. Maupin did not need to consult an archive to document his characters' reactions to AIDS because he was living through the worst of the disease in San Francisco, which was hit hard by the epidemic in its early years. Rather, he created an archive of trauma by writing his character Michael Tolliver's experience of losing his lover to AIDS and having to then move through the gay community to find ways to deal with the disease. The *Tales of the City* novels as archive become important because of their enduring presence in American popular culture and the ease with which one can access the books from libraries and bookstores.

Serial Format and the Novel

What makes the story compelling to readers then and now? I believe the answer is in the serial format. The serial began in the nineteenth century, with Charles Dickens as its most important pioneer. Jennifer Hayward attributes the medium to social and technological developments that included urbanization, higher literacy rates, and new concepts of leisure as an activity that lent itself to more reading. Hayward also found that industrialization, transportation, and advertising made it easier for audiences to become connected in shared reading experiences.[20] Sean O'Sullivan has outlined six features of a serial that characterize Maupin's original source material and the novels. These elements include:

(a) iteration through the constant return to the house at 28 Barbary Lane, binding characters to one another through this shared setting;
(b) *multiplicity*, evidenced through the presence of at least two storylines, one large and one small, that occurs simultaneously within a single novel;
(c) *momentum* that spurs the reader along through the regular use of the cliff-hanger;
(d) *world-building* as a result of Maupin romanticizing San Francisco against the historical backdrop of the 1970s and 1980s;
(e) the *personnel* include main, new, and marginal characters who are deployed to move the story along;
(f) the *design* of the serial is such that readers of the original columns might expect an entry of approximately five hundred words, while readers of the

---

[20] Jennifer Hayward, *Consuming Pleasures: Active Audiences and Serial Fictions from Dickens to the Soap Opera* (Lexington: University Press of Kentucky, 1997), 22.

novels would expect similar short chapters (with slightly longer ones later in the series) that kept readers going for at least one more chapter.[21]

The *Tales* series as an artifact employs these literary characteristics that keep readers engaged in the story that represents the aspects of urban sexuality and health in the 1970s and 1980s.

Despite the relative popularity of the original *Tales of the City* column, some readers were reluctant to admit to reading the daily installments. In 1976, Sharon Stack, a health educator and regular reader, believed that the column "glorifies San Francisco. It has to do with the San Franciscan's desire to hear about himself. … I can't say it's great literature. But it only takes about 30 seconds to read, so how could it hurt you?"[22] An additional factor in the serial's success was that Maupin incorporated local landmarks and places readers would recognize, such as Balboa Café for singles, and Grace Cathedral.[23] The desire to see one's city being reflected in a positive light and the levity that *Tales* provided to the reader opened the door to empathy and understanding especially toward the queer community that, despite making modest political and social gains, still experienced discrimination in employment, violent attacks on gays and lesbians and their businesses, and police harassment.[24]

In 1976, when Maupin began to write the serial, there was a thriving gay community that many heterosexual San Franciscans chose to keep at a distance. The community grew, especially as many more arrivals—who tended to be young, white, and male—came to the city in hopes of no longer needing to repress their sexuality.[25] Maupin's column was monitored by editors of the *San Francisco Chronicle* who were afraid of alienating readers with an explicit discussion of gay and lesbian stories and more importantly, sexual expression. As a result of editorial censorship, Maupin implied sex between two men by placing them in bed with each other, but had to skirt further exposition on the subject. Maupin was also encouraged to keep the gender identity of Anna Madrigal, the matriarch and landlady, a secret. Maupin felt that this editorial decision was rooted in transphobia, but he believed that there was some benefit to this move,

---

[21] Sean O'Sullivan, "Six Elements of Serial Narrative," *Narrative* 27, no. 1 (2019): 49–64, https://doi.org/10.1353/nar.2019.0003.
[22] Associated Press (San Francisco), "San Francisco's Newest Heroine Has Following," *Baytown Sun* 54, no. 301 (September 29, 1976).
[23] Kaliss, "Two Writers' Wry Views of Romance," 13.
[24] John D'Emilio, *Making Trouble: Essays on Gay History, Politics, and the University* (New York: Routledge, 1992), 89–93.
[25] Frances FitzGerald, "The Castro-I," *New Yorker* (July 21, 1986), https://www.newyorker.com/magazine/1986/07/21/i-the-castro.

for it built suspense and, when Anna became romantically involved with Edgar Halcyon, showed her humanity.[26] Early in the series, Madrigal treats all of her young tenants as though they were her family by frequently referring to them as her children and imparting her sage advice on them. The audience even learns in *More Tales of the City* that Mona is her biological child, which complicated the chosen family dynamic that Madrigal had established with her tenants.[27]

Some gay readers believed that by writing the serial, Armistead Maupin gave away places that the community had established as their own away from the heterosexual gaze. In fact, the story even had the rare ability to out some members of the gay community. For example, Michael Tolliver met his lover at Gay Night at a roller rink called Grand Arena; when this installment was published, Maupin was approached by a stranger who felt that he had been outed since everyone at his law office realized that he coincidentally went skating on Gay Night.[28]

Critics of the series brushed the stories off as trivial. The dean of the University of California at Berkeley's School of Journalism, Ed Bayley, showed his disdain for the series in a newspaper article about its rise in popularity. "I can remember when newspapers used to run novels in serial form. … Some of them were good. … None of them were this bad."[29] Bayley's criticisms were not elaborated upon, but the pervasiveness of queer characters and the implied sexual expression in their personal lives might have hit a nerve.

The demands of writing a daily serial involved a tremendous amount of organization and character development that threatened to elude Maupin once he became a local celebrity. However, his personal experiences and the city offered him room to create new storylines and further develop his characters. Mrs. Madrigal, as she is known to all of her residents, was based partly on Dawn Pepita Langley Hall, whose transition and marriage to an African American auto mechanic scandalized some of the elites in Charleston, South Carolina.[30] Additionally, Mrs. Madrigal drew her characteristic empathy and flair for the dramatic from Maupin's own grandmother, who believed in reincarnation and read Maupin's palms as a child; she was notably the first person in his memory who admonished someone for making a homophobic comment.[31] Even Maupin's

---

[26] Maupin, *Logical Family*, 202.
[27] Robyn R. Warhol, "Making 'Gay' and 'Lesbian' into Household Words: How Serial Form Works in Armistead Maupin's 'Tales of the City,'" *Contemporary Literature* 40, no. 3 (1999): 387–8, https://doi.org/10.2307/1208883.
[28] Maupin, *Logical Family*, 205.
[29] Associated Press (San Francisco), "San Francisco's Newest Heroine Has Following."
[30] Maupin, *Logical Family*, 131–3.
[31] D. Richards, "Maupin's World," *Dallas Voice* (June 19, 1987), sec. II, 35.

trips taken with one of his closest friends found their way into the series. Cruises to Mexico and Alaska factored into major plots in *More Tales of the City* and *Further Tales of the City*, respectively; trips to London and the island of Lesbos are also part of the plots in *Babycakes* (1984) and *Sure of You* (1989).

Perhaps the most significant installment in the series that remained intact as the story transitioned to a novel form was "Letter to Mama." The letter, like many aspects of the series, was semi-autobiographical and had protagonist Michael Tolliver writing home to come out to his mother. Michael was prompted by his parents' embrace of Anita Bryant, who rallied and led conservative opposition to a 1977 Dade County, Florida ordinance that gave gays and lesbians civil rights. The "Save Our Children" campaign maintained that gays and lesbians were engaged in an effort to recruit children into becoming homosexuals. The campaign was successful and saw the repeal of the ordinance by 71 percent.[32] Nevertheless, the letter was one of the more earnest and heartfelt parts of the early series. In this fictional setting, Maupin (1980) offered a political commentary on the humanity of gays and lesbians across the United States:

> Dear Mama,
>
> I'm sorry it's taken me so long to write. Every time I try to write to you and Papa I realize I'm not saying the things that are in my heart. That would be O.K., if I loved you any less than I do, but you are still my parents and I am still your child. ...
>
> I wouldn't have written, I guess, if you hadn't told me about your involvement in the Save Our Children campaign. That, more than anything, made it clear that my responsibility was to tell you the truth, that your own child is homosexual, and that I never needed saving from anything except the cruel and ignorant piety of people like Anita Bryant ...
>
> ... Being gay has taught me tolerance, compassion and humility. It has shown me the limitless possibilities of living. It has given me people whose passion and kindness and sensitivity have provided a constant source of strength.[33]

Upon its original publication, the letter hit home with a large segment of the San Francisco gay community, and it was later run as a regular installment in the *Chronicle* series and reproduced in *More Tales of the City*. Amidst the fervor over Anita Bryant's anti-gay campaign, Maupin read the letter aloud at a benefit for the Miami Gay Support Committee; when he finished, he said there was "a rumbling

---

[32] Kevin Michael Kruse and Julian E. Zelizer, *Fault Lines: A History of the United States since 1974*, 1st ed. (New York: W.W. Norton, 2019), 83–4.

[33] Armistead Maupin, *More Tales of the City* (New York: Harper & Row, 1980), 221–3.

that grew from a few hands clapping into a stadium-style foot-stomping frenzy as the audience rose to its feet."[34] Readers of the column revealed that they had used "Letter to Mama" as a template for their own coming out to their parents, while others took out Michael Tolliver's name and substituted their own.[35] The care and benevolence with which Maupin treated his queer characters helped the novels attain success when they were sold outside of San Francisco. Maupin believed that "the burgeoning gay and lesbian bookstores across the country were ... help[ing] me reach an audience that grew larger from year to year."[36] The reach of the texts beyond the local setting that initially inspired them is historical evidence that readers connected with the characters and stories and built community around the novels.

The serial reflected Maupin's experiences as a gay man living in San Francisco, but upon a closer reading of the characters who are incorporated into the various stories, the reader learns that they tend to lack racial and ethnic diversity. Considering the overwhelmingly white demographics of San Francisco in the 1970s and 1980s, it would seem unsurprising that such characters are absent.[37] The minority characters that do eventually appear in the story do so to highlight the racism and absurdity of several of the white, wealthy members of the cast of characters. Nevertheless, some of the characters do fall into stereotypes and jokes that a reader might find disagreeable by today's standards. One of the historian's tasks is to read these representations within the context in which they were produced, which is to say that while Maupin himself would not have been seen as "racist" in his historical context, the cultural climate would have allowed for such caricatures. This is also not to excuse such representations, but to learn how to recognize and refuse such characterizations in the future.

In *Tales of the City*, DeDe Halcyon Day, the daughter of Edgar Halcyon, the chairman of the board of the advertising agency Halcyon Communications, has an affair with Lionel Wong, a Chinese "delivery boy."[38] DeDe becomes pregnant with twins and, in *Further Tales of the City*, tells her mother to pass them off as Vietnamese orphans that she is fostering for the purpose of keeping their identity a secret.[39] Additionally, characters of color often fell into two

---

[34] Maupin, *Logical Family*, 221.
[35] Ibid., 219–21.
[36] Dick Donahue, "Armistead Maupin: Tales Worth Talking About," *Publishers Weekly* (September 11, 2000): 63, https://www.publishersweekly.com/pw/by-topic/authors/interviews/article/21206-armistead-maupin-tales-worth-talking-about.html.
[37] http://www.bayareacensus.ca.gov/counties/SanFranciscoCounty70.htm.
[38] Armistead Maupin, *Tales of the City* (New York: Harper & Row, 1978), 96–8.
[39] Maupin, *More Tales of the City*, 178.

categories: representing deceitful stereotypes, or helping white, main characters with little or no individual characterization or agency. In *Further Tales of the City*, Bambi Kanetaka was portrayed as a conniving news reporter who, despite lacking any serious skills, continues to get better assignments than Mary Ann Singleton because of her affair with Larry Kenan, the news director. She later threatens to go public with a major story to which Mary Ann had been promised exclusive access.[40] Finally, in *Babycakes* (1984), Michael Tolliver heads to London as part of an apartment swap with a dashing British sailor. There Michael meets a teenager named Wilfred who is described only as an "aborigine." He is sensitive and accompanies Michael while trying to find his friend in London. Wilfred provides levity and perspective to Michael as he tries to adjust to the recent death of his partner. However, Wilfred's story concludes when Michael flies back to the United States.

One of the more perplexing characters whose storyline took a rather unexpected twist was that of D'orothea Wilson, an African American fashion model and one of the main characters that was not stereotyped into having a submissive or secondary role. Introduced in *Tales of the City* (1978), it is later revealed that she is a white woman. Where a reader might hope to find diversity and powerful representations of African Americans in this popular series, they find that D'orothea was faking her race by taking pills meant to treat vitiligo, which turned her skin darker as she took more of the medication. Her motivation was her desire to make money, as African American models were in demand (one could read a history of fetishization of models of color in this instance). When her lover, Mona Ramsey, finds out she is white, there is little to no consequence for D'orothea, as they remain together. Maupin's motivations for this character were slightly misguided. In his memoir, Maupin maintained that all of his characters were "relentlessly lily-white," so he introduced D'orothea. He explained that one reader wrote in: "Up until now your characters have rung true, but D'orothea is nothing but a white woman in black skin."[41] Maupin's attempt at creating an African American character had failed, so he devised the vitiligo pills as a means for working himself out of this corner and highlighted the problem of creating characters of different race and ethnicity while being a white gay man.

The depictions of the queer community and ethnic minorities did much of the work of keeping the reader connected to the series. The serial and the novels

---

[40] Armistead Maupin, *Further Tales of the City* (New York: Harper & Row, 1982).
[41] Maupin, *Logical Family*, 206–7.

that resulted from it provide source material for giving historians and readers the ability to think about the past.⁴² Even though this original source material was altered by the author himself in preparation for publication as novels, the reader can still glean an insight from the past about how marginalized groups were characterized and the extent to which they acted in service to other characters in the story.

Health and HIV/AIDS in the City

Illness is one mode of building suspense for the reader and provides the characters opportunities to interact with one another in demonstrating empathy, compassion, curiosity, secrecy, disclosure, and (for added effect) death. Illness throughout the series, especially with the emergence of the AIDS epidemic, was significant because it reinforced the notion that *Tales of the City* could function as an archive by demonstrating how gay and straight people confronted death around them. Historian Allan Brandt has written about the history of venereal disease and has pointed out that we must look beyond the usual paradigm of infection and clinical response and incorporate the social meaning of disease and its associated symbols.⁴³ Sarah Chaney's examination of Victorian-era medical texts and literature on self-mutilation likewise outlines the extent to which medicine and culture can mutually reinforce one another to reflect society's values.⁴⁴ Throughout the series, illness inspires several characters to make decisions in their present and for their future, but this is complicated with the emergence of AIDS whose destruction leaves in its wake an uncertain future.

The *Tales of the City* series is rife with examples that illustrate how illness spurred the decision-making of its main cast of characters. Early in *Tales of the City* (1978), Edgar Halcyon is revealed to have failing kidneys after a visit to a faith healer. Edgar's storyline demonstrates his desire to break free of the confines of his marriage and his upper-class lifestyle, and he finds comfort in clandestine dates with Mrs. Madrigal. In the same book, Mary Ann Singleton takes a volunteer position at the Bay Area Crisis Switchboard and immediately learns that her coworker, Vincent, is prone to depression leading to self-inflected

---

⁴² Kaliss, "Two Writers' Wry Views of Romance," 12; Maupin, *Logical Family*, 224.
⁴³ Allan M. Brandt, *No Magic Bullet: A Social History of Venereal Disease in the United States since 1880* (New York: Oxford University Press, 1985), 3–6.
⁴⁴ Sarah Chaney, "'A Hideous Torture on Himself': Madness and Self-Mutilation in Victorian Literature," *Journal of Medical Humanities* 32, no. 4 (December 1, 2011): 280, 286–7, https://doi.org/10.1007/s10912-011-9152-6.

injuries, namely the amputation of his left ear and his right little finger. Both Edgar Halcyon and Vincent's storylines end with their deaths: Edgar dies from kidney failure, and Vincent commits suicide. Each man's death impacts Mrs. Madrigal's and Mary Ann's lives differently. Mary Ann, who is still very much the sheltered newcomer on the verge of returning to Ohio, experiences Vincent's death as another matter of reality that breaks her innocence. However, Mrs. Madrigal, who was one of the first transgender characters in American literature, finds acceptance and love with Edgar. The reader learns that Mrs. Madrigal is transgender considerably late in the series, after she has demonstrated the large extent of her humor and maternal guidance to the residents at 28 Barbary Lane. Mrs. Madrigal's relationship with Edgar Halcyon evolves in much the same way as they date and fall in love. Humanizing Mrs. Madrigal was important on two fronts. Historically, the transgender community began to lose its connection with the gay and feminist communities in the 1970s and thus would have needed a figure to hold the communities together.[45] Read as a historical document, Mrs. Madrigal reminds the reader of the presence of transgender individuals in society whose lives were not marked by pathology or deviance, but a certain level of ordinariness by simply trying to find love.

The effects of disease and illness come into sharper focus, however, in Michael Tolliver's experiences with the AIDS epidemic. Similar to many nonfictional stories about the gay community before and during the AIDS era, Michael's own journey begins in *More Tales of the City* (1980) when he is diagnosed as having Guillain-Barré syndrome after being unable to move while in bed with his lover, Jon Fielding. Beginning early in the series, Michael is on a never-ending quest for an affectionate and enduring relationship that seems to be resolved as Fielding, a medical doctor, remains by Michael's side through his illness. (But the relationship proves to be temporary as the reader learns in *Further Tales of the City*.)

The reader leaves Barbary Lane in *Further Tales of the City* with a sense of closure, as many of the storylines that began the book have been rectified. However, by the time *Babycakes* (1984) is published, the reader senses that a noticeable amount of time has elapsed and the mood has turned somber. The main characters have each experienced changes in their lives, but perhaps the most traumatic change was the death of Jon Fielding to AIDS-related complications. Michael Tolliver's storylines become weighed down with the sadness and frustration that many in the gay community felt about the loss

---

[45] Susan Stryker, *Transgender History* (Berkeley, CA: Seal Press, 2008), 94–101.

of life. For many, the forfeiture of sexual liberation and the need to remain safe by wearing condoms and limiting sexual contacts defined a new sense of responsibility for the larger community. At the same time, gay men also placed the responsibility of so many lost lives on the federal government's inaction in the first years of the epidemic. In many ways, Michael's stories can be read for the huge shift in sexual life before and after the onset of AIDS.

When describing how Mary Ann was dealing with the loss, Maupin explained to the reader, "Jon had been dead for over three months, but she suffered the loss more acutely now than ever before. To gain distance on the tragedy was to grasp … the terrible enormity of it."[46] Mary Ann was able to process the impact of AIDS on someone that she knew and cared about, but only after time had passed. Read within the context of the 1980s, one might conclude that Mary Ann in this instance is emblematic of the heterosexual world that distanced itself physically and emotionally from AIDS because it was a "gay disease." Mary Ann harbored no ill-will toward Jon or Michael. In fact, she cared for both men deeply and felt her own sense of loss that was often eclipsed by her professional and personal relationships. However, Michael was not afforded such distance because he was Jon's lover and because the disease was ravaging the gay community to which he belonged. Michael's initial method of dealing with his grief was to center himself within the community by volunteering with an AIDS hotline.[47]

Maupin's artistic decision to have Jon Fielding die was his way of making a point about AIDS and the gay community. Jon's death was meant to jar readers and to demonstrate "that our brightest, and finest, and loveliest people were dying." These were the people who were outspoken about their sexuality and identity, proclaiming, "'I am a fag, and I am proud of it, and I don't care, and I love my life, and I am not ashamed of sleeping around.' Those were the people who were dying and who were already my heroes."[48] This enormous loss of life overshadowed what was once a vibrant, sexually liberated community that now had to cope with grief and approached sex with an overabundance of caution.

In fact, the novels offer an index of coping mechanisms of gay men in response to their newfound loss of sexual expression. For example, in London, Michael's teenaged friend Wilfred gets into a scuffle with his father after the latter finds a sex magazine. Michael asks why he reads those magazines, and Wilfred jokingly tells Michael that the magazines are for "wanking." Michael says, "It's a lot safer

---

[46] Armistead Maupin, *Babycakes* (New York: Harper & Row, 1984), 24.
[47] Ibid., 18–21.
[48] Richard Canning, *Gay Fiction Speaks: Conversations with Gay Novelists* (New York: Columbia University Press, 2000), 174.

to have sex with a magazine. ... My friend Ned calls it periodical sex."[49] Michael also shows the reader other methods that gay men used to cordon themselves off from the spread of the virus, which included phone sex, videotaped pornography, and "JO parties" where men would come together to masturbate without any penetration or fluid exchange.[50]

In *Significant Others* (1987), Maupin takes the opportunity to demonstrate that even heterosexuals were at risk of contracting HIV. When Brian Hawkins has an affair with a woman who was recently diagnosed as having AIDS, he worries about his own sexual health and, in a moment of panic, shows how even well-intentioned straight people felt about the disease. In disclosing his predicament to Michael, he says, "Michael, there are innocents involved here," referring to his wife and adopted daughter. Michael replies, "Innocents, huh? Not like me. Not like Jon. Not like the fags. ... It's a virus. Everybody is innocent."[51] Michael believed that no one would pay attention to the disease until straight people began to contract the virus.[52] In many ways, Michael's viewpoint reflects a historical reality. Examining the impact that AIDS had on American society, and especially in the gay community, we see how the liberalism of the 1960s, in this context the gay liberation movement, and the conservatism of the 1980s clashed. President Ronald Reagan's response to AIDS was nonexistent in the early years of the epidemic, and thanks to the efforts to reduce federal spending, the administration had cut funding to the Centers for Disease Control and Prevention, which hindered the early response. When Reagan finally spoke of AIDS, he stressed abstinence instead of safer sex practices.[53] Maupin seemed to return Reagan's reticence in the *Tales* novels that spanned his presidency. The characters mention the Reagans in passing, acknowledging the context in which they are living, but not giving them undue attention. In one scene, Michael and his new lover, Thack Sweeney (introduced in *Significant Others*), are watching a censored version of *Kramer vs. Kramer* in which Dustin Hoffman's character and his son were urinating in the morning. Thack is incredulous: "Can you believe that? ... They cut out the sound of the pee! Those fuckers!"—to which Michael replies, "Must not be in keeping with Family Values." Thack registers his anger

---

[49] Maupin, *Babycakes*, 170.
[50] Armistead Maupin, *Significant Others* (New York: Perennial Library, 1987), 22, 25–7.
[51] Ibid, 67–8.
[52] Ibid., 204.
[53] Gil Troy, *Morning in America: How Ronald Reagan Invented the 1980s*, Politics and Society in Twentieth-Century America (Princeton, NJ: Princeton University Press, 2005), 19, 202; David France, *How to Survive a Plague: The inside Story of How Citizens and Science Tamed AIDS*, 1st ed. (New York: Alfred A. Knopf, 2016), 61.

at the now humorless scene with "Fuckin' Reagan" before discussion of the president fizzles out.[54]

Maupin's own resistance and frustration surfaces in *Sure of You* (1989), as evidenced by the mention of AIDS Coalition to Unleash Power (ACT-UP). Formed in New York City, this activist group used public protests to agitate for more government involvement in addressing the epidemic in the form of a national policy to address AIDS, increased funding for studies on experimental drugs, and an end to discrimination against people with AIDS (PWAs).[55] In the novel, Michael and Thack cope with being a sero-discordant, or mixed-status, couple. Michael is HIV-positive and Thack is HIV-negative. Throughout the novel, Thack becomes more militant than Michael and embraces the activism of ACT-UP. Thack feels the overwhelming need to "do something" about the price of azidothymidine (AZT) and US Senator Jesse Helms, whose homophobia was a regular display on the Senate floor. Maupin also nods to ACT-UP's "Silence=Death" campaign when Thack proposes building a trellis in the shape of a triangle with pink flowers for the purpose of provoking their homophobic neighbor.[56] While Thack and Michael never make it to an ACT-UP meeting in the novels, this part of the story simultaneously works to document the history of ACT-UP (a reader might be prompted to research what role this organization had in AIDS activism) and signals the pessimism that Michael felt about the epidemic that he embodied with his own status as HIV-positive.

Organizations such as ACT-UP produced carefully orchestrated protests and campaigns in an attempt to bring visibility to government inaction in providing medications and safer sex education to their communities. This extended to the politics of outing prominent public figures and government officials whose decisions, or lack thereof, negatively impacted the response to AIDS. Maupin himself believed that outing was one of the ways in which more attention could be brought to AIDS relief. Closeted gay men were perceived by activists to be part of the problem behind the lack of government response to AIDS, especially those men of status (celebrities, government officials). Maupin, who had maintained a friendship with Rock Hudson in his early days in San Francisco, was responsible for outing him after Hudson announced he had AIDS.[57] The practice by friends, lovers, or family members of naming the cause of death other than AIDS also

---

[54] Armistead Maupin, *Sure of You* (New York: Harper & Row, 1989), 30.
[55] France, *How to Survive a Plague*, 253.
[56] Maupin, *Sure of You*, 31, 69–70.
[57] William A. Henry, III, Andrea Sachs, and James Willwerth, "Ethics: Forcing Gays Out of the Closet: Homosexual Leaders Seek to Expose Foes of the Movement," *Time* (January 29, 1990): 67, http://content.time.com/time/subscriber/article/0,33009,969264-1,00.html.

contributed to the desire to out people for hiding their sexuality. Thack exhibits this frustration in *Sure of You* when he plays a game in which he combs through the obituaries to identify which deaths were a result of AIDS. Stumbling across the obituary of Archibald Anson Gidde (a wealthy realtor) Thack says, "This is why people don't give a shit about AIDS! Because cowardly pricks like this make it seem like it's not really happening!"[58] For Thack and Maupin himself, outing was the only way in which AIDS would be acknowledged and lives saved.

The first six novels of the *Tales of the City* series documented the lives of mostly young, white characters living in San Francisco in the 1970s and 1980s. The stories that began as light-hearted entertainment conclude somberly as the young adults who once were drawn into each other's lives by virtue of living at 28 Barbary Lane have now moved out of the house and embarked on their separate life trajectories. The most impactful of these storylines is that of Michael Tolliver's, who begins the series as a young man trying to find love and ultimately taking on a lifetime of grief once the AIDS epidemic claims his lover, friends, and the community to which he had escaped into from his conservative family. These novels leave behind an accessible archive of a period that affected a large swath of the gay community that readers today can read to begin to understand this unique period in queer history.

Conclusion

Viewing the *Tales of the City* series as an entire historical document encourages further discussion about the direction of the medical humanities and history's place within it. Maupin was a chronicler of the time and place he lived in, and through the format of a serial, he created an opportunity for readers to share those historical experiences. The novels provide traces of the past that allow the reader to imagine what life was like, compare it to their present, and envision a different future. Readers connect with characters and think through the rise and presence of disease in everyday life.

The series opens up the possibilities of being read within a large body of medical humanities scholarship that can interrogate the response to the AIDS epidemic in historical context. Medical humanities scholarship is expansive, but has taught students to read literature in the "fullest sense" by questioning what was said in the personal and social contexts in which the work was written, and has

---

[58] Maupin, *Sure of You*, 85.

also held that literature can teach moral lessons that guide medical students and doctors in the profession.[59] Wear and Nixon have postulated that reading novels provides an ability to become a "productive" reader of the text, which serves to highlight the personal connections, good or bad, that a reader has to the text.[60] Additionally, Sari Altschuler has studied the history of medical imagination in American health and literature and adeptly points out that imagination and creativity are not concepts separated from each other, but are closely related. For Altschuler, creativity opens up possibilities "of seeing and knowing that can reveal more about health and diminish human suffering."[61] Readers who are willing to think more capaciously about the content of the series and the context in which they were produced are likely to gain a significant understanding of the gay community and a sense of compassion and understanding that most outsiders have difficulty attaining.

Where previous approaches in narrative medicine have dealt with illness within the author's body[62] and medical professionals' responses to illness,[63] the series models a different form of writing about one's own experience with illness in an identity community. Maupin has talked about how the gay community's oppression has helped him to view the oppression of other groups. "If your heart is in the right place … you can learn a lot by being homosexual. You learn to appreciate other people's oppression when you recognize what it is that makes your life uncomfortable."[64] It was this sensitivity that led to his creation of fully realized queer characters who were sympathetic and earned the reader's respect. Maupin's ability to center transgender, bisexual, and lesbian characters was also important for the audience to grasp what it meant to be a member of a marginalized group.

In 1987, Maupin observed, "Til we start recording our own history, we will never be legitimized in anyone's eyes, even our own."[65] It is unclear whether he intended his work to be read as documents of the past for future readers, but the

---

[59] Anne Hudson Jones, "Why Teach Literature and Medicine? Answers from Three Decades," *Journal of Medical Humanities* 34, no. 4 (December 1, 2013): 416–18, https://doi.org/10.1007/s10912-013-9241-9.

[60] Delese Wear and Lois LaCivita Nixon, "The Fictional World: What Literature Says to Health Professionals," *Journal of Medical Humanities* 12, no. 2 (June 1, 1991): 58–60, https://doi.org/10.1007/BF01142869.

[61] Sari Altschuler, *The Medical Imagination: Literature and Health in the Early United States*, Early American Studies (Philadelphia: University of Pennsylvania Press, 2018), 202.

[62] See Arthur W. Frank, *The Wounded Storyteller: Body, Illness, and Ethics*, 2nd ed. (Chicago: University of Chicago Press, [1995] 2013).

[63] See Rita Charon, *Narrative Medicine: Honoring the Stories of Illness* (Oxford: Oxford University Press, 2006).

[64] Richards, "Maupin's World," 35.

[65] Ibid., 38.

enduring nature of the series lends some credence to the author as a historical eyewitness. Browning has read the *Tales of the City* series as an artifact of gay folk life written by an author who did not hide his sexual orientation; as such, "gay men read his books and nod their heads in acknowledgement while thinking, 'This is the story of my life.' "[66] Heterosexual readers, on the other hand, gain an insight about a community far removed from their own frame of experience.[67] The novels become "artifacts of gay customary and material folk culture" that are easy to circulate, thus opening up a part of his lived experience and cultural heritage.[68] From the vantage point of the 1990s, Browning believed this cultural heritage to be endangered by the AIDS crisis, and it very much was since many artists of the time were dying from the disease.[69] Returning to Cvetkovich, we are also reminded that this artifact functions as an archive of emotion and trauma that solidifies the author's experiences while still relating what members of the gay community experienced in the past. The reader is left with the series as an artifact and archive whose narrative functions as a means for inviting the audience in to examine the extent to which illness has been constructed and the community's reaction to it. Maupin's ability to create commonalities through effective, first-hand storytelling legitimizes the queer community even as political trends and attitudes continue to shift in American society. Consequently, *Tales of the City* provides a template for how to interpret other works of fiction as snapshots of specific moments in history.

---

[66] Jimmy D. Browning, "Something to Remember Me By: Maupin's 'Tales of the City' Novels as Artifacts in Contemporary Gay Folk Culture," *New York Folklore* 19, no. 1 (January 1, 1993): 85.
[67] Ibid.
[68] Ibid., 85.
[69] Ibid., 72.

9

The Suffering Caregiver:
Toward an Embodied Experience of
End-of-Life Pain through Literature

Benjamin Gagnon Chainey

Introduction

"Is the experience of pain preferable to the annihilation of experience?"[1] This question, posed by Hervé Guibert, a French writer who died in 1991 while HIV-positive, resounds from the darkest areas of his terminal phase. In the last pages of his personal diary, Guibert asks whether pain is the touchstone of one's end-of-life experience. In other words, Guibert wonders if pain might be the key to embracing death as a crucial life experience. For the writer, death is not a dreadful moment to abolish with overmedicalization, nor is it an obscene experience to hide and neutralize, between the walls of the hospital, positivistic discourses and practices. Guibert's question reaches to the heart of contemporary debates over physician-assisted dying, which consider the patient's experience of intolerable and irreversible pain and suffering—physical or psychological—to be the ticket to this ultimate form of care: that of a chosen and dignified death. To say that death could be a kind of care—and not the inevitable failure of life— implies a major paradigm shift regarding modern medicine's goal of healing, sometimes pursued at all costs. It therefore risks contradicting one of the most famous phrases of the Hippocratic Oath: "First do no harm," from the Latin locution *"Primum no nocere."* In the context of end of life, pain sometimes becomes so unbearable that it surpasses the relief capacity of palliative care, which consequently harms the dying patients more than its cares for them.

---

[1] Hervé Guibert, *Le mausolée des amants: Journal, 1976–1991* (Paris: Gallimard, 2001), 513. All translations from French works are by the author, unless otherwise noted.

In such an ambiguous, disturbing—but not rare—scenario, suffering patients may contemplate death as the ultimate form of care, not only to relieve their physical and psychic pain but also to preserve their dignity in this difficult yet vital process. In this vein, "Medical Assistance in Dying," also known as MAID, became legal in Canada in 2016, after a series of legal cases and national commissions beginning in the early 1990s culminated in the establishment of a "Select Committee on Dying with Dignity" in the province of Québec in 2009.[2] One of the main eligibility criteria to access MAID is to "experience unbearable physical or mental suffering from your illness, disease, disability or state of decline that cannot be relieved under conditions that you consider acceptable."[3]

The main goal of this chapter is to reflect, from literary and cultural perspectives, and in conversation with medical and ethical stances, on this crucial and complex eligibility criterion of MAID, which would implicate a capacity for the caregivers to assess, and for the patients to express, an "experience of unbearable physical or mental suffering" that would make death the most well-suited form of care. In this chapter, rather than trying to reach a single, clear, and objective answer, I will argue that we must ask ourselves if univocal and normative methodologies of assessing end-of-life pain are, to begin with, appropriate ways to face the problem.

I will show, in the first part of this chapter, that the nature of pain precedes and escapes its formation and stabilization in language. Building on this insight, I will then argue that we need to think not only of new ways of assessing pain, disease, and death but also of developing, following Matthew Ratcliffe, our ability to *experience* them within "our sense of others [involving] a bodily response that is inextricable from a distinctive way of experiencing *possibilities*."[4] End-of-life pain and suffering are played out in an intricate and cruel theater of intersubjectivity that is entangled in "our sense of others as persons," sometimes confused in a "feeling of ambiguity" inherent to every human relation.[5]

Following seminal philosophers, writers, bioethicists, literary and cultural essayists—including Sigmund Freud, Georges Canguilhem, Michel Foucault, Hervé Guibert, David J. Rothman, Elaine Scarry, and Emmanuel Levinas—I will

---

[2] National Assembly of Québec, "Commission spéciale sur la question de mourir dans la dignité" (Select Committee on Dying with Dignity), 2009, http://www.assnat.qc.ca/en/travaux-parlementaires/commissions/csmd-39-1/index.html.

[3] Canada Health, "Medical Assistance in Dying," March 18, 2021, https://www.canada.ca/en/health-canada/services/medical-assistance-dying.html#a2.

[4] Matthew Ratcliffe, "The Structure of Interpersonal Experience," in *The Phenomenology of Embodied Subjectivity*, ed. Rasmus Thybo Jensen and Dermot Moran, Contributions to Phenomenology (New York: Springer, 2013), 221, original emphasis.

[5] Ibid., 221–2.

show in the second part of the chapter how pain and death have been overlooked and hidden from collective space and speech, making them taboos that we pretend to alleviate only by not facing or experiencing them.

By focusing on aesthetic sensitivity, I will reflect, in the third part of the chapter, on the ways in which literature, through its capacity to express ambivalent, disturbing, and paradoxical sensations, emotions, and situations, can help us better experience and embody the equivocal nature of pain and dying. If pain, disease, dying, and death are phenomena that precede and/or surpass the normativity of language, then why do we confine ourselves within the frame of ethical norms and medico-legal discourses to reflect on them?

Instead, in the fourth and final part of the chapter, I will propose a methodological shift away from this interdisciplinary debate and toward the application of an aesthetic sensitivity found in literature and arts that is historically and epistemologically at the origin of the concept of empathy. I will build this final reflection on the performative power of the aesthetic sensitivity of literature by beginning with the general definition of performativity that Judith Butler gives in her *Notes toward a Performative Theory of Assembly*: performativity "characterizes first and foremost that characteristic of linguistic utterances that in the moment of making the utterance makes something happen or brings some phenomenon into being."[6] How can literature, therefore, bring the phenomenon of end-of-life pain into being, allowing caregivers, patients, and their families to better express, share, and feel the complexity of it?

Assessing Univocally or Experiencing Equivocally?

Numerous challenges bar the way toward a clear delineation of what an "unbearable physical or mental suffering" may be. This eligibility criterion of MAID, at least in Canada, is difficult to pin down with a definition that would be *univocal*, in the common sense of "having one meaning only," a sense that also "[traces] back to the Latin noun *vox*, which means 'voice.'"[7] Avoiding the limitation of suffering to a single definition matters crucially in the case of end-of-life suffering, given that a mistaken assessment would be irreversible. Yet, while the subjective and, indeed, *intersubjective* character of the evaluation of

---

[6] Judith Butler, *Notes toward a Performative Theory of Assembly* (Cambridge, MA: Harvard University Press, 2015), 28.
[7] "Univocal, adj.," *Merriam-Webster*, accessed March 31, 2021, https://www.merriam-webster.com/dictionary/univocal.

pain and the apprehension of death seems to make it improbable to reach such univocity, a clear and shared definition of the core MAID criterion is essential given the high stakes. This imperative is a paradox: caregivers and patients must join their voices and perspectives to univocally define and assess a reality—the "unbearable physical or mental suffering"—that is essentially equivocal or, more precisely, moved not only by one voice but also by a polyphonic "feeling of ambiguity" that lies at the core of human relations.[8] End-of-life care—and medically assisted dying as an ultimate form of care—forces all the human beings involved in the experience to join their voices, feelings, and perspectives together, to hopefully constitute that one voice belonging to the patient.

This fraught philosophical question, a literal life-or-death question, is influenced by the nature of suffering and pain. Of course, pain can refer to "negative" sensations, feelings, affects, and mindsets, but from a linguistic perspective, pain is also what precedes, resists, and even destroys language. As Elaine Scarry writes in *The Body in Pain*: "Physical pain does not simply resist language but actively destroys it, bringing about an immediate reversion to a state anterior to language, to the sounds and cries a human being makes before language is learned."[9] Even if Scarry refers specifically to physical pain, primal resistance to language also extends to psychic and psychological sufferings that escape materialization in the body—despair is not "X-rayable," as Scarry writes—and objectification in language. The author synthesizes the aporetic challenge of understanding pain through language: pain "is not *of* or *for* anything. It is precisely because it takes no object that it, more than any other phenomenon, resists objectification in language."[10]

In the specific context of end-of-life pain and suffering, medical, legal, and bioethical discourses dominate MAID. Even if the knowledge conveyed through those discourses follows "evidence-based" reasoning, they remain rooted in language and discursive constructions. However, as Scarry argues, no discourse can pretend to be a univocal expression when it comes to pain. Bodies in all languages can suffer from pain; all can also be surpassed by its polyphonic and ambiguous performativity. Following this reflection, it is understandable that many physicians and caregivers working in end-of-life care find their task difficult. The Dutch sociologist Roeline Pasman suggests that evaluating end-of-life suffering is at times so intricate, in part because physicians/caregivers cannot

---

[8] Ratcliffe, "The Structure of Interpersonal Experience," 222.
[9] Elaine Scarry, *The Body in Pain: The Making and Unmaking of the World* (New York: Oxford University Press, 1985), 4.
[10] Ibid., 5, original emphasis.

even *imagine* complex and unbearable suffering. Therefore, their "evidence-based" practice is far from evident.[11] End of life may be one of many complex clinical situations—albeit one every human being will face—where imagination and knowledge walk hand in hand with uncertainty and, eventually, death.

More practically, instead of demanding that patients express their pain within the bounds of medical, legal, and bioethical discourses for physicians and caregivers to assess it, could we conceive of modes of *experiencing* pain that would break free from the confines of such limiting forms of expression? By lending a more attentive ear to the words of Hervé Guibert, as a writer but also as a patient, the remainder of this chapter will provide a path toward a more resolutely empathetic experience of pain that would be anchored in the aesthetic sensitivity on which literary performativity is based. Recognizing that pain and suffering escape the confines of scientific and evidence-based discourse—while not necessarily denying it—helps us better imagine the complex and sometimes unbearable reality of the dying patient. I contend that beyond the sought-after alleviation of pain, an empathetic experience at the end of life through the aesthetic sensitivity of literature might reveal other meaningful, and often paradoxical, facets of the suffering endured by both the patient and the caregiver.

Deconfining Our Cultural Relations to Suffering, Disease, and Death

If all acts of care are relational, and if death is at times presented as an appropriate form of care for suffering, a dialogue must be established between death and suffering. Contrary to an intuitive human response to turn away from these phenomena, such a dialogue would not seek to isolate them, but would rather invite those who fight against suffering and death, namely patients and caregivers, to engage with them. This dialogue would help overcome both the difficulty we feel when hearing and looking at death and suffering, and our resistance to accompanying and supporting these experiences. It would do so by trying to understand how pain, suffering, and death find their own way to expression, or how they fail to do so. Once we attune ourselves to their different, sometimes ambiguous or even contradictory expressive modalities, which may or may not

---

[11] H. Roeline Pasman, "What Characterizes Complex Euthanasia Consultations?," in *Experiences of SCEN (Support and Consultation on Euthanasia in the Netherlands) Physicians* (Second International Conference on End of Life, Law, Ethics, Policy, and Practice), Halifax, Nova Scotia, 2017.

include clear and positive language, we may gain an enhanced, nuanced portrait of pain, suffering, and death in the care relation. Hence, to be able to experience end-of-life pain and suffering in all their polyphonic complexity, we need to release them, to let their multiple voices intertwine with the care relation, in the hope that they lead to a dialogue between caregivers, the patients, and their close ones. In that sense, writing in the year of Guibert's passing, David J. Rothman denounced the way pain and death are isolated from the stream of everyday human relations:

> To deal on a daily basis with injury, pain, disfigurement, and death is to be set apart from others. Modern society has constructed exceptionally sturdy boundaries around illness, confining it to the hospital and making it the nearly exclusive preserve of the medical profession. … To be sure, this process is not new, but it has surely accelerated over the last several decades. … The isolation of disease is certainly not complete, however.[12]

Rothman is right in pointing out that the exclusion process of pain, disease, and death is not new. His analysis of our contemporary attitude toward death resonates directly with Freud's essay "Reflections on War and Death," originally published in 1915 and translated in 1918, just at the end of the Great War. In the essay's introduction, Freud depicts a still-relevant portrayal of our ambiguous and often repressed individual and collective feelings and thoughts toward war, suffering, and death. Freud writes about the "disturbing voices" that occasionally disrupt "the enjoyment of [our] common civilization."[13] These voices remind us that war and death are "unavoidable," but, if only we listened to them, they would help us better "imagine" what these realities are and, thus, help us better prepare for when they inevitably arrive.

Freud thus reveals our individual and collective resistance to facing crucial questions about suffering and war, and our suppression of any thoughts about death's omnipresence within life, even when we keep it silent and invisible within the hospital walls or far from us, in a foreign country. However, death and violent conflicts do emerge, as they did during the production of this volume with the COVID-19 pandemic at the end of 2019, and the explosion of racial tensions following the killing of George Floyd on May 25th, 2020. Explaining

---

[12] David J. Rothman, *Strangers at the Bedside: A History of How Law and Bioethics Transformed Medical Decision Making* (New York: Basic Books, 1991), 135.
[13] Sigmund Freud, *Reflections on War and Death*, trans. A. A. Brill and Alfred B. Kuttner (New York: Moffat, Yard, 1918), 9.

how tragedies can be rampant within the social body, yet inappropriately suppressed by some authorities, Freud states:

> Shall we not admit that in our civilized attitude towards death we have again lived psychologically beyond our means? Shall we not turn around and avow the truth? Were it not better to give death the place to which it is entitled both in reality and in our thoughts and to reveal a little more of our unconscious attitude towards death which up to now we have so carefully suppressed?[14]

For Freud, the questions of suffering, individual and collective disease, and death are often "rejected as calumnies which can be ignored in the face of the assurances of consciousness, while the few signs through which the unconscious betrays itself to consciousness are cleverly overlooked."[15] My goal here is not to debate psychoanalysis and our subconscious struggle with war and death, but to stress that end-of-life suffering and death are unavoidable realities that should not be compartmentalized within one discipline, one discourse, or one place, such as the hospital or the palliative care unit. This siloing of death to protect us—for our own good?—from facing it daily, as end-of-life caregivers do for us, is not a viable or responsible solution. Death, whatever its cause, is the only certainty all human beings share, and it therefore is counterproductive to isolate ourselves from it. Hiding it from the collective eye only creates an illusion of control over it, while it ineluctably continues its work. Even if opinions diverge on the value of Freud's psychoanalytical theory, it is difficult not to agree with his suggestion that, if suffering and death are universal problems, then we ought to face them, even if it's painful and troubling, or perhaps even violent and indecent, as 2020 and early 2021 brutally proved to us.

Facing pain, suffering, and death is better than hiding or turning away from them. Therefore, in response to Guibert's question that introduced the chapter, Freud's answer might be: "It is better to experience pain than to annihilate the experience of it." Annihilating the experience of pain could result in the incapacity to experience, embody, or bear anything *at all*. Nor would it allow us to *heal* from it. Rather, clinging to language as a protective blanket could dehumanize us, offering an illusionary escape from our duty to bear human life as "death at work," with its concert of "disturbing voices." Freud similarly states:

> This may not appear a very high achievement and in some respects rather a step backwards, a kind of regression, but at least it has the advantage of taking the

---

[14] Ibid., 71.
[15] Ibid., 65.

truth into account a little more and of making life more bearable again. To bear life remains, after all, the first duty of the living. The illusion becomes worthless if it disturbs us in this.[16]

Isolation from pain and death is not a solution; it ironically prevents us from listening carefully to what is disturbing in order to face and bear it. Isolation from pain and death is the *illusion* of a solution: an artificial and repressed way of "dealing" with them, rather than a genuine attempt at reconciling our bodies, minds, and languages with these realities.

The literary and artistic work of Guibert extends the project—initiated by Rothman and Freud, but which should arguably concern all of humanity—to decompartmentalize pain and death. Well before he entered the terminal phase of AIDS at the beginning of the 1990s, Guibert was invested in exploring the experience of pain and dying, dating from his first published text in 1977, titled *La Mort propagande* in French (which I freely and literally translate into English as *Death Propaganda*). In this book, Guibert responds to a need to see and hear his own body's suffering and "death at work" within him—and in each one of us—to better understand it, even to unmask it. That being said, Guibert does not pursue this programmatic and "auto-corpographic" work, whose fantastic overtones could surpass the borders of decency for some readers, by confining his suffering in the sturdy boundaries of a book (like modern hospitals do, according to Rothman). Guibert writes his body in order to share it:

> My body, under the effect of either pleasure or pain, is put in a state of theatricality, of paroxysm, that I would like to reproduce in some way: photography, film, tape recording. As soon as a deformation occurs, as soon as my body is hysterical, I would put in place a transcription mechanism: eructation, dejection, sperm as a result of wanking, diarrhea, spit, catarrh in the mouth and in the butt. … My body is a laboratory that I offer as an exhibition, the sole actor, the sole instrument of my organic desires. Partitions on a fabric of flesh, of insanity, of pain. Observe how it operates, harvest its performance. … At the conclusion of this series of expressions, the ultimate travesty, the ultimate make-up, death. We gag it, we censor it, we attempt to drown it in bleach, to suffocate it in ice. For my part, I want to let it rise its powerful voice and sing, a diva, throughout my body. She will be my only partner, and I will be her interpreter.[17]

---

[16] Ibid., 71.
[17] Hervé Guibert, *La mort propagande* (Paris: Gallimard, [1977] 2009), 7. .

While his approach may appear exhibitionist and shocking to some audiences, Guibert's whole literary work—counting more than thirty novels, essays, photograph collections, and a film script, even though he died at 36 years of age— may be read as a humble yet total gift of a self to the Other. His investigation of his own body in every possible state—suffering, enjoying, dying, exulting, and so on—is an uncompromising work of life and death, literature and art. At the end of his diary, corresponding with the end of his life, Guibert writes: "When the time comes to disappear, I'll know I won't have kept anything to myself (isn't that 'my' experience?)."[18] Guibert was writing as he was living: without compromise on communicating and sharing even his most violent, painful, and disturbing experiences, making literature a space of absolute hospitality for expressions, sensations, and relations. Echoing this diary entry, reading Guibert could be understood as a shared literary experience of (sometimes extreme) intimacy that paradoxically defies modesty and sometimes common decency. Guibert invites us to collectively read and feel, through his literary works, the intimate and ultimate experience of pain and death in progress. When it appeared in 1977, *La Mort propagande* received praise from Michel Foucault, who found in Guibert's text direct echoes of the first volume of his seminal *History of Sexuality: The Will to Knowledge* (which had been published a year earlier, in 1976). More precisely, in the last chapter, titled "Right of Death and Power over Life," Foucault writes: "Now it is over life, throughout its unfolding, that power establishes its dominion; death is power's limit, the moment that escapes it; death becomes the most secret aspect of existence, the most 'private.'"[19]

As we listen to the conversation between Foucault and Guibert,[20] we are tempted to ask them (since they are both dead but still very much alive through their texts): How can we collectively explore and experience death, even though it appears to be "the most secret aspect of existence, the most 'private'"? How might we work *together* through language's reluctance to express the experience of death, but also through death's sometimes indecent aspects and disturbing voices?

---

[18] Guibert, *Le mausolée des amants*, 412.
[19] Michel Foucault, *The History of Sexuality*, trans. Robert Hurley, first American ed. (New York: Pantheon Books, 1978), 138.
[20] Foucault and Guibert became close friends during their lives. They shared paths until the end, as they both died due to HIV or from the complications of AIDS. Guibert died a few days after a suicide attempt made by ingesting digitalin, a heart medication. In his novel *To the Friend Who Did Not Save My Life*, the first of his "AIDS writings," Guibert refers directly to Foucault's end of life and death through the character of Muzil. First published in 1990 under the title *À l'Ami qui ne m'a pas sauvé la vie*, the novel made Guibert famous to the broader public.

Breaking Free from Ethical Norms through Aesthetic Sensitivity

An embodied experience like the one Guibert wants to share with his readers, a gift of intimacy to be lived collectively, only makes sense when it is understood through the dual prism of empathy. Empathy is not only oriented by prescriptive ethics for the giving subject's good, but also moved by the sensitivity toward the receiving subject. In counterpoint to the rigorous medical, legal, and ethical discourses surrounding end-of-life care, empathy, as a sensitive phenomenon, is not yet judged by language. In this way, empathy is reminiscent of pain, which precedes, surpasses, or even destroys language's borders, as Scarry's comment on the dilemma between "assessing univocally or experiencing equivocally suggests."[21] Felt and shared sensitive experience can be difficult to stabilize in (ethical) language or knowledge. Pain, suffering, disease, and dying, even if they are universal and "normal" experiences, often escape the normativity of language. Linguistic and epistemological norms fail to capture the suffering body's pathological performativity, with its slippages that defy attempts at categorization and classification. The ill and dying body, while seemingly offering its death in progress for clinical eyes to assess and for languages to express, also inflicts suffering on anyone attempting to make sense of it. Disease and dying are fundamentally destabilizing experiences of their own—unique in themselves while common to everyone—and resist comparison to the "normal" nature of health. Georges Canguilhem, the French physician and philosopher of science who specialized both in epistemology and biology, writes in his seminal essay *The Normal and the Pathological*:

> The patient is sick because he can admit of only one norm. To use an expression which has already been very useful to us, the sick man is not abnormal because of the absence of a norm but because of his incapacity to be normative. With this view of disease, we see how far we are from the conception of [Auguste] Comte[22] or [Claude] Bernard.[23] Disease is a positive, innovative experience in the living being and not just a fact of decrease or increase. The content of the pathological state cannot be deduced, save for a difference in format, from the

---

[21] Scarry, *The Body in Pain*, 5.
[22] French philosopher of science who developed the doctrine of positivism during the first half of the nineteenth century.
[23] French physiologist who founded and developed experimental medicine in the second half of the nineteenth century.

content of health; disease is not a variation on the dimension of health; it is a new dimension of life.[24]

If disease, suffering, and dying are to be considered "new dimensions of life," experiences preceding and escaping stabilization by preexisting norms, they absolutely need to be felt in bodies as well as languages and aesthetics. This is not to say that they must be stabilized in normative meaning; on the contrary, what is at stake is freeing them from meaning. In doing so, clinical reasoning shifts from asking "why" to asking "how" ill and suffering bodies and languages resist norms. It is not because they have none, but because they combine and juxtapose too many, often ambiguous and contradictory norms. At the extreme experience of the limits of human suffering, end-of-life pain's "incapacity to be normative" results in oscillating and uncertain bodies: human, but also aesthetic, artistic, and literary bodies. The extension of the term "bodies" to include the aesthetic, the artistic, and the literary is not only metaphorical; such bodies are also to be understood *as* suffering and dying bodies. To avoid reverting to using language as mediation and protection from experience, we may need to invert and displace Susan Sontag's notion of *illness as metaphor* and think instead of *metaphor as disease*. If a metaphor is an image constructed by playing with a second degree of language, shifting from its "normal" meaning to "nonnormal" images—in the sense that they are built outside the normativity of words and discourses—then metaphor is what escapes the "norm" of language, making it "pathological" not because metaphors are necessarily bad, but because they break free from language's first-level normalcy. Following this logic, aesthetic, artistic, and literary bodies *are* experiences of suffering and dying, to the extent that they are also living performatively, in Butler's sense of the concept. Literature is never a still life: it is a moving and a dying life.

Literary and artistic aesthetics ought also to be considered through empathy's position before and beyond the ethical. Aesthetics break free from the dichotomy between good and evil. End-of-life pain, when considered as an aesthetic phenomenon, is to be experienced outside of normative logics. In the same way as the vital necessity to decompartmentalize death was regularly asserted throughout the twentieth century—by the likes of Freud, Foucault, Guibert, and Rothman—the argument that pain must be understood through both empathy and aesthetics is not new. Even though it has yet to find its way into medical practice, this argument may be traced back

---

[24] Georges Canguilhem, *The Normal and the Pathological*, trans. Carolyn R. Fawcett (New York: Zone Books, [1978] 1989), 186.

to nineteenth- and early twentieth-century aesthetic theory, particularly to "the German notion of 'Einfühlung,' which [was] translated as 'empathy,' thus introducing the latter term into the English language."[25] When psychology and neurocognitive researchers pose the crucial and complex question, "Is there a relationship between aesthetic and interpersonal experience?" in a study on empathy, they help us realize that there is no unique, univocal answer.[26] On the contrary, they suggest that any attempt to understand the relationship must acknowledge the fundamentally dual and always oscillating movement between the aesthetic and interpersonal dimensions of shared experience. The authors thus confirm that experience lies before and beyond any stabilization of ethical norms:

> Historically, this question is motivated by the fact that experiences of both types have been accounted for in terms of the German notion of "Einfühlung." ... Accordingly, it is possible to distinguish between aesthetic and interpersonal "empathy" in English in much the same way as it is possible to distinguish between aesthetic and interpersonal "Einfühlung" in German, thereby suggesting a common psychological mechanism supposed to underlie both aesthetic and interpersonal "empathy."[27]

Coming back to Guibert, existing theories of the experience of pain thus appear to justify the French writer's conception of his own polymorphic, polyphonic, and oscillating body, escaping any normative effort at compartmentalization: alternately and at once human and literary, biological and artistic. In the second volume of his "AIDS writings," published the year of his death, in 1991, and titled *The Compassion Protocol*, Guibert discusses the use of (still unapproved) medical treatment in the case of terminally ill patients, writing:

> Today I would like to work on a dissection table. It is my soul that I dissect at each new day of toil. ... On the table, I perform all kinds of examinations, I take section snapshots, I conduct magnetic resonance investigations, endoscopies, radiographs, and scans, and I deliver the images for you to decipher on the luminous plate of your sensitivity.[28]

---

[25] Joanna Ganczarek, Thomas Hünefeldt, and Marta Olivetti Belardinelli, "From 'Einfühlung' to Empathy: Exploring the Relationship between Aesthetic and Interpersonal Experience," *Cognitive Processing* 19, no. 2 (May 1, 2018): 141, https://doi.org/10.1007/s10339-018-0861-x.
[26] Ibid.
[27] Ibid., 142.
[28] Hervé Guibert, *Le protocole compassionnel: roman* (Paris: Gallimard, 1991), 94.

However, this ambivalent and reciprocal oscillation between human and literary bodies, which Guibert would like us not to read rationally but to feel sensitively, comes at a price. There is a vital necessary risk to its embodiment, by the patient as much as by the caregiver. As Emmanuel Levinas writes, "Exposed, open like a city facing the approaching enemy, sensitivity, beneath any will, any act, any declaration, any stance—is vulnerability itself."[29] This philosophical equivalency between sensitivity and vulnerability means that when the end-of-life caregiver exposes their own sensitivity, in an attempt to empathetically assess, feel, and alleviate the suffering of the dying patient, the shared experience occurs at the limits of vulnerability and intimacy. End-of-life caregivers, whether they know it or not, necessarily put themselves at risk to that same vulnerability the dying patient is living.

For if "suffering through the other is having charge of him, supporting him, being in his place, consuming oneself through him," and if "all love and all hate of the other, as a thoughtful attitude, suppose a prior vulnerability,"[30] the place of sensitivity as part of end-of-life care becomes a tightrope walker's art: a risky performance that would at once follow the requirements of medico-legal objectivity and give way to the subjective vulnerability that is the foundation for the expression and reception of the Other's suffering. It is a painful task at the meeting point of medicine, law, arts, literature, and the humanities, but that is inescapable if one hopes to fully embrace human subjectivity. According to Levinas, writing in the year of Guibert's death:

> It is this attention to the suffering of the other that, through the cruelties of our century (despite these cruelties, because of these cruelties) can be affirmed as the very nexus of human subjectivity, to the point of being raised to the level of supreme ethical principle—the only one it is impossible to question—shaping the hopes and commanding the practical discipline of vast human groups.[31]

If the shared experience of the Other's suffering appears to be the "supreme ethical principle," following Levinas, it is also always on the verge of toppling over the edge and becoming an extreme *unethical* principle. Considering this risk, we better understand why accompanying someone through death, with an empathetic sensitivity toward their suffering, is an undeniable source of anguish

---

[29] Emmanuel Lévinas, *Humanisme de l'autre homme*, Livre de poche, Biblio essais (Montpellier: Fata Morgana, 1972), 104.
[30] Ibid., 105.
[31] Emmanuel Lévinas, *Humanism of the Other*, trans. Nidra Poller, 1st reprint ed. (Urbana: University of Illinois Press, [1972] 2006), 81.

and fear that also causes discomfort and pain for the caregiver. On the one hand, as Canguilhem tells us, it is a "positive" experience in the sense that it is a totally "new dimension of life."[32] On the other, it is not an epistemologically positive experience as it is anchored in uncertainty, in the sensitive ambiguity of meaning.

Following this oscillating path, end-of-life feelings are both univocally and equivocally shared by dying patients and their caregivers. Together, they experience the limits of sensitivity, sense, and meaning. Hence, expressing and sharing end-of-life pain, if we return to Scarry's reflection, may be one of the most ambivalent experiences of all. It is the experience of extreme vulnerability at the limits of both sensitivity and certainty. Scarry writes:

> So, for the person in pain, so incontestably and unnegotiably present is it that "having pain" may come to be thought of as the most vibrant example of what it is to "have certainty," while for the other person it is so elusive that "hearing about pain" may exist as the primary model of what it is to "have doubt." Thus, pain comes unsharably into our midst as at once that which cannot be denied and that which cannot be confirmed. Whatever pain achieves, it achieves in part through its unsharability, and it ensures this unsharability through its resistance to language.[33]

As Guibert observes caregivers at his bedside, he writes in his hospital diary: "Sometimes, they just don't know anymore, they feel their way, they sweat buckets. They're afraid."[34] Fear of being mistaken, of not knowing, fear of saying or doing the wrong thing, fear of being accused, fear of being found guilty; it goes without saying that the words and actions of caregivers who accompany the dying—both professionals and family members—are laden with meaning and heavy in consequence. The ever-oscillating ethical responsibility that befalls them is an always ambivalent burden they must carry, but that they must not—and cannot—carry alone. Not unlike the pain they help alleviate, the caregivers toiling in the space-time of the end of life, facing death daily, should also be accompanied, equipped to handle the injunction of empathy that is thrust upon them.

Empathy, before it was appropriated by medical discourses as an "ethical method" of conceiving the Other's suffering, was an aesthetic, shared, embodied, and multidimensional experience. An intersubjective and, indeed,

---

[32] Canguilhem, *The Normal and the Pathological*, 186.
[33] Scarry, *The Body in Pain*, 4.
[34] Hervé Guibert, *Cytomegalovirus: A Hospitalization Diary*, trans. Clara Orban (New York: Fordham University Press, [1996] 2016), 59.

interdisciplinary apparatus must then be (re)constructed to help caregivers become writers and artists: to help them imagine the suffering of the Other, as Pasman suggests; to decompartmentalize it, following Freud, Foucault, Guibert, and Rothman; or to learn to suffer through the Other, to take up Levinas's suggestion.[35]

The Embodied Experience of End-of-Life Pain through Literature

In the eye of end of life's ethical knot, art and literature must add their voices to the polyphonic chorus and contribute to the care of the dying and to the tools of the caregiver. More than yet another scale to evaluate pain, a dose of morphine, or a committee's approval, empathy and aesthetics are constant reminders that it is crucial not to dehumanize the suffering of the Other, even when it becomes— for the dying as well as those who witness death—difficult to bear with one's own vulnerability and sensitivity. During one of his last nights at the hospital, Guibert writes: "I get up to jot down some phrases that swim through my head, or else they'll haunt me until tomorrow. The cries of the suffering which come from nearby rooms are almost more heart-rending than one's own suffering."[36]

In the hospital environment, where Guibert finds himself during his last moments, pain and suffering are omnipresent, testing the limits of the bearable and of despair, and do not affect only the suffering patient him/herself. On the verge of death, while AIDS is gradually making him blind, Guibert realizes his deepest fear of sightlessness, reflects on his pain, embraces it, and adds: "I'm not saying I'd like to become blind, there are situations so desperate that one tries to take advantage of them, but it's something I'm not familiar with, and I always love to slip into unknown situations, no matter the consequences."[37] What Guibert affirms, as he is in the verge of losing his vision, should not be reduced to the dying man's despair as he accepts his fate, or to the macabre fantasy of an "artist of the self." Guibert is perhaps stating here the desire of the writer not only to write about suffering but also to experience and share it. Guibert's posture is an invitation to collectively dare to conceive of the inconceivable, even when it is painful; to rehabilitate sensitivity, even when it makes us vulnerable. As a

---

[35] Pasman, "What Characterizes Complex Euthanasia Consultations?"
[36] Guibert, *Cytomegalovirus*, 33.
[37] Ibid., 46.

possible response to an essay by Québec physician Alain Vadeboncœur, in which the author criticizes actors for not being able to "play dead,"[38] Guibert might respond: "Physicians, caregivers and ethicists—do they know how to die?" For if the goal of physician-assisted dying is to die better, then is there not a need to learn to die? No discourse and no actor can pretend, by themselves, to teach an experience so intricate as pain, suffering, dying, and death. Rather, we need to join the voices that resonate at the end of life, even those that may be disturbing.

"Listen to the disturbing, and take it into account," said Linda Ganzini, a psychiatrist at Oregon Health and Science University, during her keynote lecture at the Second International Conference on End of Life Law, Ethics, Policy and Practice.[39] And if Guibert is right in stating, between parentheses, at the very end of his personal diary "(One of the roles of literature is to teach death)," then it belongs to us—medical, arts, literature, and humanities scholars—to break through the partitions that keep death neatly within the bounds of the hospital, disciplines, and languages.[40] We need to take death out of the parentheses, the same parentheses that keep literature, arts, and the humanities apart from other forms of end-of-life discourse. It is only at that price, and at that risk, that we may better humanize the end of life.

---

[38] Alain Vadeboncœur, *Les acteurs ne savent pas mourir* (Montréal: Lux, 2014) .
[39] Linda Ganzini, "Empirical Studies: What Do We Know about End-of-Life Decision-Making around the World?," in *Experiences of SCEN (Support and Consultation on Euthanasia in the Netherlands) Physicians* (Second International Conference on End of Life Law, Ethics, Policy and Practice), Halifax, Nova Scotia, 2017.
[40] Guibert, *Le mausolée des amants*, 559.

Part 4

Alternatives

Introduction

The structure of the essays in this collection might be framed as a trajectory from stability to indeterminacy, or from past and present thinking to future orientations. Part 1, "Identities/Institutions," looks at how institutions, from hospitals to armies, have shaped (and continue to shape) health at an individual, identitarian level. The chapters in this first part demonstrate the ethical value of using a humanities approach—in this instance, literary studies—to elucidate structures of power that govern health and illness. Focusing more explicitly on the real-life delivery of healthcare, Part 2, "Practices," describes how such approaches have already been imported into the clinical encounter, recognizing the limitations and lacunae of existing attempts at interdisciplinarity. Part 3, "Contingencies," is even less sanguine about the application of humanities approaches to medical practice. These chapters reveal how such bodily realities as disability, terminal illness, and death not only trouble biomedical aims and assumptions but also reveal gaps in the humanities' self-knowledge, even as they propose solutions to those gaps.

Bringing this trajectory to an open-ended conclusion by way of the literary studies that opened the volume, this final part, "Alternatives," identifies and analyses the potential for creative challenges to biomedicine's dominance of the cultural sphere. Chapters by Diana Rose Newby and Anna Fenton-Hathaway highlight the potential of speculative fiction and dystopia to reach beyond the regime of medical knowledge through formal experimentation. Free from the bonds of realism, these literary genres rethink the relationship of culture with medicine, or envision another form of medicine entirely. This part exemplifies the critical and stylistic values present throughout this collection, questioning assumptions about the purpose of dystopian representation and investigating the stylistic elements of books and films that enhance their potential for analysis.

These values inform one another, as the critical lens encourages readers to look more closely at the stylistic choices and their role in shaping how we understand bodily states.

The first chapter in this part, by Newby, analyzes a recent work of speculative fiction, *Confessions of the Fox* by Jordy Rosenberg (2018), for its creative reimagination of hormone usage. Newby's analysis takes up a critical neologism by Rosenberg, "endochronology," as the starting point for an investigation of how the novel's experimental form troubles a "progress narrative of the alignment of sex hormones and subjectivity." This critique of hormonal teleology in trans studies recalls Lau's discussion of recentering care around "crip time" rather than cure, though, here, the nonbinary rather than the disabled body offers the temporal model. Rosenberg's novel is set in the eighteenth century, and it features a historical thief and prison-breaker. Rosenberg imagines this protagonist as an intersex and transgender man, whose sexual status as "chimera" is further enabled by his consumption of a mysterious "serum" that is reminiscent of exogenous testosterone (T). Newby argues that the novel's form, which intermixes scientific and supernatural early modern thinking with auto-theory and the history of medicine, is analogous to this serum in its ability to facilitate fluidity and play: "The text of *Confessions* is a compound that transforms in order to resist the many traditions from which it both draws and departs." In dialogue with modern scholarship on T as a socially constructed mythos, Newby's essay promotes the collection's ethical orientation of situating the cultural products of the humanities within a biomedical matrix. The chapter captures the critical value of the volume, too, as Newby finds in Rosenberg's speculative fiction a critique of an assumption that might be shared by hormonal biomedicine and by trans studies in the humanities: that the movement toward an aligned hormonal and subjective identity is necessarily one of progress. A possible solution is found in the novel's style: its "generic blending" promotes alternative kinds of "wide-ranging and ever-becoming narratives," in keeping with the realities of "mutable forms" of living bodies.

The final chapter in the collection, by Fenton-Hathaway, highlights the proliferation of "dystopia" as a term to describe elements of the real world and the utility of these applications, begging the question: "Whose dystopia?" The chapter traces the widespread circulation of the term throughout healthcare contexts, where it is used freely, and in the health humanities scholarly literature, where it is cited in the context of teaching. Dystopia is invoked, Fenton-Hathaway argues, in order to produce a "fear appeal" that serves a social purpose. Yet, the rhetorical power of the genre is dulled by critical and pedagogical readings that "tether" dystopian fictions to the familiar problems of the contemporary world—a blunting of the imagination that paradoxically leads to the acceptance of troubling realities. As health humanities scholars become more interested in dystopia as a teachable genre, Fenton-Hathaway's essay makes the case for a formal (in addition to a thematic) analysis of dystopian works, and ultimately to the possibility of reading genres *besides* the dystopia. In cautiously elaborating on the potential for speculative fiction to offer an alternative to the structures of biomedicine and medical knowledge, these chapters posit a need for greater curiosity and attention to developing genres. Medicine, health, and illness might be reimagined, they argue, through an attention to how literary studies engages readers around disquieting possibilities for human life and health.

10

Against "Endochronology": Hormonal Rebellion and Generic Blending in *Confessions of the Fox*

Diana Rose Newby

Alchemy is both form and content in Jordy Rosenberg's *Confessions of the Fox*. A novel that combines and thus remakes multiple generic traditions, *Confessions* also tells a story about other kinds of creative, metamorphic plurality. It's a story about fluid and excessive embodiments that resist the reductive logics of "endochronology," Rosenberg's (2018) neologism for the "progress narrative of the alignment of sex hormones and subjectivity."[1] This resistance expresses itself most obviously through the novel's protagonist and eponymous fox, Jack Sheppard, a real-life eighteenth-century thief and prison-breaker whom Rosenberg reimagines as an intersex and transgender man. The fictionalized Sheppard navigates his status as sexual "chimera"—a common term for intersex persons in the early eighteenth century, when Rosenberg's central story takes place—by imbibing a mysterious "serum,"[2] a fictional early modern version of exogenous testosterone. Yet Sheppard's is not the only act of hormonal rebellion in *Confessions*: a crew of female pirates, who establish "a Maroon Society of Freebooters" in the Western Pacific, are identified as the serum's original creators and consumers.[3] Their invention is apparently motivated not by the pirates' desire (in twenty-first century terms) to transition altogether, but rather by their interest in communal gender and sexual play—the fun of taking on some of the physical attributes of "grizzled coves," and of feeling more "Free and Liberated with each other," erotically and otherwise.[4] In the cases of both Sheppard and

---

[1] Jordy Rosenberg, *Confessions of the Fox* (New York: One World, 2018), 301.
[2] Ibid., 215.
[3] Ibid., 214.
[4] Ibid., 215, 216.

the pirates, Rosenberg's novel presents examples of recalcitrant bodily practices that reject culturally and medically normative models of sexual subjectivity. And these practices find their parallels in the novel's form, which blends the scientific and the supernatural, speculative historical fiction and auto-theory,[5] history of medicine and the drug novel, criminal confession and carceral critique. Much like the pirates' serum, the text of *Confessions* is a compound that transforms in order to resist the many traditions from which it both draws and departs.

This chapter reads the alchemical serum as a figure that consolidates hormonal rebellion and generic blending in Rosenberg's work. To trace this connection, I situate *Confessions* at the intersection of contemporary hormone studies, gender and sexuality studies, and the new materialisms, a critical juncture where scholars have theorized not only bodies but also sex hormones themselves as "material-semiotic actors" that play a complex and critical role in the biomedical and political maintenance of sexual difference.[6] Although sex hormones have long been recruited to essentializing narratives of human behavior and identity, their actual activity tends to undermine those narratives: in its material expression, testosterone in fact blurs the binary division of sex that Western culture and medicine have long labored to uphold.[7] Accordingly, as Paul B. Preciado (2016) has argued, "democratizing the consumption of hormones" would force a major reckoning with the "undeniably multiple, malleable, and mutable nature of bodies and pleasure."[8] I suggest that Rosenberg's novel pursues such a reckoning in the form of the pirates' serum, whose vagrant proliferation across human bodies collapses the boundaries that artificially demarcate such dualisms as self/other, male/female, and human/nonhuman, giving shape to a view of embodied life as porous, plural, and shared.

What's more, *Confessions* destabilizes literary and disciplinary borders out of an attentiveness to the complicity of these epistemological conventions with

---

[5] Arianne Zwartjes, for one, defines autotheory as a form that "brings together autobiography with theory and a focus on situating oneself inside a larger world," in "Autotheory as Rebellion: On Research, Embodiment, and Imagination in Creative Nonfiction," *Michigan Quarterly Review* (July 23, 2019). Notably, given the aims of this chapter, Zwartjes refers to this heterogeneous genre as "the chimera of research and imagination." Recent examples include Maggie Nelson's *The Argonauts* (2015) and Paul B. Preciado's *Testo Junkie* (2016).

[6] Donna Jeanne Haraway, *Simians, Cyborgs, and Women: The Reinvention of Nature* (New York: Routledge, 1991), 200; Celia Roberts, *Messengers of Sex: Hormones, Biomedicine, and Feminism*, Cambridge Studies in Society and the Life Sciences (New York: Cambridge University Press, 2007), 19.

[7] Rebecca M. Jordan-Young and Katrina Alicia Karkazis, *Testosterone: An Unauthorized Biography* (Cambridge, MA: Harvard University Press, 2019).

[8] Paul B. Preciado, *Testo Junkie: Sex, Drugs, and Biopolitics in the Pharmacopornographic Era*, trans. Bruce Benderson (New York: The Feminist Press at the City University of New York, 2016), 230.

the often-violent management of biological sex. At the level of experimental fictional form, Rosenberg aligns the novel's readers with its fictional pirates, whose anti-endochronological and anti-biocapitalist consumption materializes an embodied heterogeneity that eschews traditional categories.[9] In so doing, Rosenberg invites us to interrogate our own consumption practices: our participation in cultural and medical narratives that might stifle and restrict, and our potential to unwrite those stories anew.

Endocrinology's Ends

The narrativization of the activity of sex hormones could be said to have begun in 1935, when testosterone was chemically isolated and named by a group of Dutch researchers. Their work helped inaugurate the "golden age of steroid chemistry"[10]—roughly 1930–50—a period during which studies of both testosterone and estrogen were exploited to account for sex differences on a molecular level. Yet, these efforts to biologically essentialize sex had their roots in much older practices. As early as 400 BCE, Aristotle claimed to have demonstrated through experiments with birds that certain "qualities of 'maleness'" could be controlled by castration.[11] Centuries later, in or around 1771,[12] the Scottish surgeon John Hunter successfully transplanted cock testes into the abdomens of hens and documented the resulting changes in the hens' physiology: effects that proved, to Hunter's mind, that "the testis is the source of the 'male factor.'"[13] And in the late nineteenth century, Mauritian neurologist and physiologist Charles Édouard Brown-Séquard (1889) conducted a series of trials—first on nonhuman animals and then on himself—to test his hypothesis that "the weakness of old men" was due in part to "the gradually diminishing action" of the "substance or substances which, being formed by the testicles, give

---

[9] Susanne Lettow defines biocapitalism as "processes of the primary valorization of materials derived from human bodies and nonhuman living beings," "the meaning of these processes for capitalist accumulation strategies," and "related transformations of modes of labour, exploitation and subjectivation," in "Biocapitalism," *Krisis*, no. 2 (2018): 13.

[10] R. S. Vardanyan and Victor J. Hruby, *Synthesis of Best-Seller Drugs* (Amsterdam: Elsevier/AP, 2016), 460.

[11] Lynn Loriaux, *A Biographical History of Endocrinology* (Ames, IA: Wiley Blackwell, 2016), 74.

[12] As T. R. Forbes explains, there are no extant records of Hunter's experiments with testis transplantation; it's assumed that these notes were destroyed by Sir Everard Home, Hunter's executor and brother-in-law. In "Testis Transplantation Performed by John Hunter," *Endocrinology* 41, no. 4 (1947): 329–31.

[13] Loriaux, A Biographical History of Endocrinology, 74.

power to the nervous centres and other parts."[14] Brown-Séquard was determined to synthesize this "substance," and his attempts culminated in "one of the most famous auto-experiments of all time": the creation of an "elixir" composed of blood, semen, and the juices from the crushed testicle of a dog or guinea-pig, and the injection of this elixir into the 72-year-old physician's own body.[15] The outcome was such that Brown-Séquard felt convinced he had lit upon a fountain of youth; in myriad ways, his former strength and vigor were temporarily restored, confirming his theory that those purportedly essential qualities of masculinity were controlled by the spermatic glands and the fluids they produce.

As this condensed chronology attests, the commonplace story of testosterone (or "T," as it's often called) has long been shaped by widely shared beliefs about what it means to be "male." Even before it was isolated, T was imagined as the very essence of ideal masculinity, of youth, power, and virility. When modern endocrinology made possible both the study and the synthesis of T, this research was always already hitched to a social myth-making machine driven by a binary and biologically determinist understanding of gender and sex. Twentieth-century sex hormone studies, as Karkazis and Jordan-Young (2019) put it, were "a closed loop, both grounded on and apparently justifying" the expectation that sex dualism has a real, material basis in the body's chemistry.[16] Accordingly, testosterone became bound up in the medical and cultural maintenance of sexed embodiment and identity; to understand, manipulate, and manufacture T was and is to control the terms of subjectivity.[17]

Confessions locates itself within a loosely fictionalized version of this hormonal history. In both its motivation and its results, the invention of the pirates' serum shares common ground with Brown-Séquard's auto-experiment. Not unlike Brown-Séquard, the pirates hope to enhance their physical brawn; they "admired the swine," which they raised in their Maroon Society, for the pigs' "especial Meatiness"; and using swine urine, they create a "serum" that made the pirates "thicken similarly."[18] After their settlement is raided by the East India Company, however, the pirates' serum falls into the hands of Jonathan Wild, another real-life figure from the early eighteenth century: a self-fashioned "Thief-Taker General" who helped fight London's crime at the same time that he ran his

---

[14] Charles-Édouard Brown-Séquard, "Note on the Effects Produced on Man by Subcutaneous Injections of a Liquid Obtained from the Testicles of Animals," *The Lancet* 134, no. 3438 (July 20, 1889): 105, https://doi.org/10.1016/S0140-6736(00)64118-1.
[15] Jordan-Young and Karkazis, *Testosterone*, 7.
[16] Ibid., 6.
[17] Preciado, *Testo Junkie*.
[18] Rosenberg, *Confessions of the Fox*, 215.

own underworld empire. Rosenberg's fictionalized Wild sets about remaking the serum using "the nasty bits of the world's most famous rogues"[19]—that is, the testicles of incarcerated men, to whom he has access through the penal industry that he helps populate. His macabre methodology brings together the castration and transplantation experiments of Hunter with the early twentieth-century eugenics of Leo L. Stanley, who conducted or supervised thousands of testicular implantations on inmates at San Quentin Prison.[20] Motivated by the belief that an ideal masculinity is materially discoverable in the bodies of ideally masculine men, Wild emblematizes a long tradition of institutionally coordinated violence in service of establishing sex dualism as a social and medical fact. In short, his is the history of "endochronology," a tradition of discourse and praxis leveraging T toward the maintenance of a reductive model of sexual identity.

Further, Wild's plan to market the serum as a "Granulated Strength Elixir" that endows the drinker with roguish "Vitality"[21] encapsulates the capitalist thrust of sex hormone studies in their mainstream form. In the novel's reimagined early modern context, Rosenberg locates a fictional antecedent for the more contemporary phenomenon that Preciado has described as the "regular trafficking networks of biological materials among gynecologists, laboratory researchers, pharmaceutical industries, prisons, and slaughterhouses."[22] Today, these are the biocapitalist "networks" that commodify and transmit synthetic T as part of a larger "apparatus ... of subjectification"[23]: the ongoing, systemic production of the hormonal self. Through the character of Wild, *Confessions* gives shape to two interconnected facets of this apparatus, highlighting the collusion of medical and carceral institutions in the management of the self as such.

Moreover, in the novel's frame narrative, Rosenberg suggests the complicity of academia in the pharmaceutical industry's commodification of both sex hormones and the sexed body. This fictional layer is composed of the textual "annotations" of one Dr. Voth, a contemporary scholar of the eighteenth century who has recovered what appears to be Jack Sheppard's memoir—the "confessions" that form the novel's primary narrative—from the library archives of the university where he teaches. After obtaining the Sheppardian manuscript, Dr. Voth finds himself at the center of a scheme contrived by his university's

---

[19] Ibid., 296-7.
[20] Jordan-Young and Karkazis, *Testosterone*.
[21] Rosenberg, *Confessions of the Fox*, 294.
[22] Preciado, *Testo Junkie*, 163.
[23] Ibid., 161.

"Dean of Surveillance"[24] and the marketing director of an organization called P-Quad Publishers and Pharmaceuticals, who together plan to market the manuscript as "the earliest authentic confessional transgender memoirs in Western history"[25] alongside an "organic, humane, bioidentical open-source testosterone."[26] Structurally, *Confessions* draws an implicit connection between the biocapitalist machinations of P-Quad and Wild, establishing each figure at either pole of a timeline that begins and ends with the "scientific Management of the body" for political and economic gain.[27]

The forces of biocapitalism engender a pivotal tension in the manuscript's narrative, as Sheppard's desire to transform his body through consumption of the pirates' serum comes into ideological conflict with Wild's grisly methods and coercive intentions for reproducing the drug. When Sheppard begins regularly consuming the stolen serum, he becomes fairly addicted, thrilled by its unifying, enlivening effects on his body and attendant sense of self. Yet, Sheppard's girlfriend and coconspirator, Bess Khan, recognizes the danger of preserving the serum, which Wild will use, as she puts it, to "finance and embolden his entire factory of Policing."[28] For Rosenberg's eighteenth-century characters and contemporary readers alike, this conflict raises important questions: What are the political and ethical tradeoffs of consuming sex hormones that have been produced by a system whose aims are to subjugate bodies and accumulate capital? And what are the possibilities for modes of production and consumption that circumvent or even obstruct this system's control? The answer to the second of these questions, in particular, is made available in the rebellious activity of the pirates' original serum, which gives expression to the indiscriminate and vagrant agency of T, allowing the hormone to tell a new story about sex, selfhood, and community.

Becoming Vagrant

The story of the pirates' serum begins with the pirates themselves, whose short subplot only occupies a handful of pages in *Confessions*, but whose semiotic force is central to the novel's biocapitalist critique. After overtaking an East

---

[24] Rosenberg, *Confessions of the Fox*, 119.
[25] Ibid., 122.
[26] Ibid., 121.
[27] Ibid., 138.
[28] Ibid., 223.

India Company ship called the *Katherine* off the coast of India, the pirates are joined by mutinying members of the *Katherine*'s crew, who "swear Allegiance to piracy" and enthusiastically agree to form "the new Freebooter society."[29] At least through the late eighteenth century, "freebooter" was a common term for pirates or "any person who goes about in search of plunder."[30] In *Confessions*, however, the word accrues fresh valences from the founding mission of the pirates' society: once they join forces with the mutineers, their shared goal simply becomes "living free of the East India Company."[31] For the newly formed crew, such freedom translates not to a life of "plundering"—which was precisely the project of the East India Company itself—but rather to fully renouncing the political and economic trappings of empire. This objective takes them to the Java Sea, where they throw anchor "far from any coast" and establish a fully self-sufficient community in which "everything was held in common and every soul Valu'd and loved,"[32] from "the female pirates, some Anglo Englishmen, several Tahitian Islanders, Africans, French Protestants, and lascars," to "a small Band of chickens and swine they had liberated from a Dutch ship (cautious to escort off only those animals who walked willingly alongside, not wanting to 'press-gang' any creatures into labor)."[33] In short, the Freebooter commons is an anti-capitalist utopia. Here, the terms of subjectivity aren't contingent on production or conducive to alienation; instead, labor is given freely; the fruits of that labor—including the serum—are widely and equally enjoyed, and inhabitants of all races and even species are granted equal value and the right to be loved.

These tenets of social equity and nonviolence find material expression in the creation of the pirates' serum. Whereas Wild's "Granulated Strength Elixir" is a product of biocapitalist brutality against human bodies, the pirates' serum has a very different origin. It's made not from the genitals of executed men, or even from those of murdered or tortured nonhuman animals, but through a "Subtle" and anodyne process that the pirates develop after "many gentle Experiments with the animals and plants" that also hold membership in the peaceful society.[34] The pirates first learn to distill swine urine with fruit pectin in order to form a "stiff jelly," to which they then apply "a complex combination of herbs, fruits,

---

[29] Ibid., 213, 214.
[30] "Freebooter, n.," in *OED Online* (Oxford University Press), accessed April 26, 2021, http://www.oed.com/view/Entry/74384.
[31] Rosenberg, *Confessions of the Fox*, 214.
[32] Ibid.
[33] Ibid., 214. As it's used in the Sheppardian manuscript, "lascar" refers to any person of South Asian descent; more traditionally, it designated "a South Asian sailor in service to the East India Company," in ibid., 27.
[34] Ibid., 215.

mashing Techniques, and an ineffable *Something else:* exposure to certain strains of Starlight."[35] A benign and natural procedure, it also verges on the absurd. The fifth step in the process, for example, requires that the creator "mash together 4 ounces (or thereabouts) liquorice and parsley root" with a variety of other ingredients "and place in a pot covered with swine milk harvested through a gentle coaxing that involves the adept Imitation of baby swinedom by the smallest Member of the community, mewling and crawling about," an operation for which "some training in baby swine Thespianship may be necessary."[36] Clearly, Rosenberg is having fun here, but the playfulness serves a point. As originally conceived, the recipe is "frankly Inimitable"[37]: at once bloodless and irrational, it can't be replicated according to standard scientific practices.

Through the indefinite and fanciful language of the serum recipe, the novel offers an incisive epistemic critique. *Confessions* takes place toward the tail end of Europe's Scientific Revolution, a period during which the precepts of the scientific method were refined and entrenched. Among the method's axioms is the insistence that experimentation should rely on precise measurements and reproducible techniques—two rules to which the free-wheeling pirates obviously don't adhere. In its "inimitability," the serum thus eschews the conventional mode of knowledge production in the Western sciences, at the same time that it materializes a more intimate and yet more capacious epistemology: a way of knowing by noticing, hesitating, feeling, and becoming. Making the serum requires recognizing that the swine "are very fond of rubbing their hindquarters" on "the Amorphophallus plant" and collecting the swine's urine when it is accidentally deposited in the flower's "deep pockets," rather than attempting to "extort the swine of their urine by force."[38] It involves sensing, not calculating, the sufficient weight of "several" ounces of this urine, in combination with "handfuls" of leaves, twigs, and "white lily flowers, bruised."[39] And it demands imitating "baby swinedom," possibly to the point of being nursed by a sow. It's an altogether messy, intuitive, and boundary-crossing enterprise, collapsing the flimsy limits that separate both animal from plant (as the swine masturbate with *Amorphophallus titanium*, or the so-called corpse flower, whose carrion-scented flesh is coupled with a markedly phallic spadix and a meat-hued spathe) and human animal from nonhuman animal (as the pirates perform as newborn pigs).

[35] Ibid.
[36] Ibid., 312.
[37] Ibid., 313.
[38] Ibid., 311.
[39] Ibid., 312.

It's worth stressing here that the creative intention behind the pirates' serum is about more than mere animal performance. In Rosenberg's phrasing, the pirates "admired the swine" and "wished to thicken similarly"—in other words, to become truly swinelike, not merely in behavior but at the level of embodied being. The pirates' serum thus enacts an ontological as well as an epistemological break with Enlightenment-era scientific orthodoxy. Against the prevailing trends of natural history, which increasingly dedicated its efforts to taxonomizing plant and animal life, both the process and the product of the serum give rise to bodily experiences and identities that defy easy categorization. As Gilles Deleuze and Felix Guattari write in *A Thousand Plateaus* (1980), natural history was intently preoccupied with the question of how to understand "the relationships between animals," and its primary approach to this question was to think in terms of "the sum and value of differences," the qualities that distinguish one animal from another according to "series and structure."[40] What Deleuze and Guattari propose instead—and what the pirates' serum also invokes—is an ontology of becoming: an understanding of life as characterized by the passage of affective intensities among bodies, and the ongoing, mutual transformations that this passage stimulates.[41] From this perspective, life can't be classified according to distinctions and differences; rather, it can only be understood in terms of affinities and reciprocities, the zones that are contiguous and shared. "Becoming," they suggest, "is to extract particles between which one establishes the relations of movement and rest, speed and slowness that are closest to what one is becoming, and through which one becomes."[42] Put another way, becoming is necessarily "molecular," involving the very real communication of particulate matter across the porous boundaries of living forms, an exchange that takes place on the basis of both proximity and desire.[43] We become, that is, through contact with the bodies close to ours, and through sheer longing for those bodies. Longing to be them, to be *with* them: an indistinguishable continuum.

A version of Deleuzian ontology gains purchase not only in the practical procedure that brings the pirates' serum into being but also in the serum's

---

[40] Gilles Deleuze and Felix Guattari, *A Thousand Plateaus: Capitalism and Schizophrenia*, trans. Brian Massumi (Minneapolis: University of Minnesota Press, [1980] 2005), 234.

[41] The frame narrative of *Confessions* makes explicit the Deleuzian influence that runs implicitly throughout the novel's main narrative. Although Voth does not draw directly on Deleuze and Guattari's formulation of becoming, he does discuss at length their adjacent concept of the body without organs, which Voth interprets in the following terms: "Making love is not really about getting your organs serviced. Rather, when you're making love, the organs that have been forced into [an] Oedipal narrative get *rearranged*" (ibid., 203).

[42] Deleuze and Guattari, A Thousand Plateaus, 272.

[43] Ibid.

impact on the Maroon Society. Both politically and erotically, enhanced freedom of being and behavior follows the serum's integration into the daily life of the community, suggesting an increased blurring of social, sexed, and sexual boundaries between the bodies of its inhabitants. In the erasure of difference that it yields, the serum helps the pirates realize their aspirations toward a radical model of political subjectivity, which replaces the traditional Western notion of a single, self-contained subject with a more dispersed and multitudinous understanding of identity. Much of what makes the recipe "Inimitable" is that it singularly derives from the group's synergistic energies, drawing on the "collective knowledge" produced by the pirates through their work as "eager amateur Scientists," astronomers, farmers, and gardeners.[44] The serum and its effects are thus material manifestations of a multiplicity of bodies brought into close, productive proximity by their mutual desire for new forms of knowing and being in the world—for "fragmented and fugitive" approaches to individual and social existence,[45] ways of being in "excess" of the biocapitalist institutions that manage human life.[46] We might call it a desire for vagrancy: a common term in the early modern context, and one that recurs throughout *Confessions*, designating bodies that can't or won't be bound by normative social and legal protocols.[47] Through the pirates, Rosenberg evokes a Deleuzian reclamation of vagrancy in spite or perhaps *because* of its criminal connotations. To be vagrant, in this sense, is to be undisciplined and uncontained—to exceed the boundaries of institutions, of individual bodies, of all restrictive categories.

Vagrancy as such crucially defines the forms of rebellion that the novel imagines for its protagonist. Within the world of the manuscript, the progress of Wild's plot gets thwarted not only by Sheppard's theft of the serum but also through the jail-breaker's own excessive embodiment. Near the novel's conclusion, Sheppard discovers that he is the "rogue" whose "nasty bits" Wild most ardently wants to appropriate; the latent irony of this scene, of course, emerges from the gap between what Wild believes and what the reader understands about Sheppard's sex. Although Rosenberg is careful to refuse readerly access to intimate details about his protagonist's genitalia—an authorial withholding that enacts its own

---

[44] Rosenberg, *Confessions of the Fox*, 313.
[45] Ibid., 301.
[46] Ibid., 267.
[47] In the legal language of the period, to be vagrant was to be criminally "wandering" and "idle," to "run away" from "Wives or Children," to use "subtle Craft, or unlawful Games or Plays," and to live without "any visible means of subsistence, and not giving a good account" of oneself (quotes from Rosenberg, ibid., 21). Rosenberg takes these definitions more or less word for word from Parliament's 1714 Vagrancy Act.

discursive critique—we're given enough information to know that Sheppard doesn't possess the exact anatomy that Wild has in mind.[48] Sheppard's intersex and transgender status accordingly shores up the tendency of real, living bodies to exceed the strictures of a biocapitalist model that takes sex dualism as its premise: a tendency to be, or to become, multiple things at once.

The motif of vagrant excess is further realized in the novel's conclusion, as Sheppard and Bess escape London for the wild Fenlands of Eastern England, where they plan to found a new utopian society and remake the serum based on the pirates' recipe.[49] Their flight parallels the vagrancy of Voth, who leaves town with the Sheppardian manuscript in order to obstruct P-Quad's marketing scheme. He joins a secret community dedicated to archiving the stories of those whose bodies and lives have transcended sexual categories—including the stories of both Sheppard and Voth, who is also intersex and trans. And in another utopian gesture, the location of this community turns out to be a literally otherworldly library that exists in a different space and "at a different timescale" than ours[50]; in this place known as "the Stretches," its inhabitants document "the history of how we exceeded our own limits,"[51] producing "fragmented and fugitive" narratives that balk the reductive logics of endochronology. The novel thus cements the affinities between Sheppard and Voth through this formally paired achievement of rebellious vagrancy. With and through their unbounded bodies, both characters exceed their own limits, effectively resisting the medical and cultural structures that discipline and contain.

Undisciplining the Academy

At the same time that it tightly aligns the vagrancy of Sheppard and Voth, *Confessions* also amplifies the symbolic resonance between the pirates' serum and the Sheppardian manuscript itself. As Voth slowly discovers, "there is no

---

[48] Rosenberg's discretion on this subject pointedly rejects a long tradition of medical writing about intersex anatomy, which has been repeatedly subjected to invasive and often violent scrutiny in both clinical and narrative treatments. See, for example, the medical dossier appended to the memoir of nineteenth-century French intersex person: Michel Foucault, ed., *Herculine Barbin: Being the Recently Discovered Memoirs of a Nineteenth-Century French Hermaphrodite*, trans. Richard McDougall, vintage books ed. (New York: Pantheon Books, [1980] 2010).

[49] It's worth noting that the Fenlands present another variation on the novel's recurring themes of boundary-crossing and blurred taxonomies: the Fens are marshland, ecologically rich and wild, where land and water intermix indistinguishably, and where mired dead plant matter never fully decays.

[50] Rosenberg, *Confessions of the Fox*, 266.

[51] Ibid., 267.

(one) body" in the "archive" of the confessions, and "no one subject either"[52]; far from a typical memoir, the manuscript is a work of "collective diary-keeping,"[53] a communal palimpsest produced by many writers over many years. In one chapter, for instance, Voth recognizes a passage from an 1872 speech by Frederick Douglass attributed to a surviving member of the Freebooter Society. This instance of anachronistic narrative pastiche recalls for Voth a past conversation with a former graduate student, who hinted at her participation in a movement to "decolonize" texts "under ownership of university libraries" by editing and revising them.[54] Voth suspects that the Sheppardian manuscript is one of those texts "improved upon" through this practice,[55] a theory that would help explain the ahistorical addition of the Douglass quote. Moreover, after Voth takes up residence in the so-called Stretches, he learns about a group named the "'CEO' (Chimera Emancipation Organization, 1977–1990, approx.)," which carried out a similar "decolonizing" project that specifically sought to remedy the representation of intersex persons in academic literature.[56] Speculating that the manuscript bears the traces of the CEO's touch as well, Voth registers the impossibility of determining which scenes are "original to the text"[57] and which were added after its initial composition: a realization that explodes his scholarly commitment to establishing the document's authenticity as *the* Sheppardian memoir. Just as there is no one subject, so, too, is there no one author; the manuscript, like the serum, is a multiplicity.

In stressing the multiauthored status of the fictional Sheppardian manuscript, Rosenberg calls attention to the multitudinous nature of the novel itself. A plurality of subjects and authors comprises *Confessions*, its layered narrative a crowded patchwork of literary allusions and scholarly intertexts; "P-Quad," for one, clearly nods to *Pequod*, Captain Ahab's whaling ship in Herman Melville's *Moby Dick*, while the motley crew of Rosenberg's Maroon Society draws implicit inspiration from Peter Linebaugh and Marcus Rediker's (2000) *The Many-Headed Hydra: Sailors, Slaves, Commoners, and the Hidden History of the Revolutionary Atlantic*. According to certain metrics, this heterogeneous and frequently pedagogic form might be considered a stylistic shortcoming, as it prevents the novel from cohering into a neatly linear story and around natural-seeming characters. Elisabeth Sheffield (2019) suggests as much in her review

---

[52] Ibid., 259.
[53] Ibid.
[54] Ibid., 261.
[55] Ibid..
[56] Ibid., 268.
[57] Ibid.

of *Confessions*, noting that both Sheppard and his girlfriend Bess "feel rather like didactic avatars, or criticocartoons, for Voth's theoretical inclinations."[58] This is an especially apt description of Bess, who is given to jarringly modern pronouncements on a range of subjects, from biocapitalism to discipline and punishment. In one scene that will feel prescient for contemporary readers, Bess addresses a crowded pub on the social consequences of epidemic, vainly attempting to persuade her comparatively obtuse audience that the state is using plague to raise "a *securitizational furor*" in order "to police us further."[59]

It strikes me as fully in line with Rosenberg's critical project, however, that his subjects don't achieve strict verisimilitude but instead help to constellate the novel's many ideological strands. By making Bess the mouthpiece for multiple "theoretical inclinations," Rosenberg enacts another version of the transhistorical pastiche whereby he attributes the words of Frederick Douglass to a fictional "freeloader." Further, he prompts readers to interrogate the assumptions that might lead us to view the character and the beliefs of someone like Bess— namely, a woman of color and a sex worker—as necessarily anachronistic. A work of radical historical and political rewriting in the vein of *The Many-Headed Hydra* and *The Undercommons*,[60] *Confessions* presents an exploration of alternative possibilities, of the stories that very well might have been, beyond the purview of too-narrow chronologies. With both Bess and Sheppard, Rosenberg presents not single characters but what we might call archives: a term that Voth, paraphrasing the French philosopher Jacques Derrida, defines as "less a record of what has been said, and more an ongoing problem of what cannot be."[61] Approaching the novel as an archive in the Derridean sense highlights the political significance of plurality for Rosenberg. Becoming multiple in authorship and in form has clear decolonial implications, insofar as it opposes the canonizing structures of academic epistemology, which are traditionally shaped by logics of individualism, competition, and hierarchy. Rosenberg shows us this opposition not only in the Sheppardian manuscript, which radically revises the standard account of its protagonist's embodied life and identity, but also in the polyvocal and multigeneric texture of *Confessions* as a whole. The novel itself is an archive, host to a multiplicity of stories that have been "forgotten, repressed,

---

[58] Elisabeth Sheffield, "An Uneven Luxuriance," *American Book Review* 40, no. 6 (2019): 18, https://doi.org/10.1353/abr.2019.0102.
[59] Rosenberg, *Confessions of the Fox*, 117, original emphasis.
[60] Stefano Harney and Fred Moten, in *The Undercommons: Fugitive Planning & Black Study* (New York: Minor Compositions, 2013), critically assess the history, structures, and praxes of the academy through the lens of the Black radical tradition.
[61] Rosenberg, *Confessions of the Fox*, 84.

disallowed" by the standard narratives that literary history tells.[62] Through its superabundance of representational modes, *Confessions* provides an aesthetic model for its own anti-endochronological politics of multiplicity.

In formalist terms, some literary critics might feel tempted to call this model "hybrid," a now-classic term for texts in which "elements of two or more genres are combined," sometimes "to form a new genre or subgenre" altogether.[63] Yet, the concept of generic hybridity is riddled with notable limitations, both in application to *Confessions* and more generally. As Martina Allen has pointed out, hybridity has its roots in a discourse of genetics that maintains a view of biological classifications as essentially fixed. According to this discourse, a hybrid organism does not "undermine or even explode traditional categories," but instead is readily "integrated into … a place between the two parental species," effectively reinforcing "the existing taxonomical system."[64] Hence hybridity's problematic place in colonial discourses, where it was long used to define racial identity in ways that reasserted the hierarchical distinction "between colonizer and colonized."[65] To these crucial objections, I would add that "hybrid" has historically been used as a pejorative for intersex persons in medical literature,[66] further affirming Allen's observation that hybridity relies on "a binary, essentialist model" of biological identity.[67] In these ways, the term represents much of what Rosenberg's novel actively works to resist, and it also falls short as a label for literary works in a broader sense. Although systems of classification such as the academic canon might suggest otherwise, we would be hard-pressed to fit many fictional texts into rigid taxonomies. Much like the living body, the novel is always already a porous, heterogeneous form—and language itself is nothing if not alchemical.

A more appropriate descriptor for *Confessions*, I propose, is generic blending, which Allen offers up as an alternative to hybridity. "Blending" avoids essentialist pitfalls by privileging "process" over "artefact," training our focus on what a text is doing and how, rather than diagnosing what a text "is."[68] To think in terms of blending is also to recognize generic mixing as a phenomenon that

---

[62] Ibid.
[63] David Duff, "Key Concepts," in *Modern Genre Theory*, ed. David Duff, Longman Critical Readers (Oxfordshire: Routledge, 2000), xiv.
[64] Martin Allen, "Against 'Hybridity' in Genre Studies: Blending as an Alternative Approach to Generic Experimentation," *Trespassing Journal* 2 (2013): 5.
[65] Ibid., 7.
[66] Elizabeth Reis, "Divergence or Disorder? The Politics of Naming Intersex," *Perspectives in Biology and Medicine* 50, no. 4 (2007): 535–43, https://doi.org/10.1353/pbm.2007.0054.
[67] Allen, "Against 'Hybridity' in Genre Studies," 8.
[68] Ibid., 12.

regularly occurs in plural and "partial" ways, and which is often "unobtrusive" and "covert," only noted when attention is called to it, or when it calls attention to itself.[69] It's thus a fitting framework for appraising both the structure and the content of *Confessions*, a novel that self-reflexively indexes at the level of narrative form its investment in becoming vagrant, its recuperation of bodies at once plural and partial, its reveling in the playful, messy blendings of life. "The body is written," Voth reflects, "(like a book is written)—or rewritten—in the process of making love"[70]: an active process of combining with other bodies, other possibilities, in mutually transformative exchange. By calling attention to its own excessive, endlessly processural textuality, Rosenberg's work offers a "frankly Inimitable" but nonetheless vital recipe for experimental storytelling— for new epistemologies that intentionally leverage the praxes and politics of generic blending toward more generous ways of knowing, and therefore being, in the world.

Such experiments, I would venture, include the transdisciplinary work of the health humanities. A nascent field that continues to resist neat classification, the health humanities productively chafe against the adjacent province of the medical humanities, which we might call "hybrid" inasmuch as it has tended to preserve disciplinary organization by generally centering medicine. In contrast, the health humanities' motivating project is one of "inclusiveness and expansiveness."[71] Arguably giving precedence to neither medicine nor the humanities, the discourse at once combines and interrogates the two methodologies, working to undiscipline some of the conventions that structure and contain academic work. In turn, and as with *Confessions*, this self-reflexively blended genre enables less bounded, more wide-ranging, and ever-becoming narratives. Under the rubrics of the health humanities, space can be made for new stories about living bodies, in all their vagrant experiences and multiple, mutable forms.

---

[69] Ibid.
[70] Rosenberg, *Confessions of the Fox*, 203.
[71] Therese Jones, Delese Wear, and Lester D. Friedman, "Introduction: The Why, the What, and the How of the Medical/Health Humanities," in *Health Humanities Reader*, ed. Therese Jones, Delese Wear, and Lester D. Friedman (New Brunswick, NJ: Rutgers University Press, 2014), 7.

11

Whose Dystopia?

Anna Fenton-Hathaway

Emergency physician Leana Wen is a research professor of health policy and management at George Washington University Milken School of Public Health, and a public health advocate appearing frequently on news programs. She has also served as the Health Commissioner for the City of Baltimore (2015–18) and the president/CEO of Planned Parenthood (2018–19). After a research trip assessing the health system in China, Wen delivered a TEDx talk in 2014 titled "Liberty, Democracy, Equity and Justice in Health Care." The title of a spinoff article in *Psychology Today*, however, more closely matched the talk's framing: "What Does a Health Care Dystopia Look Like?"

"Imagine a world," Wen opens—"a *different* world. Your eight-year-old daughter has diabetes. She needs one shot of insulin a day, but you can only afford one shot a week. She has a seizure. You bring her to the hospital, but they turn her away because you're $5.00 short."[1] In the same world, she continues, "If you have lots of money, you can get just about anything you want. An MRI or two, no problem. A kidney? That can be managed too."[2] According to Wen, this dystopic world "is China today"—and unless we change course here in the United States, she warns, this is exactly where we're headed.[3]

Wen's overt call to action evokes Rob McAlear's rhetorical model of dystopia, in which dystopian fiction employs "what rhetoricians call a 'fear appeal' in an attempt to persuade their readers of the necessity of intervention in the present to avoid the possible horrors of the future."[4] In this essay I grant that *dystopia*—both

---

[1] My warm thanks to Arden Hegele, Anna Terwiel, Dan Gleason, Mary J. Dudas, and Sara V. Press for their insightful comments on early drafts of this essay.
Leana Wen, *Liberty, Democracy, Equity, and Justice in Healthcare*, TEDx video (University of Nevada, 2014), 00:19–00:39.
[2] Ibid., 01:12–01:23.
[3] Ibid., 02:45–02:54.
[4] Rob McAlear, "The Value of Fear: Toward a Rhetorical Model of Dystopia," *Interdisciplinary Humanities* 27, no. 2 (2010): 24.

the literary genre and its invocation in commentary like Wen's—has political expedience. In recent years, for instance, reproductive rights groups across the United States have staged protests in costumes out of Margaret Atwood's (and Hulu's) *The Handmaid's Tale*.[5] When an advisor to President Donald Trump claimed the right to "alternative facts" in 2017, American citizens ran to George Orwell's *Nineteen Eighty-Four*.[6] And Ayn Rand's *Atlas Shrugged* has been a touchstone and a motivation for American libertarians for decades, credited with inspiring new candidates for office during the Obama administration in particular, when sales of the book rose sharply.[7] Yet, I also see evidence of a new response to dystopia, one that is the phenomenological opposite of what McAlear's rhetorical form intends. This reaction perceives the dystopic "future" as something that is already regrettably, perhaps even infuriatingly, happening— to others—at some distance from the reader herself. That is, readers may be approaching dystopias as veiled versions of the known rather than as harbingers of the "new," an approach that blunts the impact of the fear appeal. Drawing on insights into the dystopia genre from McAlear, Lyman Tower Sargent, Tom Moylan, and Raffaella Baccolini, I seek to demonstrate this peculiar groove of reader response and explore its possible causes.

Identifying this kind of reader response is newly useful in a health humanities context following arguments such as Phillip Barrish's "Health Policy in Dystopia" (2016), Tod Chambers's "Eating One's Friends: Fiction as Argument in Bioethics," also from 2016, and Evie Kendal's 2018 "Utopian Literature and Bioethics: Exploring Reproductive Difference and Gender Equality." In his essay, Barrish names three fictional dystopias "defined by issues of health care access, distribution and funding" that "offer fresh, unexpected vantage points on our own ... collective health care 'story,'" and which help crystallize the "possibilities as well as difficulties involved in effecting structural reform in a health care system with many moving parts."[8] Barrish is careful to distinguish the dystopic texts that are useful in this regard, however, and this care is exhibited as well by Chambers and Kendal. Indeed, one of Kendal's key insights concerns text selection. She argues that bioethicists overrely on a reductive version of Aldous Huxley's *Brave New World* (1932) in debates on technologies that would enable

---

[5] Christine Hauser, "A Handmaid's Tale of Protest," *New York Times* (June 30, 2017), sec. U.S., https://www.nytimes.com/2017/06/30/us/handmaids-protests-abortion.html.
[6] Michael Schaub, "Not an 'Alternative Fact': George Orwell's *1984* Tops Amazon's Bestseller List," *Los Angeles Times* (January 25, 2017), sec. Books.
[7] George Will, "Running Not Shrugging," *Townhall* (May 27, 2010), https://townhall.com/columnists/georgewill/2010/05/27/running-not-shrugging-n1064485.
[8] Phillip Barrish, "Health Policy in Dystopia," *Literature and Medicine* 34, no. 1 (2016): 106, 126–7.

fetal gestation outside the female body (or "ectogenesis"), contrasting how often Huxley's dystopia is name-checked in such discussions—259—to the number of times Marge Piercy's 1976 feminist utopia *Woman on the Edge of Time*, which depicts such technologies as enabling gender equality, appears—seven. This disparity, Kendal concludes, produces a disproportionately negative view of ectogenesis and its potential social effects.

Chambers's choice of generically unsettling speculative fiction—all with dystopic elements, none canonical—further supports Kendal's argument about text selection. According to Chambers, who recommends using speculative rather than realist fiction in ethics and literature and medicine courses, "in many ways it is the extreme anti-realist examples that stand to help bioethics most."[9] These arguments share a fundamental question: What genres or texts will be most pedagogically, ethically, or practically effective for bioethics or policy deliberations? In all three, dystopia demands consideration as a viable answer.

These discussions predate the SARS-CoV-2 pandemic, of course. In April 2020, Iro Filippaki placed this question in our new context:

> As I teach narrative medicine in the midst of Covid-19, I've come to realize that to address urgency, which is a constant in the work of healthcare teams, we need to teach texts that re-create a sense of urgency in the classroom. Although it has been argued that exposure to narrative medicine and storytelling in particular improves working conditions, teaches empathy, and ultimately makes "better doctors," recent events show clearly that perhaps we also need to ask what kind of text would enable physicians and nurses to better understand and work within increasingly *illiberal* surroundings.
>
> In short: what do we have to gain by convincing medical schools to shelve William Carlos Williams' collected works, and instead teach (distinctly non-medical) texts like Melville's "Bartleby the Scrivener"?[10]

Though Filippaki does not advocate specifically for the use of dystopias, as Barrish does, she joins him, Chambers, and Kendal in seeking texts that will produce both new insights about healthcare and a specific affect (in this case urgency) in their readers. Understanding and anticipating currents of reader response that might short-circuit those effects is thus worthwhile. Such an understanding would enable physicians like Dr. Wen to make more compelling appeals for changes to our healthcare system, help medical educators to select

---

[9] Tod Chambers, "Eating One's Friends: Fiction as Argument in Bioethics," *Literature and Medicine* 34, no. 1 (2016): 102.
[10] Iro Filippaki, "COVID-19 and the Future of Narrative Medicine," *SYNAPSIS* (April 1, 2020).

more powerful texts for their students to engage with, and, in the case of dystopia at least, free readers to seek out other genres with which to make sense of the world.

Imagining Real Worlds

In her TEDx talk, Wen states outright her aim in using dystopia rhetoric. But except for her opening cue—that the world she asks us to imagine is necessarily a "different" one—my first reaction to the talk is not one of fear but one of identification. Aren't some of these scenarios already happening in the United States? True, an emergency room would be unlikely to turn away a young girl experiencing a seizure—but not having enough money to buy the proper course of medicine seems more than plausible. (A quick search for "assistance with the cost of insulin" turns up numerous hits, a patchwork of organizations offering help that bespeaks a widespread problem of affordability; an American Diabetes Association working group on the rising out-of-pocket costs of insulin confirms the problem.[11]) Wen's chain of logic linking wealth to access to higher-quality care and/or overutilization, too, feels less like a specter than an absolute fact of American life.

In the early part of the talk, before the revelation that this different world is contemporary China, Wen asks her audience what world *they* are imagining, anticipating that "the cynics among us will say that this mess is health care in the U.S." In this answer, we see her awareness of the response she wants to avoid. In its position—the first of several responses she ventriloquizes—we see her awareness of its likelihood.

To better understand the tradition Wen's "healthcare dystopia" draws on, it is useful to touch on dystopia's history and criteria. The term "utopia" was originally coined by Thomas More in the sixteenth century to mean an impossibly perfect society; he created the term by combining the Greek words *ou* ("no, not") and *topos* ("place") to make "no-place," which in turn punned on the Greek *eu* or "good."[12] To describe more straightforward depictions of idealized societies and

---

[11] William T. Cefalu et al., "Insulin Access and Affordability Working Group: Conclusions and Recommendations," *Diabetes Care* 41, no. 6 (June 1, 2018): 1299–311, https://doi.org/10.2337/dci18-0019.

[12] "Utopia, s.v.," *Merriam Webster Dictionary*, accessed May 3, 2021, https://www.merriam-webster.com/dictionary/utopia; Lyman Tower Sargent, "The Three Faces of Utopianism Revisited," *Utopian Studies* 5, no. 1 (1994): 5.

avoid the irony embedded in More's term, some critics prefer the term *eutopia*. *Dystopia* simply replaces eutopia's "good" with the Greek "bad."

Of dystopia's many definitions, most resemble the capsule history above in that they depend on other categories or genres for their meaning. Dystopia is often defined relationally or extratextually; the form is widely understood to comment on the contemporaneous society of the author, for instance. Dystopia is distinguished from literary eutopia by conjuring a "terrible new world" rather than a wonderful one as its setting, although the two have been called "generic siblings" and may be aligned in their aim to shape the future (either by aspiration or prevention).[13] It is distinguished from apocalyptic or post-apocalyptic literature by its attention to organized social and political relations rather than what happens after their obliteration.[14] And it is distinguished from anti-utopia by its intention—which is not, as it is in anti-utopia, to critique any specific eutopia or utopian project or to direct suspicion toward utopianism in general.[15] This last distinction is the one that tends to get collapsed outside of the academy. In an article for the *New Yorker*, for example, the historian Jill Lepore refers approvingly to Gregory Claeys's *Dystopia: A Natural History*, yet proceeds to blur this division, one he (somewhat grudgingly) maintains. According to Claeys, "It is clear that not all dystopias are anti-utopias as such"[16]; in Lepore's summary, a modern dystopia "can be apocalyptic, or post-apocalyptic, or neither, but it has to be anti-utopian, a utopia turned upside down, a world in which people tried to build a republic of perfection only to find that they had created a republic of misery."[17] While I believe Lepore is overgeneralizing, her version of dystopia suggests one critique against their use in medical education and bioethics: it stacks the deck against change. If the very genre argues that all reformist efforts end up in ruins, why seek to improve anything?

Wen's dystopia does not participate in this kind of conservatism. It ticks dystopia's other definitional boxes, though—it encompasses social and political relations (by charting the political decisions that led China to its current healthcare system), describes that world negatively, and does not blame utopianism (in this case communism) for the problem. And while it fails to

---

[13] Raffaella Baccolini and Tom Moylan, "Introduction: Dystopias and Histories," in *Dark Horizons: Science Fiction and the Dystopian Imagination*, ed. Raffaella Baccolini and Tom Moylan (New York: Routledge, 2003), 5, 4.
[14] Gregory Claeys, *Dystopia: A Natural History: A Study of Modern Despotism, Its Antecedents, and Its Literary Diffractions* (Oxford: Oxford University Press, 2017), 270.
[15] Sargent, "The Three Faces of Utopianism Revisited," 8.
[16] Claeys, *Dystopia*, 284.
[17] Jill Lepore, "A Golden Age for Dystopian Fiction," *New Yorker* (May 29, 2017), https://www.newyorker.com/magazine/2017/06/05/a-golden-age-for-dystopian-fiction.

meet the influential definition introduced by Sargent in 1994 that dystopia is a "*non-existent* society described in considerable detail," it still insists on the term, converting reality into fiction by applying the genre's tropes.[18] One such trope is how empty language facilitates and reveals a society's deeper ills: in this vein, Wen recounts hearing a class of Chinese medical students reciting the Hippocratic Oath, but repeating their professor's name—"I, Professor Wu, ..."— instead of their own names when it was time for each to speak.[19] Another is the sinister imagery and plotlines, well explored in science fiction and Hollywood alike, summoned by the claim that "a kidney ... can be managed" as long as the price is right.

The twenty-first century use of "dystopia"-as-label has, in many ways, eclipsed the formal criteria established in the 1990s. See, for example, Cato Institute senior fellow and surgeon Jeffrey A. Singer's use of the term—and quoting of Rand—in "Toward Medical Dystopia" (2013), where the suggested dystopia results from government-led standardization and reform, or his 2020 post, cowritten with Patrick Eddington, titled "The War on Opioids: Digital Dystopia Edition."[20] On the other end of the political spectrum, the *British Medical Journal*'s GP commentator Des Spence locates "Medicine's Dystopian Future" emerging from the influence of Big Pharma.[21] In each of these cases, the dystopia in question is direct commentary on the present, with just the lightest literary dressing. Singer is particularly fond of describing a bureaucratic practice outlandishly and punctuating it with the familiar reveal: "This would form a good basis for a dystopian science fiction novel—except it's true ... [/] If all of this sounds somewhat terrifying, that's because it is."[22]

This rhetorical blending of fiction with future is not so far off from the way novelist and short-story author Junot Díaz employs the concept: "Certainly we are at peak dystopia. ... It has become, along with apocalyptic narrative, the default narrative of the generation. ... We are making the genre in which we are living."[23] Díaz may invoke literary terminology like "narrative" and "genre,"

---

[18] Sargent, "The Three Faces of Utopianism Revisited," 9, emphasis added.
[19] Wen, *Liberty, Democracy, Equity, and Justice in Healthcare*, 13:14–13:38.
[20] See Jeffrey A. Singer, "Toward Medical Dystopia," *Journal of Trauma and Acute Care Surgery* 75, no. 3 (August 31, 2013): 517–19; Jeffrey A. Singer and Patrick Eddington, "The War on Opioids: Digital Dystopia Edition," Cato Institute (June 17, 2020).
[21] See Des Spence, "Medicine's Dystopian Future," *British Medical Journal* 345, no. 7882 (November 10, 2012): 47.
[22] Singer and Eddington, "The War on Opioids."
[23] Junot Díaz and Avni Majithia-Sejpal, "Global Dystopias, Critical Dystopias: A Podcast with Junot Díaz," *BR: A Political and Literary Podcast* (October 31, 2016)

but his thrust is that "dystopia" is an extraliterary, and accurate, way to describe contemporary reality.

What I am suggesting here is that gambits like Wen's and assertions like Díaz's may be starting to produce the opposite of their intended purpose. Instead of alarming people into behavior change, that is, the ubiquity of the label "dystopia"—as well as its sometimes-dubious application—may be grooming readers to greet each new claim with a kind of rueful knowingness, if not outright resignation.

Imagination vs. Redescription

One problem with applying the label of dystopia is that, as McAlear observes, "dystopia is the possibility of redescribing *any* system as fearful."[24] This insight is a rebuke to the credibility of any one dystopia (and is supported by the recent book-buying patterns of Americans under each new presidential administration).[25] Two examples, both about policies governing end-of-life care in the United States, illustrate McAlear's point. The first centers on the Affordable Care Act's proposed reimbursement for physician discussions about the cessation of a patient's life support—and the interpretation of that prospect as creating "death panels" that assign certain populations to be euthanized.[26] "Death panels" was the term used by Sarah Palin in her August 7, 2009, "Statement on the Current Healthcare Debate," posted to Facebook. Having gained national recognition as John McCain's running mate during his unsuccessful 2008 presidential campaign, Palin used her prominence to portray "the thinking of ... president [Obama]'s health care advisor" as "Orwellian" and to pronounce: "The America I know and love is not one in which my parents or my baby with Down Syndrome will have to stand in front of Obama's 'death panel' so his bureaucrats can decide, based on a subjective judgment of their 'level of productivity in society,' whether they are worthy of health care. Such a system is downright evil."[27] Palin's claim was eventually deemed PolitiFact's "Lie of the Year"—but it nonetheless circulated

---

[24] McAlear, "The Value of Fear," 37, emphasis added.
[25] See Lauren Fields, "Why Americans Are Reading Dystopian Classics to Understand President Trump," *Deseret News* (February 5, 2017); "*Atlas Shrugged* Sets a New Record!," The Ayn Rand Institute (January 20, 2010).
[26] Angie Drobnic Holan, "PolitiFact—PolitiFact's Lie of the Year: 'Death Panels,'" *PolitiFact* (December 18, 2009), sec. National.
[27] Sarah Palin, "Statement on the Current Health Care Debate," Facebook (August 7, 2009), https://www.facebook.com/notes/sarah-palin/statement-on-the-current-health-care-debate/11385 1103434/.

widely and became, if not a Republican talking point, at least a pointed ellipsis: even if death panels themselves were a fiction, "Orwellian" agents were likely establishing a path to such things in the current legislation.[28] In an effort to sink real-world healthcare policy, Palin reached immediately for a famous writer of dystopias and an enduring dystopic trope.[29]

Palin's portrayal of an end-of-life discussion as a plot to kill off the "unproductive" is a stark example of McAlear's dystopic redescription. The next example also comes from a political struggle over healthcare, although this one contains no explicit statement that either the policy in question or its absence is "dystopic." The scene is from the 2011 documentary *How to Die in Oregon*, which follows patients and families pursuing physician-assisted dying and juxtaposes those experiences with debates about expanding the Death with Dignity Act to states beyond Oregon; the perspective it introduces invites the reader to reassess the earlier, positive depiction of such a death that opens the documentary.

The scene comes in the middle of the film, just after a series of media clips featuring different pundits, physicians, and "Death with Dignity" proponents arguing over the legislation. The last voice before the shift of scene is a radio show caller with this point: "When you're talking about someone living with a chronic disease, when you talk about poor people, and when you offer someone death versus living, I think we all need to take notice."[30] The next visual on the screen is a Dexter, Oregon residence with a camper on posts, a rusted oil barrel, and cinder blocks in the foreground. As we learn more about Randy Stroup, the subject of this segment, we realize we are in fact following the caller's advice—"taking notice" of a poor person with advanced cancer who is offered the option of assisted dying. Stroup recounts that after a diagnosis of advanced prostate cancer, a failed course of chemotherapy, and the expectation that he would only live a few months, his physician said he might try a "stronger chemotherapy." Stroup continues: "Well, the Oregon Health Plan (OHP) decided that as long as it didn't increase my life for five years, then they didn't want to pay for it"—but they *would* pay "for comfort and palliative care, including a doctor-assisted suicide." As he sees it, "they don't care. It still just appalls me. No man has got the right to offer money to have somebody else killed. ... To think they could ...

---

[28] Holan, "PolitiFact—PolitiFact's Lie of the Year."
[29] For evidence that forced euthanasia, particularly of the old, is a frequent trope in dystopias dating as far back as the 1600s, see Sara D. Schotland, "Forced Execution of the Elderly: Old Law, Dystopia, and the Utilitarian Argument," *Humanities* 2, no. 2 (2013): 160–75.
[30] Peter Richardson, *How to Die in Oregon*, videorecording (Portland, OR: Clearcut Productions, 2010), 51:40–51:55.

send me a letter saying they'd pay to kill me—but won't pay to help me."[31] Written credits inform the viewer that OHP reversed its decision after Stroup went public with his story; he died four weeks later, having received the chemotherapy OHP initially said it would not cover.

Although the bulk of the film seems to be "on the side" of aid-in-dying, it treats Stroup's suspicion about its legislative and insurer motivations evenhandedly. Stroup is an outlier among the cast of people the documentary has been following thus far, seated in their comfortable apartments and garden-ringed houses alongside family or physicians, some even driving their own cars. In contrast, our first image of Stroup is him hunched over exposed ignition wires, his rough hands working on a fix. Other signs of class difference appear: the camera lingers on Stroup's Bud Lite t-shirt, his belt buckle and hat with a bald eagle overlaying the Stars and Stripes, his mud-splattered van's decals of the Confederate flag and the words "Shut Up and Fish." Even though he starts off by telling us that he has two sons and five grandchildren and his mother lives in a facility nearby, there are no people besides him in the scene. It is possible to read this outlier status as somehow invalidating, as if Stroup's reading of the OHP's offer is a deliberate, Palinesque misconstrual. But the economic frame provided by the radio caller—and, I would argue, the presence of the Confederate flag, which prompted at least this viewer to recognize that there were no Black people or other people of color in the entire documentary[32]—led me into a series of questions about whose dystopia this might be.[33]

In terms of Stroup, his apparent poverty, likely isolation, and deep mistrust of the OHP add up to a kind of dystopic lens through which the viewer can suddenly resee earlier scenes. In particular, it drove me back to the scene before the opening credits, where an older white man goes through with the procedure in front of massive windows overlooking a dense forest, surrounded by friends and family for whom he expresses love and gratitude. He sings and thanks the voters of Oregon for making this good death possible; he lays down and is caressed and murmured to as he dies.[34] The scene emphasizes control, choice, and material comfort, and it depicts a robust network of care. What Stroup does,

---

[31] Ibid., 51:57–55:10.
[32] For a discussion of Oregon's history of racial violence and exclusion, see Walidah Imarisha's "Why Aren't There More Black People in Oregon? A Hidden History," *PDXTalks* (October 23, 2015). Imarisha is also the coeditor, with Adrienne Maree Brown, of the influential *Octavia's Brood: Science Fiction Stories from Social Justice Movements* (Chico, CA: AK Press, 2015).
[33] The science-fiction writer Cadwell Turnbull's "Dystopia Isn't Sci-Fi—For Me, It's the American Reality," *Wired* (July 19, 2020), neatly conveys the view of America as a dystopia for Black people. Turnbull's essay is a brief illustration of a much broader engagement with this concept.
[34] Richardson, How to Die in Oregon, 03:28–04:23.

then, is make me ask for whom that earlier version of aided dying is available, and what volume and quality of healthcare options preceded it. Might a single law be a tool for choice and comfort for one population—and a form of targeted, mercenary euthanasia for another? And if so, is that difference not inherently dystopic?

This moment of questioning was, for me, a different experience altogether than my response to Dr. Wen's lecture or Palin's post. Stroup believes he is living in a system that wishes to dispose of him—and by avoiding calling it a "dystopia," he makes that belief feel immediate, even plausible: this "terrible new world" does not lurk sometime in the future or recall some past atrocity; it is *here*, simultaneously with the nonterrible present world, the flipside in all respects of that opening scene.[35] The absence of the label gives me the room to discover a dystopia rather than accept or reject the one on offer.

The Impulse to Restore Order

Here I want to call attention to a different effect of McAlear's claim: not just that any system can be described as dystopic (and thus could be described otherwise, depending on a different political or social orientation), but that such systems are being *re*described. In other words, a social system or government or historical period exists prior to its dystopification through fiction; dystopias may be intended as warnings about the future of the reader's own society, but they do not engage her in "social dreaming" the way utopias do.[36] Working via redescription, dystopias instead ask their readers to become sleuths: What is the social system/historical period/government to which the dystopia refers? Building on critical insights into the targeted nature of dystopia,[37] I observe that mentally mapping one's possible future onto someone else's present or past does two things: it confirms the current position of the reader as necessarily nondystopic, and it converts what might be a shocking jolt to the imagination into knowing recognition.

---

[35] The notion of a "flipside" revealing an initially unrecognized evil in an apparently positive society harks back to H. G. Wells's 1895 *The Time Machine*, where the appearance of a peaceful symbiosis between two races gives way to the reality that one is preying on the other.
[36] Sargent, "The Three Faces of Utopianism Revisited," 1.
[37] See, for example, Darko Suvin's description of dystopia as either "explicitly designed to refute a currently proposed eutopia" or an "open extrapolation or subtle analogy to human relations and power structures in the writer's reality" in Darko Suvin, "Theses on Dystopia 2001," in *Dark Horizons: Science Fiction and the Dystopian Imagination*, ed. Raffaella Baccolini and Tom Moylan (New York: Routledge, 2003), 189, 196.

In *About Time*, Mark Currie analyzes a passage from Paul Ricoeur's *Time and Narrative*, suggesting that experimental configurations of narrative time (Currie's own examples include Graham Swift's 1943 *Waterland*, and Martin Amis's 1999 *Time's Arrow*) may end up reinforcing, rather than upsetting, a reader's sense of time as "rectilinear succession." As Currie writes:

> It would be foolish to assume that the detours and loops involved in the narration of *Waterland* present any real challenge to the predominance of chronology as a model of time. In fact it would be safer to claim that the active efforts of a reader in the reconstruction of a time line function to reinforce linear causality in a novel like *Waterland*, the active reconstruction of causation and succession being more participatory than the passive mode in which the reader receives a linear plot.[38]

Ricoeur and Currie both have a great deal more to say about the capacity of fiction to create or configure temporality. But the counterintuitive effect named here chimes well with my concerns about the current experience of reading dystopias, and suggests to me that we think carefully before incorporating them into medical or bioethics training.

The sense that dystopias are redescriptions of the already known rather than potential futures is often fostered by writers of dystopias themselves. "I would not put any events into the book that had not already happened in what James Joyce called the 'nightmare' of history, nor any technology not already available," insists Atwood in a piece about composing *The Handmaid's Tale*.[39] While her claim is meant to increase the credibility of the novel's Republic of Gilead, thus establishing a firmer cause for readerly fear, it also teaches readers that even the most arresting aspects of the dystopia are already accounted for. Indeed, it might encourage them to mimic that accounting by hunting out dystopia's specific historical or contemporary sources. As a *Synapsis* article on contemporary dystopia, in which body markings are used to discriminate against groups of inhabitants, puts it, "If these events sound familiar—either through hyperboles of the present or indices of history that I track in my endnotes—they should."[40] Recall the familiar refrain: "*... except it's true.*"[41]

---

[38] Mark Currie, *About Time: Narrative, Fiction and the Philosophy of Time*, Frontiers of Theory (Edinburgh: Edinburgh University Press, 2012), 93.
[39] Margaret Atwood, "Margaret Atwood on What *The Handmaid's Tale* Means in the Age of Trump," *New York Times* (March 10, 2017), sec. Books, https://www.nytimes.com/2017/03/10/books/review/margaret-atwood-handmaids-tale-age-of-trump.html.
[40] Salvador Herrera, "Skin Deep: Biometrics and Containment in Sabrina Vourvoulias's INK," *SYNAPSIS* (November 29, 2019).
[41] Singer and Eddington, "The War on Opioids," emphasis added.

An anecdote: I'm teaching an elective seminar for first-year medical students on speculative fiction and bioethics, and one group gives a presentation on Charlie Brooker's anthology TV series *Black Mirror*—the "Men against Fire" episode from 2016. The episode features soldiers who are outfitted with neural implants to distort how they see an indigenous population; the implants make these hungry, terrorized people appear to the soldiers as horrific, infective, superhuman "roaches."[42] When the protagonist's implant starts malfunctioning, he glimpses reality without this overlay; in an eventual confrontation with the military psychologist, he learns that the military resorted to the use of implants due to high failure-to-fire rates in past wars.[43] In class, a student quickly observes that the same thing was basically done to Myanmar's Rohingya population, via military intervention but also through dehumanizing, violent propaganda spread on the social media: in this parallel, Facebook is a less dramatic (and noninvasive) counterpart of *Black Mirror*'s implant, but no less effective a technology of distortion.[44]

There are nods in class and a request for the student to explain more about the atrocities taking place in Myanmar. Still, and more relevant to the present argument, the class seemed more settled after this moment. In shifting us from dystopia to the real world, the student's observation effectively neutralized any potential fear appeal for our Chicago classroom.

There are, of course, several ways to handle momentary impasses in class discussion; I could have pointed out that the episode predated the genocide, for one, or else shifted us from the concrete to the abstract via the thought experiment posed at the end of the show.[45] I bring the story up here, though, because the student's impulse so closely mirrored my own initial response to the episode. *What were the origins of the argument about the failure-to-fire*

---

[42] The term *inyenzi* (cockroaches) was used by Hutu propagandists and militias to refer to the Tutsi population in the lead-up to the genocide of 1994. See Kennedy Ndahiro, "In Rwanda, We Know All about Dehumanizing Language," *The Atlantic* (April 13, 2019). Thanks to Molly Lindberg for pointing out this connection.

[43] Evidence for these rates, and the military's apprehensiveness about them, is taken from *Men against Fire: The Problem of Battle Command*, the controversial history of the Second World War by S. L. A. Marshall. See Charlie Brooker and Annabel Jones, "Men against Fire," in *Inside Black Mirror* (New York: Crown Archetype, 2018).

[44] See Steve Stecklow, "Hatebook: Inside Facebook's Myanmar Operation. A Reuters Special Report," Reuters (August 15, 2018), https://www.reuters.com/investigates/special-report/myanmar-facebook-hate/.

[45] The thought experiment in question is a twist on Robert Nozick's "experience machine." Here's my paraphrase of *Black Mirror*'s version: if you knew that you were dehumanizing and doing violence to a group of people in real life—but had little hope of stopping the violence if you retained your grip on reality (yet would certainly suffer from the knowledge of your complicity)—might you opt instead for a false version of experience where you perceived your actions as noble?

rate, and what war was it associated with primarily? Where has the specific term "roaches" been used to dehumanize groups of people before? Like Currie's reader reassembling traditional chronology from an experimental depiction of time, I react to the imaginary future worlds of *Black Mirror* by ferreting out their historical or present-day bases.

I assume that this impulse is not the only, and maybe not even the primary, reaction for today's readers of dystopian fiction and viewers of dystopian films. But considering the recent interest in the genre from health humanities scholars, it is prudent to explore objections to its uses. These objections may come from scholarly analyses of its deployment in bioethical debate, certainly.[46] But they might also come from a careful reflection on our own experience of reading.

* * *

Borrowing from the 1980s notion of the "critical utopia" and coined in 1994 by Sargent, the "critical dystopia" stands distinct from the standard or traditional dystopia. Where a traditional dystopia forecloses hope within the story—with all of its resistant characters dead or co-opted, as in *Nineteen Eighty-Four*—or else neglects to imagine the steps leading from the reader's present to the present of the story, as in many Hollywood dystopias—the "critical dystopia" both depicts the events leading from the real world to the imagined one and seeds some hope within the story. Yet, as Baccolini points out in "The Persistence of Hope in Dystopian Science Fiction," "Genres change in relation to the times."[47]

In our current time, I argue, the future possibilities held out by the critical dystopia are increasingly being defused by a critical dystopia *reader*, one who reacts to the rhetorical model by reading past the form. As the medical definition of dystopia—"malposition," "faulty or abnormal position of a part or organ"[48]—calls for the physician to reposition what's out of place, dystopias today seem to ask of readers a similar repositioning: to identify correspondences with the known world and tether any "social dreaming" to historical or present-day events. If this is the case often enough, we should be asking which genres *besides* the dystopia the health humanities might use to engage such readers anew.

---

[46] See Ruth Levy Guyer and Jonathan D. Moreno, "Slouching toward Policy: Lazy Bioethics and the Perils of Science Fiction," *American Journal of Bioethics* 4, no. 4 (September 1, 2004): W14–17; Evie Kendal, "Utopian Literature and Bioethics: Exploring Reproductive Difference and Gender Equality," *Literature and Medicine* 36, no. 1 (2018): 56–84.
[47] Raffaella Baccolini, "The Persistence of Hope in Dystopian Science Fiction," *PMLA*, Special Topic: Science Fiction and Literary Studies: The Next Millennium, 119, no. 3 (2004): 520.
[48] "Dystopia," *The Free Dictionary* (Farlex), https://medical-dictionary.thefreedictionary.com/dystopia.

Coda

Roanne Kantor

The core project of this volume has been to share ideas in a "department without walls." In putting this space together, our editors Rishi Goyal and Arden Hegele imagined a "dialogue in the space occupied by different perspectives." For me, one of the most essential but challenging aspects of this project has been the cultivation of our mutual vulnerability, our openness to being reshaped by the encounter with other methods, other fields, and, fundamentally, other bodies. And it is the negotiation of such vulnerability that the essays in this volume address from a variety of perspectives.

In his exploration of AIDS narratives, for example, John A. Carranza reflects that reading *Tales of the City*, "in the 'fullest sense' " must include a consideration of "personal and social contexts in which the work was written," as well as "moral lessons for medical students and doctors." Aspects of this approach are shared in the essays by Alicia Andrzejewski, Livia Arndal Woods, and Kristina Fleuty, all of whom, in various ways, try to recover what Benjamin Gagnon Chainey calls "ambivalent and reciprocal oscillation between human and literary bodies."

The irony is that this kind of "oscillatory" reading "in the fullest sense" is the opposite of how I was trained to read as a literary critic. The utilitarian pursuit of "personal and social contexts," to say nothing of "moral lessons," is the habit of the untrained, the uninitiated—"bad" readers, in short.[1] Here, following Merve Emre, I mean bad readers as "individuals socialized into the practice of readerly identification, emotion, action, and interaction"—in other words, everything we hope that literature can do for medicine and health![2]

---

[1] Merve Emre, *Paraliterary: The Making of Bad Readers in Postwar America* (Chicago: The University of Chicago Press, 2017).
[2] Ibid., 3.

These include experiences of, say, a student interested in entering the field of clinical psychiatry who reads "emotionally," identifying the modernist literary style as a symptom of psychological distress; a student preparing for medical school who reads "interactionally" to improve her communication with future patients; a student working in health policy who "identifies" in literary characters the experiences of care work in her own ethnic community; and a student transitioning from "interaction" to "identification" as she uses literature to relate to her own experience of progressively going blind. All of these and many more have come into my classroom and shaken up my doxa about "good" reading and its relationship to "critique," surfacing a different reading of literature as interpersonal relation that, in turn, requires a different orientation to time.

It was Joshua Franklin's piece on the role of medical anthropology in medical training that most clearly reflected this experience to me. The essay opens on a scene of paralysis in which Franklin's deep training in writing as critique falters in its encounter with writing as a practical, urgent tool within medicine: the patient chart. The failure to account for this other use of writing, Franklin reflects, reveals an underlying problem in the attitude of medical anthropology as a field: "The expectation that anthropological critique will transform medical practice, *and not the other way around*" (emphasis added). I would go further to say that the risk of interdisciplinarity in fields like medical and health humanities is the reification of this unequal relation: one field makes use, and the other makes do. The history of medical humanities is one in which, as Franklin, Diana Rose Newby, Travis Chi Wing Lau, and others remind us, medicine has set the terms and the humanities have had to "accommodate" (Lau). But this volume also points to the potential for overcorrection: a critical stance from the humanities that risks saying to other disciplines—echoing the harrowing scene of "treatment" for traumatic mutism in Pat Barker's *Regeneration*—"You must speak, but I shall not listen."[3]

The privilege of literary scholars is that we aim our critique at people who are mostly dead. Through a cute poststructuralist trick, even living writers are "dead" to literary criticism.[4] The reader–writer relationship might suggest a conversational aspect to reading, but in practice, it is figurative, infinitely deferred. This could not be more different from the everyday practice of medicine, which is an interpersonal endeavor. My concern is that if we in the humanities do not sometimes agree to be moved by our objects of critique, we

---

[3] Pat Barker, *Regeneration* (New York: Penguin, [1991] 2019), 319.
[4] Roland Barthes, *Image, Music, Text*, trans. Stephen Heath (New York: Hill and Wang, [1977] 2009).

risk placing a cordon sanitaire around "health humanities." By reinstating a true dialogue of our different perspectives, including sometimes allowing opposing positions to rub up against one another, this volume invites us to interrogate the limits of critique in this particular space.

Several essays seemed to circle this question in quite an unexpected way, in terms of the relationship between critique and time. One of my favorite books in the field of health humanities is Michael Davidson's *Concerto for the Left Hand: Disability and the Defamiliar Body*. The idea of defamiliarization on which Davidson draws is central to many different "good" ways of reading literature.[5] To defamiliarize is to look in detail, to reexamine what we take for granted and hold dear (i.e., to critique), all of which is explicitly linked to the idea of slowing down. That slowness does much good: it allows us both to use language to describe the experience of health and illness with greater precision while, at the same time, forcing us to confront the unresolvable limits of language as the vehicle for that experience (Gagnon Chainey). It also engages ideas like "crip time" (Lau) to challenge the very conventions of education and employment that define our students' relationship to a potential future career in medicine.

But slowness is not everything. My students also remind me, as they do to Franklin, that there is a role for urgency. In the final essay of the collection, Anna Fenton-Hathaway quotes Iro Filippaki in calling for texts that "re-create a sense of urgency in the classroom," that mirrors the urgency that is "a constant in the work of healthcare teams."[6] Fenton-Hathaway casts a duly critical eye on the search for this urgency within dystopian fiction, calling on us, once again, to slow down our desire to resolve these fictional futures by tying them to a safely historical referent, to linger, instead, in the realm of speculation. But I am reminded that literary scholars' tendency to overvalue ambiguity and undecidability is not always compatible with the temporality of medicine.[7] Our students, whether in medicine, in policy, or even in their own engagements with these systems as recipients of "care," have set out on a path where they often have to act quickly and decisively. It is my hope that we can continue slowing them down while also finding a way to honor their occasional need for speed.

---

[5] Michael Davidson, *Concerto for the Left Hand: Disability and the Defamiliar Body*, Corporealities (Ann Arbor: University of Michigan Press, 2008).

[6] Iro Filippaki, "COVID-19 and the Future of Narrative Medicine," *SYNAPSIS* (April 1, 2020), https://medicalhealthhumanities.com/2020/04/01/covid-19-and-the-future-of-narrative-medicine/.

[7] Timothy Richard Aubry, *Guilty Aesthetic Pleasures* (Cambridge, MA: Harvard University Press, 2018).

References

Adelman, Janet. *Suffocating Mothers: Fantasies of Maternal Origin in Shakespeare's Plays, "Hamlet" to "The Tempest"*. New York: Routledge, 1992. https://doi.org/10.4324/9780203420652.

Ahmed, Sara. "Orientations: Toward a Queer Phenomenology." *GLQ: A Journal of Lesbian and Gay Studies* 12, no. 4 (2006): 543–74.

Aitken, R. C. "Measurement of Feelings Using Visual Analogue Scales." *Proceedings of the Royal Society of Medicine* 62, no. 10 (October 1969): 989–93.

Allen, Martin. "Against 'Hybridity' in Genre Studies: Blending as an Alternative Approach to Generic Experimentation." *Trespassing Journal* 2 (2013): 3–21.

Altschuler, Sari. *The Medical Imagination: Literature and Health in the Early United States*. Early American Studies. Philadelphia: University of Pennsylvania Press, 2018.

American College of Obstetricians and Gynecologists. "Optimizing Postpartum Care." Committee Opinion. Washington, DC: American College of Obstetricians and Gynecologists, May 2018. https://www.acog.org/en/Clinical/Clinical Guidance/Committee Opinion/Articles/2018/05/Optimizing Postpartum Care.

Angst, Martin S., William G. Brose, and John B. Dyck. "The Relationship between the Visual Analog Pain Intensity and Pain Relief Scale Changes during Analgesic Drug Studies in Chronic Pain Patients." *Anesthesiology* 91, no. 1 (July 1, 1999): 34–41. https://doi.org/10.1097/00000542-199907000-00009.

Asan, Onur, Paul D. Smith, and Enid Montague. "More Screen Time, Less Face Time—Implications for EHR Design." *Journal of Evaluation in Clinical Practice* 20, no. 6 (2014): 896–901. https://doi.org/10.1111/jep.12182.

Ashcroft, Lord. *The Veterans' Transition Review*, n.p., 2014.

Associated Press. "San Francisco's Newest Heroine Has Following." *Baytown Sun* 54, no. 301 (September 29, 1976).

Atkinson, Sarah, Bethan Evans, Angela Woods, and Robin Kearns. " 'The Medical' and 'Health' in a Critical Medical Humanities." *Journal of Medical Humanities* 36, no. 1 (2015): 71–81.

Atkinson, Sarah, Jane Macnaughton, Jennifer Richards, Anne Whitehead, and Angela Woods. *The Edinburgh Companion to the Critical Medical Humanities*. Edinburgh: Edinburgh University Press, 2016.

Atwood, Margaret. "Margaret Atwood on What *The Handmaid's Tale* Means in the Age of Trump." *New York Times*, March 10, 2017. https://www.nytimes.com/2017/03/10/books/review/margaret-atwood-handmaids-tale-age-of-trump.html.

Aubry, Timothy Richard. *Guilty Aesthetic Pleasures*. Cambridge, MA: Harvard University Press, 2018.

Auerbach, Nina. *Our Vampires, Ourselves*. Chicago: University of Chicago Press, 1995.

Aull, Felice. "Health Humanities Reader." *LitMed: Literature, Arts, Medicine Database*, October 30, 2014. https://medhum.med.nyu.edu/view/15463.

The Ayn Rand Institute. "*Atlas Shrugged* Sets a New Record!" January 20, 2010. https://ari.aynrand.org/press-releases/atlas-shrugged-sets-a-new-record/.

Baccolini, Raffaella. "The Persistence of Hope in Dystopian Science Fiction." *PMLA* (Special Topic: Science Fiction and Literary Studies—The Next Millennium) 119, no. 3 (2004): 518–21.

Baccolini, Raffaella, and Tom Moylan. "Introduction: Dystopias and Histories." In *Dark Horizons: Science Fiction and the Dystopian Imagination*, edited by Raffaella Baccolini and Tom Moylan, 1–12. New York: Routledge, 2003.

Banner, Olivia. "Introduction: For Impossible Demands." In *Teaching Health Humanities*, edited by Olivia Banner, Nathan Carlin, and Thomas R. Cole, 1–18. New York: Oxford University Press, 2019. https://doi.org/10.1093/med/9780190636890.003.0001.

Banner, Olivia, Nathan Carlin, and Thomas R. Cole, eds. *Teaching Health Humanities*. New York: Oxford University Press, 2019.

Barker, Pat. *Regeneration*. New York: Penguin, [1991] 2019.

Barrish, Phillip. "Health Policy in Dystopia." *Literature and Medicine* 34, no. 1 (2016): 106–31. https://doi.org/10.1353/lm.2016.0006.

Barthes, Roland. *Image, Music, Text*, translated by Stephen Heath. New York: Hill and Wang, [1977] 2009.

Baynton, Paul C. "Disability and the Justification of Inequality in American History." In *The New Disability History: American Perspectives*, edited by Paul K. Longmore and Lauri Umansky, 33–57. The History of Disability Series. New York: New York University Press, 2001.

Beecher, Henry K. *Measurement of Subjective Responses: Quantitative Effects of Drugs*. New York: Oxford University Press, 1959.

Benjamin, Regina. "Finding My Way to Electronic Health Records." *New England Journal of Medicine* 363, no. 6 (August 5, 2010): 505–6. http://dx.doi.org.ezproxy.cul.columbia.edu/10.1056/NEJMp1007785.

Berg, Marc, and Geoffrey Bowker. "The Multiple Bodies of the Medical Record: Toward a Sociology of an Artifact." *Sociological Quarterly* 38, no. 3 (1997): 513–37.

Berlant, Lauren Gail. *Cruel Optimism*. Durham, NC: Duke University Press, 2011.

Billone, Amy Christine. *The Future of the Nineteenth-Century Dream-Child: Fantasy, Dystopia, Cyberculture*. Children's Literature and Culture. New York: Routledge, 2016.

Bleakley, Alan. *Medical Humanities and Medical Education: How the Medical Humanities Can Shape Better Doctors*. Routledge Advances in the Medical Humanities. Abingdon: Routledge, 2015. https://doi.org/10.4324/9781315771724.

Bond, M. R., and I. Pilowsky. "Subjective Assessment of Pain and Its Relationship to the Administration of Analgesics in Patients with Advanced Cancer." *Journal of Psychosomatic Research* 10, no. 2 (1966): 203–8. https://doi.org/10.1016/0022-3999(66)90064-X.

Bordo, Susan. *Unbearable Weight: Feminism, Western Culture, and the Body*. Berkeley: University of California Press, 1993.

Bowker, Geoffrey C., and Susan Leigh Star. *Sorting Things Out: Classification and Its Consequences*, first MIT Press paperback ed. Inside Technology. Cambridge, MA: MIT Press, 2000.

Bradley, Beatrice, and Tanya Pollard. "Tragicomic Conceptions: The *Winter's Tale* as Response to Amphitryo." *English Literary Renaissance* 47, no. 2 (March 1, 2017): 251–69. https://doi.org/10.1086/693893.

Brandt, Allan M. *No Magic Bullet: A Social History of Venereal Disease in the United States since 1880*. New York: Oxford University Press, 1985.

Brody, Lauren Smith. *The Fifth Trimester: The Working Mom's Guide to Style, Sanity, and Success after Baby*. New York: Doubleday, 2017.

Brooker, Charlie, and Annabel Jones. "Men against Fire." In *Inside Black Mirror*, 192–203. New York: Crown Archetype, 2018.

Brown-Séquard, Charles-Édouard. "Note on the Effects Produced on Man by Subcutaneous Injections of a Liquid Obtained from the Testicles of Animals." *The Lancet* 134, no. 3438 (July 20, 1889): 105–7. https://doi.org/10.1016/S0140-6736(00)64118-1.

Browning, Jimmy D. "Something to Remember Me By: Maupin's *Tales of the City* Novels as Artifacts in Contemporary Gay Folk Culture." *New York Folklore* 19, no. 1 (January 1, 1993): 71–87.

Buntin, Melinda Beeuwkes, Matthew F. Burke, Michael C. Hoaglin, and David Blumenthal. "The Benefits of Health Information Technology: A Review of the Recent Literature Shows Predominantly Positive Results." *Health Affairs* 30, no. 3 (March 2011): 464–71.

Butler, Judith. *Notes toward a Performative Theory of Assembly*. Cambridge, MA: Harvard University Press, 2015.

Caddick, Nick, Linda Cooper, Lauren Godier-McBard, and Matt Fossey. "Hierarchies of Wounding: Media Framings of 'Combat' and 'Non-Combat' Injury." *Media, War & Conflict*, January 13, 2020. https://doi.org/10.1177/1750635219899110.

Caddick, Nick, and Brett Smith. "The Impact of Sport and Physical Activity on the Well-Being of Combat Veterans: A Systematic Review." *Psychology of Sport and Exercise* 15, no. 1 (January 1, 2014): 9–18. https://doi.org/10.1016/j.psychsport.2013.09.011.

Canada Health. "Medical Assistance in Dying." End-of-Life Care, March 18, 2021. https://www.canada.ca/en/health-canada/services/medical-assistance-dying.html#a2.

Canguilhem, Georges. *The Normal and the Pathological*, translated by Carolyn R. Fawcett. New York: Zone Books, [1978] 1989.

Canning, Richard. *Gay Fiction Speaks: Conversations with Gay Novelists.* New York: Columbia University Press, 2000.

Carr, David. *Experience and History: Phenomenological Perspectives on the Historical World*. New York: Oxford University Press, 2014.

Carter, Albert Howard, III. "Health Humanities." *LitMed: Literature, Arts, Medicine Database*, October 20, 2016. https://medhum.med.nyu.edu/view/16593.

Cefalu, William T., Daniel E. Dawes, Gina Gavlak, Dana Goldman, William H. Herman, Karen Van Nuys, Alvin C. Powers, Simeon I. Taylor, and Alan L. Yatvin. "Insulin Access and Affordability Working Group: Conclusions and Recommendations." *Diabetes Care* 41, no. 6 (June 1, 2018): 1299–311. https://doi.org/10.2337/dci18-0019.

Chambers, Tod. "Eating One's Friends: Fiction as Argument in Bioethics." *Literature and Medicine* 34, no. 1 (2016): 79–105.

Chaney, Jen. "The Pregnancies in 'Breaking Dawn' and 'American Horror Story': A Comparative Study." *Washington Post*, November 22, 2011. https://www.washingtonpost.com/blogs/celebritology/post/the-pregnancies-of-bella-in-breaking-dawn-and-vivien-on-american-horror-story-a-comparative-study/2011/11/21/gIQA6nADlN_blog.html.

Chaney, Sarah. "'A Hideous Torture on Himself': Madness and Self-Mutilation in Victorian Literature." *Journal of Medical Humanities* 32, no. 4 (December 1, 2011): 279–89. https://doi.org/10.1007/s10912-011-9152-6.

Charise, Andrea. "Resemblance, Diversity, and Making Age Studies Matter." In *Teaching Health Humanities*, edited by Olivia Banner, Nathan Carlin, and Thomas R. Cole. New York: Oxford University Press, 2019.

Charon, Rita. *Narrative Medicine: Honoring the Stories of Illness*. Oxford: Oxford University Press, 2006.

Charon, Rita, Sayantani DasGupta, Nellie Hermann, Craig Irvine, Eric R. Marcus, Edgar Rivera Colón, Danielle Spencer, and Maura Spiegel. *The Principles and Practices of Narrative Medicine*. New York: Oxford University Press, 2016.

Chi, Jeffrey, and Abraham Verghese. "Clinical Education and the Electronic Health Record: The Flipped Patient." *JAMA* 312, no. 22 (December 10, 2014): 2331–2. https://doi.org/10.1001/jama.2014.12820.

Cimino, James J. "Improving the Electronic Health Record—Are Clinicians Getting What They Wished For?" *JAMA* 309, no. 10 (March 13, 2013): 991–2. https://doi.org/10.1001/jama.2013.890.

Claeys, Gregory. *Dystopia. A Natural History: A Study of Modern Despotism, Its Antecedents, and Its Literary Diffractions*. Oxford: Oxford University Press, 2017.

Clarke, Adele E., Janet K. Shim, Laura Mamo, Jennifer Ruth Fosket, and Jennifer R. Fishman. "Biomedicalization: Technoscientific Transformations of Health, Illness, and U.S. Biomedicine." *American Sociological Review* 68, no. 2 (2003): 161–94. https://doi.org/10.2307/1519765.

Cole, Thomas R., Ronald A. Carson, and Nathan S. Carlin. *Medical Humanities: An Introduction*. Cambridge: Cambridge University Press, 2014.

Coleridge, Samuel Taylor. "Christabel." In *Norton Anthology of English Literature*, edited by Stephen Greenblatt, 10th ed., 2:277–91. New York: W.W. Norton, [1816] 2018.

Conley, Garrard. "Utopia of the Flesh; Confessions of the Fox." *New York Times Book Review*, July 29, 2018.

Conrad, Peter. "The Shifting Engines of Medicalization." *Journal of Health and Social Behavior* 46, no. 1 (2005): 3–14.

Cooper, Nick Caddick, Lauren Godier, Alex Cooper, and Matt Fossey. "Transition from the Military into Civilian Life: An Exploration of Cultural Competence." *Armed Forces & Society* 44, no. 1 (2016): 156–77. https://doi.org/10.1177/0095327X1 6675965.

Cooper, Owens, and Deirdre Benia. *Medical Bondage: Race, Gender, and the Origins of American Gynecology*. Athens: University of Georgia Press, 2017.

Couser, G. Thomas. "What Disability Studies Has to Offer Medical Education." *Journal of Medical Humanities* 32, no. 1 (March 1, 2011): 21–30. https://doi.org/10.1007/s10 912-010-9125-1.

Crawford, Paul. "Introduction: Global Health Humanities and the Rise of Creative Public Health." In *The Routledge Companion to Health Humanities*, edited by Andrea Charise, B. J. Brown, and Paul Crawford, 3. Routledge Companions to Literature Series. Abingdon: Routledge, 2020.

Crawford, Paul, Brian Brown, Charley Baker, Victoria Tischler, and Brian Adams. *Health Humanities*. London: Palgrave Macmillan, 2015.

Cree, Alice, and Nick Caddick. "Unconquerable Heroes: Invictus, Redemption, and the Cultural Politics of Narrative." *Journal of War & Culture Studies* 13, no. 3 (2020): 258–78. https://doi.org/10.1080/17526272.2019.1615707.

Currie, Mark. *About Time: Narrative, Fiction and the Philosophy of Time*. Frontiers of Theory. Edinburgh: Edinburgh University Press, 2012.

Cvetkovich, Ann. *An Archive of Feelings: Trauma, Sexuality, and Lesbian Public Cultures*. Durham, NC: Duke University Press, 2003.

Czernik, Zuzanna, and C. T. Lin. "Time at the Bedside (Computing)." *JAMA* 315, no. 22 (June 14, 2016): 2399–400. https://doi.org/10.1001/jama.2016.1722.

Dao, Diane K., Adeline L. Goss, Andrew S. Hoekzema, Lauren A. Kelly, Alexander A. Logan, Sanjiv D. Mehta, Utpal N. Sandesara, Michelle R. Munyikwa, and Horace M. DeLisser. "Integrating Theory, Content, and Method to Foster Critical Consciousness in Medical Students: A Comprehensive Model for Cultural Competence Training." *Academic Medicine* 92, no. 3 (March 2017): 335–44. https://doi.org/10.1097/ACM.0000000000001390.

Davidson, Michael. *Concerto for the Left Hand: Disability and the Defamiliar Body*. Ann Arbor: University of Michigan Press, 2008.

Davis, Lennard J. "Introduction: Normality, Power, and Culture." In *The Disability Studies Reader*, edited by Lennard J. Davis, 4th ed., 1–16. New York: Routledge, 2013.

Deleuze, Gilles, and Felix Guattari. *A Thousand Plateaus: Capitalism and Schizophrenia*, translated by Brian Massumi. Minneapolis: University of Minnesota Press, [1980] 2005.

D'Emilio, John. *Making Trouble: Essays on Gay History, Politics, and the University*. New York: Routledge, 1992.

De Preester, Helena. "Technology and the Body: The (Im)Possibilities of Re-Embodiment." *Foundations of Science* 16, no. 2 (2010): 119–37. https://doi.org/10.1007/s10699-010-9188-5.

DeTora, Lisa M., and Stephanie M. Hilger. "Introduction: Bodies and Transitions in the Health Humanities." In *Bodies in Transition in the Health Humanities: Representations of Corporeality*, 1–8. Abingdon: Routledge, 2019. https://doi.org/10.4324/9781351128742.

Dhaliwal, Gurpreet, and Allan S. Detsky. "The Evolution of the Master Diagnostician." *JAMA* 310, no. 6 (August 14, 2013): 579–80. https://doi.org/10.1001/jama.2013.7572.

Díaz, Junot, and Avni Majithia-Sejpal. "Global Dystopias, Critical Dystopias: A Podcast with Junot Díaz." *BR: A Political and Literary Podcast*, 2016. http://bostonreview.net/podcast/global-dystopias-critical-dystopias-podcast-junot-d%C3%ADaz.

Dickens, Charles. *David Copperfield*, edited by Nina Burgis. The Clarendon Dickens. Oxford: Clarendon Press, [1850] 1981.

DiGangi, Mario. *Sexual Types: Embodiment, Agency, and Dramatic Character from Shakespeare to Shirley*. Philadelphia: University of Pennsylvania Press, 2011.

Dillard-Wright, Jessica. "Electronic Health Record as a Panopticon: A Disciplinary Apparatus in Nursing Practice." *Nursing Philosophy* 20, no. 2 (2019). https://doi.org/10.1111/nup.12239.

Don, Katherine. "Bringing Up Baby: The Terrifying, Transformational Birth Scene Showdown: *Twilight* vs. *Game of Thrones*." *Bitch Media*, November 22, 2011. https://www.bitchmedia.org/post/bringing-up-baby-the-terrifying-transformational-birth-scene-showdown-twilight-v-game-of-throne.

Donahue, Dick. "Armistead Maupin: Tales Worth Talking About." *Publishers Weekly*, September 11, 2000. https://www.publishersweekly.com/pw/by-topic/authors/interviews/article/21206-armistead-maupin-tales-worth-talking-about.html.

Dorwart, Laura. "What the World Gets Wrong about My Quadriplegic Husband and Me." *Catapult*, December 6, 2017. https://catapult.co/stories/what-the-world-gets-wrong-about-my-quadriplegic-husband-and-me.

Dreger, Ralph Mason. "A Simple Course Evaluation Scale." *Journal of Experimental Education* 22, no. 2 (1953): 145–53.

Dror, Otniel E. "De-Medicalizing the Medical Humanities." *European Legacy* 16, no. 3 (2011): 317–26.

Duff, David. "Key Concepts." In *Modern Genre Theory*, edited by David Duff, x–xvi. Longman Critical Readers. Oxfordshire: Routledge, 2000.

Dunn, Emma. "Good Vampires Don't Eat: Anorexic Logic in Stephenie Meyer's *Twilight* Series." *Jeunesse: Young People, Texts, Cultures* 10, no. 1 (June 22, 2018): 109–34.

"Dystopia." In *The Free Dictionary*. Farlex. https://medical-dictionary.thefreedictionary.com/dystopia.

Edelman, Elazer R., and Brittany N. Weber. "Tenuous Tether." *New England Journal of Medicine* 373, no. 23 (2015): 2199–201. https://doi.org/10.1056/NEJMp1509265.

Egger, Emilie. "Five Decades of 'Semiotic' Fetal Imagery in the US: Parts 1 and 2." *SYNAPSIS*, 2019. https://medicalhealthhumanities.com/2019/10/19/five-decades-of-semiotic-fetal-imagery-in-the-ust-part-1/.

Emani, Srinivas, David Y. Ting, Michael Healey, Stuart R. Lipsitz, Andrew S. Karson, and David W. Bates. "Physician Beliefs about the Meaningful Use of the Electronic Health Record: A Follow-Up Study." *Applied Clinical Informatics* 8, no. 4 (2017): 1044–53. https://doi.org/10.4338/ACI-2017-05-RA-0079.

Emre, Merve. *Paraliterary: The Making of Bad Readers in Postwar America*. Chicago: University of Chicago Press, 2017.

Engward, Hilary, Kristina Fleuty, and Matt Fossey. "The Family Perspective on Living with Limb Loss." Veterans and Families Institute for Military Social Research, 2018, 115.

Evans, Jennifer. "'Gentle Purges Corrected with Hot Spices, Whether They Work or Not, Do Vehemently Provoke Venery': Menstrual Provocation and Procreation in Early Modern England." *Social History of Medicine: The Journal of the Society for the Social History of Medicine* 25, no. 1 (February 1, 2012): 2–19. https://doi.org/10.1093/shm/hkr021.

Factor, James S., and Harald Azuma. "Visual Analog Scale and Method of Use for the Diagnosis and/or Treatment of Physical Pain." United States US6258042B1, filed September 17, 1999, and issued July 10, 2001. https://patents.google.com/patent/US6258042B1/en.

Fanestil, Bradley D. "The Tyranny of the Measuring Cup." *JAMA* 301, no. 15 (April 15, 2009): 1515–16. https://doi.org/10.1001/jama.2009.137.

Farrar, Jennifer. "Tyranny Drives 'Winter's Tale.'" *The Blade*, July 27, 2011. https://www.toledoblade.com/a-e/music-theater-dance/2011/07/28/Tyranny-drives-searing-Winter-s-Tale/stories/201107280029.

"Fashion, n." In *OED Online*. Oxford University Press. http://www.oed.com/view/Entry/68389.

Feldman, Ellen. "The Day the Computer Tried to Eat My Alligator." *JAMA* 304, no. 24 (2010): 2679. https://doi.org/10.1001/jama.2010.1805.

Fields, Lauren. "Why Americans Are Reading Dystopian Classics to Understand President Trump." *Deseret News*, February 5, 2017. https://www.deseret.com/2017/2/5/20605363/why-americans-are-reading-dystopian-classics-to-understand-president-trump.

Filippaki, Iro. "COVID-19 and the Future of Narrative Medicine." *SYNAPSIS*, April 1, 2020. https://medicalhealthhumanities.com/2020/04/01/covid-19-and-the-future-of-narrative-medicine/.

FitzGerald, Frances. "The Castro-I." *New Yorker*, July 21, 1986. https://www.newyorker.com/magazine/1986/07/21/i-the-castro.

Foley, James. *FIFTY SHADES FREED Trailer 3*. KinoCheck International, 2018.

Forbes, T. R. "Testis Transplantation Performed by John Hunter." *Endocrinology* 41, no. 4 (1947): 329–31. https://doi.org/10.1210/endo-41-4-329.

Forces in Mind Trust. "The Transition Mapping Study." August 2013.

Foucault, Michel. *The Birth of the Clinic: An Archaeology of Medical Perception*, translated by Alan Sheridan. Routledge Classics. London: Routledge, [1973] 2003.

Foucault, Michel. *Discipline and Punish: The Birth of the Prison*, translated by Alan Sheridan, 2nd vintage ed. New York: Vintage Books, [1977] 1995.

Foucault, Michel, ed. *Herculine Barbin: Being the Recently Discovered Memoirs of a Nineteenth-Century French Hermaphrodite*, translated by Richard McDougall, vintage books ed. New York: Pantheon Books, [1980] 2010.

Foucault, Michel. *The History of Sexuality*, translated by Robert Hurley, 1st American ed. New York: Pantheon Books, 1978.

Foucault, Michel. *Security, Territory, Population: Lectures at the Collège de France, 1977–78*, edited by Michel Senellart, François Ewald, and Alessandro Fontana, translated by Graham Burchell. Basingstoke: Palgrave Macmillan, 2007.

France, David. *How to Survive a Plague: The Inside Story of How Citizens and Science Tamed AIDS*, 1st ed. New York: Alfred A. Knopf, 2016.

Frank, Jason R., et al. "Competency-Based Medical Education: Theory to Practice." *Medical Teacher* 32, no. 8 (2010): 638–45, https://doi.org/10.3109/0142159X.2010.501190.

Frankovich, Jennifer, Christopher A. Longhurst, and Scott M. Sutherland. "Evidence-Based Medicine in the EMR Era." *New England Journal of Medicine* 365, no. 19 (November 10, 2011): 1758–9. https://doi.org/10.1056/NEJMp1108726.

"Freebooter, n." In *OED Online*. Oxford University Press. http://www.oed.com/view/Entry/74384.

Freud, Sigmund. *Reflections on War and Death*, translated by A. A. Brill and Alfred B. Kuttner. New York: Moffat, Yard, 1918.

Frey, John J. "At a Loss for Words." *JAMA* 297, no. 16 (April 25, 2007): 1751–2. https://doi.org/10.1001/jama.297.16.1751.

Freyd, Max. "The Graphic Rating Scale." *Journal of Educational Psychology* 14, no. 2 (1923): 83–102. https://doi.org/10.1037/h0074329.

Freyd, Max. "A Method for the Study of Vocational Interests." *Journal of Applied Psychology* 6, no. 3 (1922): 243–54. https://doi.org/10.1037/h0072563.

Friedberg, Mark W., Peggy G. Chen, Kristin R. Van Busum, Frances Aunon, Chau Pham, John Caloyeras, Soeren Mattke, Emma Pitchforth, Denise D. Quigley,

Robert H. Brook, F. Jay Crosson, and Michael Tutty. "Factors Affecting Physician Professional Satisfaction and Their Implications for Patient Care, Health Systems, and Health Policy." *Rand Health Quarterly* 3, no. 4 (2013): 1.

Gabbe, Steven G., Jennifer R. Niebyl, Joe Leigh Simpson, Mark B. Landon, Henry L. Galan, Eric R. M. Jauniaux, Deborah A. Driscoll, Vincenzo Berghella, and William A. Grobman. *Obstetrics: Normal and Problem Pregnancies*, 7th ed. Philadelphia, PA: Elsevier, [1986] 2017.

Ganczarek, Joanna, Thomas Hünefeldt, and Marta Olivetti Belardinelli. "From 'Einfühlung' to Empathy: Exploring the Relationship between Aesthetic and Interpersonal Experience." *Cognitive Processing* 19, no. 2 (May 1, 2018): 141–5. https://doi.org/10.1007/s10339-018-0861-x.

Ganzini, Linda. "Empirical Studies: What Do We Know about End-of-Life Decision-Making around the World?" In *Experiences of SCEN (Support and Consultation on Euthanasia in the Netherlands) Physicians*, Halifax, Nova Scotia, 2017.

Garland-Thomson, Rosemarie. "The Case for Conserving Disability." *Journal of Bioethical Inquiry* 9, no. 3 (September 1, 2012): 339–55. https://doi.org/10.1007/s11673-012-9380-0.

Gedye, J. L., R. C. B. Aitken, and Helen M. Ferres. "Subjective Assessment in Clinical Research." *British Medical Journal* 1, no. 5242 (June 24, 1961): 1828.

Gélis, Jacques. *History of Childbirth: Fertility, Pregnancy, and Birth in Early Modern Europe*, translated by Rosemary Morris. Cambridge, MA: Polity Press, [1991] 2005.

Gill-Peterson, Julian. *Histories of the Transgender Child*. Minneapolis: University of Minnesota Press, 2018.

Gillum, Richard F. "From Papyrus to the Electronic Tablet: A Brief History of the Clinical Medical Record with Lessons for the Digital Age." *American Journal of Medicine* 126, no. 10 (October 1, 2013): 853–7. https://doi.org/10.1016/j.amjmed.2013.03.024.

Giummarra, Michael, Loretta Vocale, and Matthew King. "Efficacy of Non-surgical Management and Functional Outcomes of Partial ACL Tears: A Systematic Review of Randomized Trials," BMC Musculoskeletal Disorders 23, no. 332 (April 8, 2022). https://doi.org/10.1186/s12891-022-05278-w.

Godfrey, Richard, Simon Lilley, and Joanna Brewis. "Biceps, Bitches and Borgs: Reading Jarhead's Representation of the Construction of the (Masculine) Military Body." *Organization Studies* 33, no. 4 (April 1, 2012): 541–62. https://doi.org/10.1177/0170840612443458.

Goldfarb, Stanley. "Take Two Aspirin and Call Me by My Pronouns." *Wall Street Journal*, September 12, 2019, sec. Opinion. https://www.wsj.com/articles/take-two-aspirin-and-call-me-by-my-pronouns-11568325291.

Good, Byron J., and Mary-Jo DelVecchio Good. "'Learning Medicine': The Constructing of Medical Knowledge at Harvard Medical School." In *Knowledge,*

Power, and Practice: The Anthropology of Medicine and Everyday Life, edited by Shirley Lindenbaum and Margaret Lock, 81–107. Comparative Studies of Health Systems and Medical Care. Berkeley: University of California Press, 1993.

Goroll, Allan H. "Emerging from EHR Purgatory—Moving from Process to Outcomes." *New England Journal of Medicine* 376, no. 21 (May 25, 2017): 2004–6. http://dx.doi.org.ezproxy.cul.columbia.edu/10.1056/NEJMp1700601.

Gowing, Laura. *Common Bodies: Women, Touch and Power in Seventeenth-Century England*. New Haven, CT: Yale University Press, 2003.

Griffin, Gail B. "'Your Girls That You All Love Are Mine': 'Dracula' and the Victorian Male Sexual Imagination." *International Journal of Women's Studies* 3, no. 5 (September 1, 1980): 454–65.

Guibert, Hervé. *A l'ami qui ne m'a pas sauvé la vie: roman*. Paris: Gallimard, 1990.

Guibert, Hervé. *Cytomegalovirus: A Hospitalization Diary*, translated by Clara Orban. New York: Fordham University Press, [1996] 2016.

Guibert, Hervé. *Cytomégalovirus: journal d'hospitalisation*. Paris: Editions du Seuil, 1992.

Guibert, Hervé. *La mort propagande*. Paris: Gallimard, [1977] 2009.

Guibert, Hervé. *Le mausolée des amants: Journal, 1976–1991*. Paris: Gallimard, 2001.

Guibert, Hervé. *Le protocole compassionnel: roman*. Paris: Gallimard, 1991.

Guyer, Ruth Levy, and Jonathan D. Moreno. "Slouching toward Policy: Lazy Bioethics and the Perils of Science Fiction." *American Journal of Bioethics* 4, no. 4 (September 1, 2004): W14–17. https://doi.org/10.1080/15265160490908022.

Halamka, John D., and Micky Tripathi. "The HITECH Era in Retrospect." *New England Journal of Medicine* 377, no. 10 (2017): 907–9. https://doi.org/10.1056/NEJMp1709851.

Hanson, Clare. *A Cultural History of Pregnancy: Pregnancy, Medicine, and Culture, 1750–2000*. Houndmills: Palgrave Macmillan, 2004.

Haraway, Donna Jeanne. *Simians, Cyborgs, and Women: The Reinvention of Nature*. New York: Routledge, 1991.

Harney, Stefano, and Fred Moten. *The Undercommons: Fugitive Planning & Black Study*. New York: Minor Compositions, 2013.

Hartzband, Pamela, and Jerome Groopman. "Medical Taylorism." *New England Journal of Medicine* 374, no. 2 (2016): 106–8. https://doi.org/10.1056/NEJMp1512402.

Hartzband, Pamela, and Jerome Groopman. "Off the Record—Avoiding the Pitfalls of Going Electronic." *New England Journal of Medicine* 358, no. 16 (April 17, 2008): 1656–8. http://dx.doi.org.ezproxy.cul.columbia.edu/10.1056/NEJMp0802221.

Hauser, Christine. "A Handmaid's Tale of Protest." *New York Times*, June 30, 2017, sec. U.S. https://www.nytimes.com/2017/06/30/us/handmaids-protests-abortion.html.

Hayes, Mary H. S., and Donald G. Paterson. "Experimental Development of the Graphic Rating Method." *Psychological Bulletin* 18 (1921): 98–9.

Hayles, Katherine. *How We Became Posthuman: Virtual Bodies in Cybernetics, Literature, and Informatics*. Chicago: University of Chicago Press, [1999] 2010.

Hayward, Jennifer. *Consuming Pleasures: Active Audiences and Serial Fictions from Dickens to the Soap Opera*. Lexington: University Press of Kentucky, 1997.

Henry III, William A., Andrea Sachs, and James Willwerth. "Ethics: Forcing Gays Out of the Closet: Homosexual Leaders Seek to Expose Foes of the Movement." *Time*, January 29, 1990. http://content.time.com/time/subscriber/article/0,33009,969264-1,00.html.

Herndl, Diane Price. "Disease versus Disability: The Medical Humanities and Disability Studies." *PMLA* 120, no. 2 (2005): 593–8.

Herrera, Salvador. "Skin Deep: Biometrics and Containment in Sabrina Vourvoulias's INK." *SYNAPSIS*, November 29, 2019. https://medicalhealthhumanities.com/2019/11/29/skin-deep-biometrics-and-containment-in-sabrina-vourvoulias-ink/.

Hirschtick, Robert E. "Copy-and-Paste." *JAMA* 295, no. 20 (2006): 2335–6.

Hirschtick, Robert E. "John Lennon's Elbow." *JAMA* 308, no. 5 (2012): 463–4.

Hise, Joseph Henry. "And Then Came the PACS." *JAMA* 318, no. 4 (July 25, 2017): 331. https://doi.org/10.1001/jama.2017.5991.

Holan, Angie Drobnic. "PolitiFact—PolitiFact's Lie of the Year: 'Death Panels.'" *PolitiFact*, December 18, 2009, sec. National. https://www.politifact.com/article/2009/dec/18/politifact-lie-year-death-panels/.

Holden, Richard. "Digital." *Oxford English Dictionary* (blog). August 16, 2012. https://public.oed.com/blog/word-stories-digital/.

Holmes, Martha Stoddard. "Embodied Storytellers: Disability Studies and Medical Humanities." *Hastings Center Report* 45, no. 2 (2015): 11–15. https://doi.org/10.1002/hast.426.

Holmes, Seth M., and Maya Ponte. "En-Case-Ing the Patient: Disciplining Uncertainty in Medical Student Patient Presentations." *Culture, Medicine, and Psychiatry* 35, no. 2 (June 2011): 163–82.

Howard, Brody. *Stories of Sickness*, 2nd ed. Oxford: Oxford University Press, 2003.

Imarisha, Walidah. *Why Aren't There More Black People in Oregon? A Hidden History*. PDXTalks, 2015.

Irani, Jihad S., Jennifer L. Middleton, Ruta Marfatia, Evelyn T. Omana, and Frank D'Amico. "The Use of Electronic Health Records in the Exam Room and Patient Satisfaction: A Systematic Review." *Journal of the American Board of Family Medicine* 22, no. 5 (September 1, 2009): 553–62. https://doi.org/10.3122/jabfm.2009.05.080259.

James, E. L. *Fifty Shades Freed*. New York: Vintage, 2012.

Jamison, Leslie. *The Empathy Exams*. Minneapolis, MN: Graywolf Press, 2015.

Jankowski, Theodora A. "… in the Lesbian Void: Woman-Woman Eroticism in Shakespeare's Plays." In *A Feminist Companion to Shakespeare*, edited by

Dympna Callaghan, 318–38. Chichester: John Wiley & Sons, 2016. https://doi.org/10.1002/9781118501221.ch16.
Jeffries, Stuart. "Friedrich Kittler and the Rise of the Machine." *The Guardian*, 2011, sec. Opinion. http://www.theguardian.com/commentisfree/2011/dec/28/friedrich-kittler-rise-of-the-machine.
Jeffries, Stuart. *Grand Hotel Abyss: The Lives of the Frankfurt School*. London: Verso, 2016.
Jenkins, Keith. *Re-thinking History*. London: Routledge, 1991.
Johnson, Merri Lisa, and Robert McRuer. "Cripistemologies: Introduction." *Journal of Literary & Cultural Disability Studies* 8, no. 2 (2014): 127–47.
Jones, Anne Hudson. "Why Teach Literature and Medicine? Answers from Three Decades." *Journal of Medical Humanities* 34, no. 4 (December 1, 2013): 415–28. https://doi.org/10.1007/s10912-013-9241-9.
Jones, Therese, Delese Wear, and Lester D. Friedman. "Introduction: The Why, the What, and the How of the Medical/Health Humanities." In *Health Humanities Reader*, edited by Therese Jones, Delese Wear, and Lester D. Friedman, 1–9. New Brunswick, NJ: Rutgers University Press, 2014.
Jordan-Young, Rebecca M., and Katrina Alicia Karkazis. *Testosterone: An Unauthorized Biography*. Cambridge, MA: Harvard University Press, 2019.
Joy, Michelle, Timothy Clement, and Dominic Sisti. "The Ethics of Behavioral Health Information Technology: Frequent Flyer Icons and Implicit Bias." *JAMA* 316, no. 15 (October 18, 2016): 1539–40. https://doi.org/10.1001/jama.2016.12534.
Jutel, Annemarie. "Sociology of Diagnosis: A Preliminary Review." *Sociology of Health & Illness* 31, no. 2 (March 1, 2009): 278–99. https://doi.org/10.1111/j.1467-9566.2008.01152.x.
Kafer, Alison. *Feminist, Queer, Crip*. Bloomington: Indiana University Press, 2013.
Kahn, Michael W., Sigall K. Bell, Jan Walker, and Tom Delbanco. "Let's Show Patients Their Mental Health Records." *JAMA* 311, no. 13 (April 2, 2014): 1291–2. https://doi.org/10.1001/jama.2014.1824.
Kaliss, J. "Two Writers' Wry Views of Romance." *Noe Valley Voice*, July 1986.
Keeling, Mary. "Stories of Transition: US Veterans' Narratives of Transition to Civilian Life and the Important Role of Identity." *Journal of Military, Veteran and Family Health* 4, no. 2 (2018): 28–36. https://doi.org/10.3138/jmvfh.2017-0009.
Kendal, Evie. "Utopian Literature and Bioethics: Exploring Reproductive Difference and Gender Equality." *Literature and Medicine* 36, no. 1 (2018): 56–84. http://dx.doi.org.ezproxy.cul.columbia.edu/10.1353/lm.2018.0002.
Khanna, Raman R., Robert M. Wachter, and Michael Blum. "Reimagining Electronic Clinical Communication in the Post-Pager, Smartphone Era." *JAMA* 315, no. 1 (January 5, 2016): 21–2. https://doi.org/10.1001/jama.2015.17025.
Kim, Eunjung. *Curative Violence: Rehabilitating Disability, Gender, and Sexuality in Modern Korea*. Durham, NC: Duke University Press Books, 2017.

King, Jennifer, Vaishali Patel, Eric W. Jamoom, and Michael F. Furukawa. "Clinical Benefits of Electronic Health Record Use: National Findings." *Health Services Research* 49, no. 1, pt. 2 (2014): 392–404. https://doi.org/10.1111/1475-6773.12135.

Kittler, Friedrich A. *Discourse Networks 1800/1900*, translated by Michael Metteer and Chris Cullens. Stanford, CA: Stanford University Press, 1990.

Kittler, Friedrich A. *Gramophone, Film, Typewriter*, translated by Geoffrey Winthrop-Young and Michael Wutz. Writing Science. Stanford, CA: Stanford University Press, 1999.

Klass, Perri. "Disconnected." *New England Journal of Medicine* 362, no. 15 (April 15, 2010): 1358–61. https://doi.org/10.1056/NEJMp0911193.

Kleinman, Arthur, and Peter Benson. "Anthropology in the Clinic: The Problem of Cultural Competency and How to Fix It." *PLoS Medicine* 3, no. 10 (October 24, 2006): e294. https://doi.org/10.1371/journal.pmed.0030294.

Kleykamp, Meredith, and Crosby Hipes. "Coverage of Veterans of the Wars in Iraq and Afghanistan in the U.S. Media." *Sociological Forum* 30, no. 2 (2015): 348–68.

Klugman, Craig M. "How Health Humanities Will Save the Life of the Humanities." *Journal of Medical Humanities* 38, no. 4 (2017): 419–30. https://doi.org/10.1007/s10912-017-9453-5.

Kommer, Curtis G. "Good Documentation." *JAMA* 320, no. 9 (September 4, 2018): 875–6. https://doi.org/10.1001/jama.2018.11781.

Kruger, Steven F. *AIDS Narratives: Gender and Sexuality, Fiction and Science*. New York: Routledge, [1996] 2011.

Kruse, Kevin Michael, and Julian E. Zelizer. *Fault Lines: A History of the United States since 1974*, 1st ed. New York: W.W. Norton, 2019.

Kudlick, Catherine. "Comment: On the Borderland of Medical and Disability History." *Bulletin of the History of Medicine* 87, no. 4 (2013): 540–59. https://doi.org/10.1353/bhm.2013.0086.

Kullmann, Thomas. "Shakespeare's *Winter's Tale* and the Myth of Childhood Innocence." *Poetica* 46, nos. 3/4 (2014): 317–30.

Kumagai, Arno K. "From Competencies to Human Interests: Ways of Knowing and Understanding in Medical Education." *Academic Medicine* 89, no. 7 (2014): 978–83.

Lambrew, Jeanne. "More than Half of Doctors Now Use Electronic Health Records Thanks to Administration Policies." *White House President Barack Obama* (blog), May 23, 2013.

Langley, G. B., and H. Sheppeard. "The Visual Analogue Scale: Its Use in Pain Measurement." *Rheumatology International* 5, no. 4 (July 1, 1985): 145–8. https://doi.org/10.1007/BF00541514.

Le Fanu, Joseph Sheridan. "Carmilla." In *In a Glass Darkly*, edited by Robert Tracy, 243–319. Oxford World's Classics. Oxford: Oxford University Press, [1872] 1999.

Lepore, Jill. "A Golden Age for Dystopian Fiction." *New Yorker*, May 29, 2017. https://www.newyorker.com/magazine/2017/06/05/a-golden-age-for-dystopian-fiction.

Lettow, Susanne. "Biocapitalism." *Krisis*, no. 2 (2018): 13–14.
Lévinas, Emmanuel. *Humanism of the Other*, translated by Nidra Poller, 1st reprint ed. Urbana: University of Illinois Press, [1972] 2006.
Lévinas, Emmanuel. *Humanisme de l'autre homme*. Livre de poche, Biblio essais. Montpellier: Fata Morgana, 1972.
Lifflander, Anne Lucy. "Hard Times and Hard Stops." *JAMA* 321, no. 9 (March 5, 2019): 837–8. https://doi.org/10.1001/jama.2019.1208.
Linker, Beth. "On the Borderland of Medical and Disability History: A Survey of the Fields." *Bulletin of the History of Medicine* 87, no. 4 (2013): 499–535. https://doi.org/10.1353/bhm.2013.0074.
Liu, Jialin, Li Luo, Riu Zhang, and Tingting Huang. "Patient Satisfaction with Electronic Medical/Health Record: A Systematic Review." *Scandinavian Journal of Caring Sciences* 27, no. 4 (2013): 785–91. https://doi.org/10.1111/scs.12015.
Livingston, Julie. "Comment: On the Borderland of Medical and Disability History." *Bulletin of the History of Medicine* 87, no. 4 (2013): 560–4. https://doi.org/10.1353/bhm.2013.0078.
Loriaux, Lynn. *A Biographical History of Endocrinology*. Ames, IA: Wiley Blackwell, 2016.
Luttfring, Sara D. *Bodies, Speech, and Reproductive Knowledge in Early Modern England*. Routledge Studies in Renaissance Literature and Culture 26. New York: Routledge, 2016.
Malone, Cynthia Northcutt. "Near Confinement: Pregnant Women in the Nineteenth-Century British Novel." *Dickens Studies Annual* 29 (2000): 367–85.
Markham, Gervase. *The English Husbandman: The First Part: Contayning the Knowledge of the True Nature of Euery Soyle within this Kingdome: How to Plow It; and the Manner of the Plough, and Other Instruments Belonging Thereto. Together with the Art of Planting, Grafting, and Gardening after Our Latest and Rarest Fashion. A Worke Neuer Written before by Any Author: And Now Newly Compiled for the Benefit of this Kingdon*. London: Thomas Snodham, 1613.
Masuda, Akihiko, Steven C. Hayes, Michael P. Twohig, Claudia Drossel, Jason Lillis, and Yukiko Washio. "A Parametric Study of Cognitive Defusion and the Believability and Discomfort of Negative Self-Relevant Thoughts." *Behavior Modification* 33, no. 2 (March 1, 2009): 250–62. https://doi.org/10.1177/0145445508326259.
Maupin, Armistead. *Babycakes*. New York: Harper & Row, 1984.
Maupin, Armistead. *Further Tales of the City*. New York: Harper & Row, 1982.
Maupin, Armistead. *Logical Family: A Memoir*. New York: Harper-Collins, 2017.
Maupin, Armistead. *More Tales of the City*. New York: Harper & Row, 1980.
Maupin, Armistead. *Significant Others*. New York: Perennial Library, 1987.
Maupin, Armistead. *Sure of You*. New York: Harper & Row, 1989.
Maupin, Armistead. *Tales of the City*. New York: Harper & Row, 1978.
May, Molly Caro. *Body Full of Stars: Female Rage and My Passage into Motherhood*. Berkeley, CA: Counterpoint, 2018.

Mazzoni, Cristina. *Maternal Impressions: Pregnancy and Childbirth in Literature and Theory*. Ithaca, NY: Cornell University Press, 2002.

McAlear, Rob. "The Value of Fear: Toward a Rhetorical Model of Dystopia." *Interdisciplinary Humanities* 27, no. 2 (2010): 24–42.

McCoy, Richard C. *Faith in Shakespeare*. Oxford: Oxford University Press, [2013] 2015.

McKinlay, John B., and Lisa D. Marceau. "The End of the Golden Age of Doctoring." *International Journal of Health Services: Planning, Administration, Evaluation* 32, no. 2 (2002): 379–416. https://doi.org/10.2190/JL1D-21BG-PK2N-J0KD.

McNeill, William H. *Hutchins' University: A Memoir of the University of Chicago, 1929–1950*, illustrated ed. Chicago: University of Chicago Press, 2007.

McRuer, Robert. *Crip Theory: Cultural Signs of Queerness and Disability*. Cultural Front. New York: New York University Press, 2006.

Meggs, Philip B., and Alston W. Purvis. *Meggs' History of Graphic Design*, 5th ed. Hoboken, NJ: Wiley, 2012.

Messinger, Seth D. "Getting Past the Accident: Explosive Devices, Limb Loss, and Refashioning a Life in a Military Medical Center." *Medical Anthropology Quarterly* 24, no. 3 (2010): 281–303.

Metzl, Jonathan M., and Helena Hansen. "Structural Competency: Theorizing a New Medical Engagement with Stigma and Inequality." *Social Science & Medicine* (Structural Stigma and Population Health) 103 (February 1, 2014): 126–33. https://doi.org/10.1016/j.socscimed.2013.06.032.

Meyer, Stephenie. *Breaking Dawn*. New York: Little, Brown, 2008.

Meyer, Stephenie. *New Moon*. New York: Little, Brown Books for Young Readers, 2006.

Meyer, Stephenie. "The Story of Twilight & Getting Published." *Stephenie Meyer* (blog). https://stepheniemeyer.com/the-story-of-twilight-getting-published/.

Meyerhoefer, Chad D., Susan A. Sherer, Mary E. Deily, Shin-Yi Chou, Xiaohui Guo, Jie Chen, Michael Sheinberg, and Donald Levick. "Provider and Patient Satisfaction with the Integration of Ambulatory and Hospital EHR Systems." *Journal of the American Medical Informatics Association* 25, no. 8 (2018): 1054–63. https://doi.org/10.1093/jamia/ocy048.

Mikk, Katherine A., Harry A. Sleeper, and Eric J. Topol. "The Pathway to Patient Data Ownership and Better Health." *JAMA* 318, no. 15 (October 17, 2017): 1433–4. https://doi.org/10.1001/jama.2017.12145.

Minot, Leslie Ann. "Vamping the Children: The 'Bloofer Lady,' the 'London Minotaur' and Child-Victimization in Late-Nineteenth-Century England." In *Victorian Crime, Madness and Sensation*, edited by Andrew Maunder and Grace Moore. The Nineteenth Century Series. Aldershot: Ashgate, 2004.

Minton, Eric. "Trust the Bard, for His Magic Is True." PlayShakespeare: Free Shakespeare Resource, September 11, 2012. https://www.playshakespeare.com/the-winters-tale-reviews/theatre-reviews/trust-the-bard-for-his-magic-is-true.

Mishra, Abhay Nath, Catherine Anderson, Corey M. Angst, and Ritu Agarwal. "Electronic Health Records Assimilation and Physician Identity Evolution: An Identity Theory Perspective." *Information Systems Research* 23, no. 3 (2012): 738–60.

Mitchell, Lisa Meryn. *Baby's First Picture: Ultrasound and the Politics of Fetal Subjects*. Toronto: University of Toronto Press, 2001.

Moffie, D. J. "The Validity of Self-Estimated Interests." *Journal of Applied Psychology* 26, no. 5 (1942): 606–13. https://doi.org/10.1037/h0056402.

Morgan, Jennifer L. *Laboring Women: Reproduction and Gender in New World Slavery*. Early American Studies. Philadelphia: University of Pennsylvania Press, 2004.

Muñoz, José Esteban. *Cruising Utopia: The Then and There of Queer Futurity*. Sexual Cultures. New York: New York University Press, 2009.

Munroe, Jennifer. "It's All about the Gillyvors: Engendering Art and Nature in *The Winter's Tale*." In *Ecocritical Shakespeare*, edited by Lynne Bruckner and Dan Brayton, 139–54. Farnham: Routledge, 2011.

Nadesan, Majia Holmer. *Governmentality, Biopower, and Everyday Life*. Routledge Studies in Social and Political Thought 57. New York: Routledge, [2008] 2011.

National Assembly of Québec. "Commission spéciale sur la question de mourir dans la dignité." Select Committee on Dying with Dignity, 2009. http://www.assnat.qc.ca/en/travaux-parlementaires/commissions/csmd-39-1/index.html

Ndahiro, Kennedy. "In Rwanda, We Know All about Dehumanizing Language." *The Atlantic*, April 13, 2019. https://www.theatlantic.com/ideas/archive/2019/04/rwanda-shows-how-hateful-speech-leads-violence/587041/.

Nethercot, Arthur H. "Coleridge's 'Christabel' and Lefanu's 'Carmilla.'" *Modern Philology* 47, no. 1 (1949): 32–8.

Obermeyer, Ziad, and Thomas H. Lee. "Lost in Thought: The Limits of the Human Mind and the Future of Medicine." *New England Journal of Medicine* 377, no. 13 (2017): 1209–11. https://doi.org/10.1056/NEJMp1705348.

O'Connell, Meaghan. *And Now We Have Everything: On Motherhood before I Was Ready*, 1st ed. New York: Little, Brown, 2018.

Oliver, Kelly. *Knock Me Up, Knock Me Down: Images of Pregnancy in Hollywood Films*. New York: Columbia University Press, 2012.

O'Sullivan, Sean. "Six Elements of Serial Narrative." *Narrative* 27, no. 1 (2019): 49–64. https://doi.org/10.1353/nar.2019.0003.

Palin, Sarah. "Statement on the Current Health Care Debate." Facebook, August 7, 2009. https://www.facebook.com/notes/sarah-palin/statement-on-the-current-health-care-debate/113851103434/.

Parker, Harry. *Anatomy of a Soldier*. New York: Alfred A. Knopf, 2016.

Pasman, H. Roeline. "What Characterizes Complex Euthanasia Consultations?" In *Experiences of SCEN (Support and Consultation on Euthanasia in the Netherlands) Physicians*, Halifax, Nova Scotia, 2017.

Paster, Gail Kern. *The Body Embarrassed: Drama and the Disciplines of Shame in Early Modern England*, illustrated ed. Ithaca, NY: Cornell University Press, 1993.

Patel, Jayshil J. "The Things We Say." *JAMA* 319, no. 4 (2018): 341–2. https://doi.org/10.1001/jama.2017.20545.

Patel, Jayshil J. "Writing the Wrong." *JAMA* 314, no. 7 (August 18, 2015): 671–2. https://doi.org/10.1001/jama.2015.5281.

Paterson, Donald G. "The Scott Company Graphic Rating Scale." *Journal of Personnel Research: Official Publication of Personnel Research Federation* 1, nos. 8–9 (1923): 361–76.

Peterson, M. Jeanne. *The Medical Profession in Mid-Victorian London*. Berkeley: University of California Press, 1978.

Peterson, Kaara L. *Popular Medicine, Hysterical Disease, and Social Controversy in Shakespeare's England*. Literary and Scientific Cultures of Early Modernity. Burlington, VT: Ashgate, 2010. https://doi.org/10.4324/9781315601373.

Polak, Kate. *Ethics in the Gutter: Empathy and Historical Fiction in Comics*. Columbus: The Ohio State University Press, 2017.

Pollock, Linda A. "Embarking on a Rough Passage: The Experience of Pregnancy in Early-Modern Society." In *Women as Mothers in Pre-Industrial England*, edited by Valerie Fildes, 39–67. London: Routledge, 1990.

Preciado, Paul B. *Testo Junkie: Sex, Drugs, and Biopolitics in the Pharmacopornographic Era*, translated by Bruce Benderson. New York: The Feminist Press at the City University of New York, 2016.

The Presidents of Northwestern. "Walter Dill Scott, Northwestern University Archives." 2009. http://exhibits.library.northwestern.edu/archives/exhibits/presidents/scott.html.

Raglan, Greta B., Benyamin Margolis, Ronald A. Paulus, and Jay Schulkin. "Electronic Health Record Adoption among Obstetrician/Gynecologists in the United States: Physician Practices and Satisfaction." *Journal for Healthcare Quality* 39, no. 3 (2017): 144–52. https://doi.org/10.1111/jhq.12072.

Ratcliffe, Matthew. "The Structure of Interpersonal Experience." In *The Phenomenology of Embodied Subjectivity*, edited by Rasmus Thybo Jensen and Dermot Moran, 221–38. Contributions to Phenomenology. New York: Springer, 2013.

Reeves, Byron, and Clifford Ivar Nass. *The Media Equation: How People Treat Computers, Televisions, and New Media as Real People and Places*. CSLI Lecture Notes, no. 63. Stanford, CA: Center for the Study of Language and Information, Cambridge University Press, 1996.

Reich, Adam. "Disciplined Doctors: The Electronic Medical Record and Physicians' Changing Relationship to Medical Knowledge." *Social Science & Medicine* 74, no. 7 (April 1, 2012): 1021–8. https://doi.org/10.1016/j.socscimed.2011.12.032.

Reis, Elizabeth. "Divergence or Disorder? The Politics of Naming Intersex." *Perspectives in Biology and Medicine* 50, no. 4 (2007): 535–43. https://doi.org/10.1353/pbm.2007.0054.

Reynolds, L. A., and E. M. Tansey, eds. *Innovation in Pain Management*. London: QMUL History C20Medicine, 2004.

Reynolds, Paige Martin. "Sin, Sacredness, and Childbirth in Early Modern Drama." *Medieval & Renaissance Drama in England* 28 (2015): 30–48.

Richards, D. "Maupin's World." *Dallas Voice*, June 19, 1987, sec. II.

Richardson, Peter. *How to Die in Oregon* (videorecording). Portland, OR: Clearcut Productions, 2010.

Rigg, Melvin G. "Favorable versus Unfavorable Propaganda in the Enjoyment of Music." *Journal of Experimental Psychology* 38, no. 1 (1948): 78–81. https://doi.org/10.1037/h0056077.

Roberts, Celia. *Messengers of Sex: Hormones, Biomedicine, and Feminism*. Cambridge Studies in Society and the Life Sciences. New York: Cambridge University Press, 2007.

Roberts, Dorothy E. *Killing the Black Body: Race, Reproduction, and the Meaning of Liberty*. 1st ed. Black Women Writers. New York: Pantheon Books, 1997.

Roberts, Julie. *The Visualised Foetus: A Cultural and Political Analysis of Ultrasound Imagery*. Theory, Technology and Society. Abingdon: Routledge, 2012. http://ebookcentral.proquest.com/lib/columbia/detail.action?docID=1068864.

Rosenbaum, Lisa. "Living Unlabeled—Diagnosis and Disorder." *New England Journal of Medicine* 359, no. 16 (2008): 1650–3. https://doi.org/10.1056/NEJMp0804984.

Rosenbaum, Lisa. "The Not-My-Problem Problem." *New England Journal of Medicine* 380, no. 9 (February 28, 2019): 881–5. https://doi.org/10.1056/NEJMms1813431.

Rosenbaum, Lisa. "Transitional Chaos or Enduring Harm? The EHR and the Disruption of Medicine." *New England Journal of Medicine* 373, no. 17 (2015): 1585–8. https://doi.org/10.1056/NEJMp1509961.

Rosenberg, Daniel, and Anthony Grafton. *Cartographies of Time*. 1st ed. New York: Princeton Architectural Press, 2010.

Rosenberg, Jordy. *Confessions of the Fox*. New York: One World, 2018.

Rosenfield, Kirstie Gulick. "Nursing Nothing: Witchcraft and Female Sexuality in *The Winter's Tale*." *Mosaic: An Interdisciplinary Critical Journal* 35, no. 1 (March 2002): 95–112.

Rosenthal, David I., and Abraham Verghese. "Meaning and the Nature of Physicians' Work." *New England Journal of Medicine* 375, no. 19 (2016): 1813–15. https://doi.org/10.1056/NEJMp1609055.

Rothman, David J. *Strangers at the Bedside: A History of How Law and Bioethics Transformed Medical Decision Making*. New York: Basic Books, 1991.

Rudin, Robert S., David W. Bates, and Calum MacRae. "Accelerating Innovation in Health IT." *New England Journal of Medicine* 375, no. 9 (September 1, 2016): 815–17. https://doi.org/10.1056/NEJMp1606884.

Sadjadi, Sahar. "The Endocrinologist's Office—Puberty Suppression: Saving Children from a Natural Disaster?" *Journal of Medical Humanities* 34, no. 2 (June 2013): 255–60. https://doi.org/10.1007/s10912-013-9228-6.

Safder, Taimur. "The Name of the Dog." *New England Journal of Medicine* 379, no. 14 (October 4, 2018): 1299–301. https://doi.org/10.1056/NEJMp1806388.

Salam, Maya. "For Serena Williams, Childbirth Was a Harrowing Ordeal. She's Not Alone." *New York Times*, January 11, 2018, sec. Sports. https://www.nytimes.com/2018/01/11/sports/tennis/serena-williams-baby-vogue.html.

Sargent, Lyman Tower. "The Three Faces of Utopianism Revisited." *Utopian Studies* 5, no. 1 (1994): 1–37.

Scarry, Elaine. *The Body in Pain: The Making and Unmaking of the World.* New York: Oxford University Press, 1985.

Schaffner, Anna Katharina. *Exhaustion: A History.* New York: Columbia University Press, 2016.

Schaub, Michael. "Not an 'Alternative Fact': George Orwell's *1984* Tops Amazon's Bestseller List." *Los Angeles Times*, January 25, 2017, sec. Books. https://www.latimes.com/books/jacketcopy/la-et-jc-george-orwell-20170125-story.html.

Scheper-Hughes, N. "Three Propositions for a Critically Applied Medical Anthropology." *Social Science & Medicine (1982)* 30, no. 2 (1990): 189–97. https://doi.org/10.1016/0277-9536(90)90079-8.

Schiff, Gordon D., and David W. Bates. "Can Electronic Clinical Documentation Help Prevent Diagnostic Errors?" *New England Journal of Medicine* 362, no. 12 (March 25, 2010): 1066–9. https://doi.org/10.1056/NEJMp0911734.

Schotland, Sara D. "Forced Execution of the Elderly: Old Law, Dystopia, and the Utilitarian Argument." *Humanities* 2, no. 2 (2013): 160–75. http://dx.doi.org.ezproxy.cul.columbia.edu/10.3390/h2020160.

Scott, Walter Dill. *Die psychologie der triebe historisch-kritisch betrachtet.* Leipzig, 1900.

Scott, Walter Dill. *The Theory of Advertising: A Simple Exposition of the Principles of Psychology in Their Relation to Successful Advertising.* Boston: Small, Maynard, 1903.

Shakespeare, Tom. "The Social Model of Disability." In *The Disability Studies Reader*, by Lennard J. Davis, 4th ed., 214–21 New York: Routledge, 2013.

Shakespeare, William. *Titus Andronicus*, edited by Jonathan Bate. Arden Shakespeare, 3rd ser. London: Bloomsbury, 1995.

Shakespeare, William. *The Winter's Tale*, edited by John Pitcher. Arden Shakespeare, 3rd ser. London: Bloomsbury, 2010.

Shakespeare, William. *The Winter's Tale: The Oxford Shakespeare*, edited by Stephen Orgel. Oxford: Oxford University Press, 2008.

Shapin, Steven. *The Scientific Revolution*, 2nd ed. Science–Culture. Chicago: The University of Chicago Press, [1996] 2018.

Shapiro, Johanna, Jack Coulehan, Delese Wear, and Martha Montello. "Medical Humanities and Their Discontents: Definitions, Critiques, and Implications." *Academic Medicine* 84, no. 2 (February 2009): 192–8. https://doi.org/10.1097/ACM.0b013e3181938bca.

Sheffield, Elisabeth. "An Uneven Luxuriance." *American Book Review* 40, no. 6 (2019): 18. https://doi.org/10.1353/abr.2019.0102.

Shields, Duncan M., David Kuhl, Kevin Lutz, Jesse Frender, Niki Baumann, and Phillip Lopresti. "Mental Health and Well-Being of Military Veterans during Military to Civilian Transition: Review and Analysis of the Recent Literature," Canadian Institute for Military and Veteran Health Research & Scientific Authority, Veterans Affairs Canada, 2016.

Siebers, Tobin. *Disability Theory*. Ann Arbor: University of Michigan Press, 2008. https://doi.org/10.3998/mpub.309723.

Singer, Jeffrey A. "Toward Medical Dystopia." *Journal of Trauma and Acute Care Surgery* 75, no. 3 (August 31, 2013): 517–19. https://doi.org/10.1097/TA.0b013 e3182a040f6.

Singer, Jeffrey A., and Patrick Eddington. "The War on Opioids: Digital Dystopia Edition." Cato Institute, June 17, 2020. https://www.cato.org/commentary/war-opio ids-digital-dystopia-edition.

Singh, Hardeep, and Mark L. Graber. "Improving Diagnosis in Health Care—The Next Imperative for Patient Safety." *New England Journal of Medicine* 373, no. 26 (December 24, 2015): 2493–5. https://doi.org/10.1056/NEJMp1512241.

Snyder, Susan. "Mamillius and Gender Polarization in *The Winter's Tale*." *Shakespeare Quarterly* 50, no. 1 (1999): 1–8. https://doi.org/10.2307/2902108.

Sontag, Susan. *Illness as Metaphor; and, AIDS and Its Metaphors*, first Picador USA ed. New York: Picador, [1989] 2001.

Spade, Dean. "Resisting Medicine, Re/Modeling Gender." *Berkeley Journal of Gender, Law & Justice* 18, no. 1 (2003): 15–37. https://doi.org/10.15779/z38nk3645g.

Spence, Des. "Medicine's Dystopian Future." *British Medical Journal* 345, no. 7882 (November 10, 2012): 47.

Stecklow, Steve. "Hatebook: Inside Facebook's Myanmar Operation. A Reuters Special Report." Reuters, August 15, 2018. https://www.reuters.com/investigates/special-rep ort/myanmar-facebook-hate/.

Steedman, Carolyn. "To Middlemarch: Without Benefit of Archive." In *Dust: The Archive and Cultural History*, 89–111. Encounters. New Brunswick, NJ: Rutgers University Press, 2002.

Stevens, Dana. "*Twilight: Breaking Dawn*, Part I Is One Seriously Sick Little Blockbuster." *Slate Magazine*, November 18, 2011. https://slate.com/cult ure/2011/11/twilight-breaking-dawn-part-i-is-one-seriously-sick-little-blockbus ter.html.

Stoker, Bram. *Dracula*, edited by Nina Auerbach and David J. Skal. New York: W.W. Norton, [1897] 1996.

Stonington, Scott D., Seth M. Holmes, Helena Hansen, Jeremy A. Greene, Keith A. Wailoo, Debra Malina, Stephen Morrissey, Paul E. Farmer, and Michael G. Marmot. "Case Studies in Social Medicine—Attending to Structural Forces in Clinical Practice." *New England Journal of Medicine* 379, no. 20 (November 15, 2018): 1958–61. https://doi.org/10.1056/NEJMms1814262.

Stryker, Susan. *Transgender History*. Berkeley, CA: Seal Press, 2008.

Sulik, Gayle A. "Managing Biomedical Uncertainty: The Technoscientific Illness Identity." *Sociology of Health & Illness* 31, no. 7 (2009): 1059–76. https://doi.org/1 0.1111/j.1467-9566.2009.01183.x.

Suvin, Darko. "Theses on Dystopia 2001." In *Dark Horizons: Science Fiction and the Dystopian Imagination*, edited by Raffaella Baccolini and Tom Moylan, 187–202. New York: Routledge, 2003.

Taylor, Janelle S. *The Public Life of the Fetal Sonogram: Technology, Consumption, and the Politics of Reproduction*. Studies in Medical Anthropology. New Brunswick, NJ: Rutgers University Press, 2008. https://ezproxy.cul.columbia.edu/login?qurl=https%3a%2f%2fsearch.ebscohost.com%2flogin.aspx%3fdirect%3dt rue%26db%3de025xna%26AN%3d246041%26site%3dehost-live%26scope%3dsite.

Toll, Elizabeth. "278.00 Obesity, Not Otherwise Specified." *JAMA* 309, no. 11 (March 20, 2013): 1123–4. https://doi.org/10.1001/jama.2013.1241.

Toll, Elizabeth. "The Cost of Technology." *JAMA* 307, no. 23 (June 20, 2012): 2497–8. https://doi.org/10.1001/jama.2012.4946.

Tomkins, Silvan S. *Affect, Imagery, Consciousness*, edited by Bertram P. Karon, 4 vols. New York: Springer, 1962.

Tosh, John. *The Pursuit of History: Aims, Methods and New Directions in the Study of Modern History*. 5th ed. Harlow: Longman, [1984] 2010.

Tousignant, Noémi. "The Rise and Fall of the Dolorimeter: Pain, Analgesics, and the Management of Subjectivity in Mid-Twentieth-Century United States." *Journal of the History of Medicine and Allied Sciences* 66, no. 2 (2011): 145–79.

Traub, Valerie. *The Renaissance of Lesbianism in Early Modern England*. Cambridge Studies in Renaissance Literature and Culture 42. Cambridge: Cambridge University Press, 2002.

Troy, Gil. *Morning in America: How Ronald Reagan Invented the 1980s*. Politics and Society in Twentieth-Century America. Princeton, NJ: Princeton University Press, 2005.

Turnbull, Cadwell. "Dystopia Isn't Sci-Fi—For Me, It's the American Reality." *Wired*, July 19, 2020. https://www.wired.com/story/dystopia-isnt-sci-fi-for-me-its-the-ameri can-reality/.

Turner, Bryan S. "Body." *Theory, Culture & Society* 23, nos. 2–3 (2006): 223–9. https://doi.org/10.1177/0263276406062576.

"Univocal, adj." In *Merriam-Webster*. https://www.merriam-webster.com/dictionary/univocal.

Upstone, Sara. "Beyond the Bedroom: Motherhood in E. L. James's *Fifty Shades of Grey* Trilogy." *Frontiers: A Journal of Women Studies* 37, no. 2 (2016): 138–64. https://doi.org/10.5250/fronjwomestud.37.2.0138.

Vadeboncœur, Alain. *Les acteurs ne savent pas mourir*. Montréal: Lux, 2014.

Vardanyan, R. S., and Victor J. Hruby. *Synthesis of Best-Seller Drugs.* Amsterdam: Elsevier/AP, 2016.

Verghese, Abraham. "Culture Shock—Patient as Icon, Icon as Patient." *New England Journal of Medicine* 359, no. 26 (December 25, 2008): 2748–51. https://doi.org/10.1056/NEJMp0807461.

Viney, William, Felicity Callard, and Angela Woods. "Critical Medical Humanities: Embracing Entanglement, Taking Risks." *Medical Humanities* 41, no. 1 (June 1, 2015): 2–7. https://doi.org/10.1136/medhum-2015-010692.

Wang, C. Jason. "Medical Documentation in the Electronic Era." *JAMA* 308, no. 20 (November 28, 2012): 2091–2. https://doi.org/10.1001/jama.2012.14849.

Wang, C. Jason, and Andrew T. Huang. "Integrating Technology into Health Care: What Will It Take?" *JAMA* 307, no. 6 (February 8, 2012): 569–70. https://doi.org/10.1001/jama.2012.102.

Warhol, Robyn R. "Making 'Gay' and 'Lesbian' into Household Words: How Serial Form Works in Armistead Maupin's 'Tales of the City.'" *Contemporary Literature* 40, no. 3 (1999): 378–402. https://doi.org/10.2307/1208883.

Washington, Harriet A. *Medical Apartheid: The Dark History of Medical Experimentation on Black Americans from Colonial Times to the Present.* New York: Doubleday, 2006.

Washington, Vindell, Karen DeSalvo, Farzad Mostashari, and David Blumenthal. "The HITECH Era and the Path Forward." *New England Journal of Medicine* 377, no. 10 (September 7, 2017): 904–6. https://doi.org/10.1056/NEJMp1703370.

Wear, Delese, and Lois LaCivita Nixon. "The Fictional World: What Literature Says to Health Professionals." *Journal of Medical Humanities* 12, no. 2 (June 1, 1991): 55–64. https://doi.org/10.1007/BF01142869.

Wehling, Peter. "The 'Technoscientization' of Medicine and Its Limits: Technoscientific Identities, Biosocialities, and Rare Disease Patient Organizations." *Poiesis & Praxis* 8, no. 2 (2011): 67–82. https://doi.org/10.1007/s10202-011-0100-3.

Weizenbaum, Joseph. "ELIZA—A Computer Program for the Study of Natural Language Communication between Man and Machine." *Communications of the ACM* 9, no. 1 (January 1, 1966): 36–45. https://doi.org/10.1145/365153.365168.

Wen, Leana. *Liberty, Democracy, Equity, and Justice in Healthcare* (TEDx video). University of Nevada, 2014. https://www.youtube.com/watch?v=xKSWaCt3fqM.

Wen, Leana. "What Does a Health Care Dystopia Look Like?" *Psychology Today* (blog), February 3, 2014. http://www.psychologytoday.com/blog/the-doctor-is-listening/201402/what-does-health-care-dystopia-look.

White, Amina, and Marion Danis. "Enhancing Patient-Centered Communication and Collaboration by Using the Electronic Health Record in the Examination Room." *JAMA* 309, no. 22 (June 12, 2013): 2327–8. https://doi.org/10.1001/jama.2013.6030.

White, Hayden V. "The Burden of History." *History and Theory* 5, no. 2 (1966): 111–34. https://doi.org/10.2307/2504510.

White, Hayden V. *Metahistory: The Historical Imagination in Nineteenth-Century Europe*. Baltimore, MD: Johns Hopkins University Press, 1973.

Whitehead, Anne. *Medicine and Empathy in Contemporary British Fiction: An Intervention in Medical Humanities*. Edinburgh: Edinburgh University Press, 2017.

Wiegman, Robyn. *Object Lessons*. Next Wave. Durham, NC: Duke University Press, 2012.

Will, George. "Running Not Shrugging." Townhall, May 27, 2010. https://townhall.com/columnists/georgewill/2010/05/27/running-not-shrugging-n1064485.

Wilson, Elizabeth A. *Affect and Artificial Intelligence. In Vivo: The Cultural Mediations of Biomedical Science*. Seattle: University of Washington Press, 2010. http://www.columbia.edu/cgi-bin/cul/resolve?clio14020718.

Wilson, James C. "Making Disability Visible: How Disability Studies Might Transform the Medical and Science Writing Classroom." *Technical Communication Quarterly* 9, no. 2 (March 1, 2000): 149–61. https://doi.org/10.1080/10572250009364691.

Wolpaw, Daniel R. "Seeing Eye to Eye." *New England Journal of Medicine* 365, no. 22 (December 1, 2011): 2052–3. https://doi.org/10.1056/NEJMp1108469.

Wolpaw, Daniel R., and Dan Shapiro. "The Virtues of Irrelevance." *New England Journal of Medicine* 370, no. 14 (April 3, 2014): 1283–5. https://doi.org/10.1056/NEJMp1315661.

Woods, Livia Arndal. "Generations in, Generations of: Pregnancy in Jane Austen." *Women's Writing* 26, no. 2 (April 3, 2019): 132–48.

Woods, Livia Arndal. "Mothers, Memoir, and Medicine." *SYNAPSIS*, May 12, 2019. https://medicalhealthhumanities.com/2019/05/12/mothers-memoir-and-medicine/.

Woods, Livia Arndal. "'Mrs. Grey Will See You Now': The Legacy of Victorian Pregnancy." *SYNAPSIS*, February 13, 2018. https://medicalhealthhumanities.com/2018/02/13/mrs-grey-will-see-you-now/.

Woods, Livia Arndal. "Now You See It: Concealing and Revealing Pregnant Bodies in 'Wuthering Heights' and 'The Clever Woman of the Family.'" *Victorian Network* 6, no. 1 (May 3, 2015): 32–54. https://doi.org/10.5283/vn.54.

Woods, Livia Arndal. "Vampire Dearest: Maternal Bodies and the Female Vampire." *SYNAPSIS*, July 19, 2018. https://medicalhealthhumanities.com/2018/07/19/vampire-dearest-maternal-bodies-and-the-female-vampire/.

Woodward, Rachel, and K. Neil Jenkings. "Military Identities in the Situated Accounts of British Military Personnel." *Sociology* 45, no. 2 (2011): 252–68. https://doi.org/10.1177/0038038510394016.

Wu, David. "Virtual Grief." *JAMA* 308, no. 20 (November 28, 2012): 2095–6. https://doi.org/10.1001/jama.2012.14169.

Yao, Lu Feng, Hai Qing Wang, Feng Zhang, Li Ping Wang, and Jiang Hui Dong. "Minimally Invasive Treatment of Calcaneal Fractures via the Sinus Tarsi Approach Based on a 3D Printing Technique." *Mathematical Biosciences and Engineering* 16, no. 3 (February 26, 2019): 1597–610. https://doi.org/10.3934/mbe.2019076.

Zulman, Donna M., Nigam H. Shah, and Abraham Verghese. "Evolutionary Pressures on the Electronic Health Record: Caring for Complexity." *JAMA* 316, no. 9 (September 6, 2016): 923–4. https://doi.org/10.1001/jama.2016.9538.

Zwartjes, Arianne. "Autotheory as Rebellion: On Research, Embodiment, and Imagination in Creative Nonfiction." *Michigan Quarterly Review*, July 23, 2019. https://sites.lsa.umich.edu/mqr/2019/07/autotheory-as-rebellion-on-research-embodiment-and-imagination-in-creative-nonfiction/.

Contributors

Alicia Andrzejewski, PhD, is an assistant professor in the College of William & Mary's English Department. Her current book project, *Queer Pregnancy in Shakespeare's Plays*, argues for the transgressive force of pregnancy in his oeuvre and the expansive ways in which early modern people thought about the pregnant body.

Kamna S. Balhara, MD, MA, is an assistant professor and assistant residency program director in the Department of Emergency Medicine at the Johns Hopkins University School of Medicine. As a practicing physician and educator, she codirects the initiative for Health Humanities at Hopkins Emergency Medicine. Her work focuses on the integration of Health Humanities across the continuum of medical education.

John A. Carranza, PhD, is a historian of science and medicine and specializes in public health and disability history. He will be a postdoctoral fellow with the Institute for Historical Studies at the University of Texas at Austin in 2022–3.

Anna Fenton-Hathaway, PhD, is the managing editor of *Literature and Medicine*, published by Johns Hopkins University Press and sponsored by the University of Illinois at Chicago. She teaches seminars on science fiction and bioethics to first- and second-year medical students at Northwestern University.

Kristina Fleuty, MA, is a research assistant at the Veterans and Families Institute for Military Social Research, based at Anglia Ruskin University in the United Kingdom.

Joshua Franklin, MD, PhD, is a medical anthropologist and psychiatry resident at the University of Pennsylvania. His work focuses on the medicalization of childhood and on care for transgender and gender-nonconforming youth in Philadelphia.

Benjamin Gagnon Chainey, PT, PhD, is a physical therapist and a postdoctoral fellow at the Medical Humanities—HEALS program at Dalhousie University.

In early 2022, he completed a PhD in French-language literature jointly at Université de Montréal and Nottingham Trent University. His PhD work conducts comparative analyses of the embodied experience of illness and of the upheaval of care relationship in both symbolist and decadent literature from the end of the nineteenth century, and in AIDS literature from the end of the twentieth century.

Rishi Goyal, MD, PhD, is director of the medical humanities major at the Institute for Comparative Literature and Society at Columbia University, an associate professor in the Department of Emergency Medicine at Columbia University Irving Medical Center, and a visiting professor at the University of Southern Denmark in Odense.

Arden Hegele, PhD, is lecturer in the discipline of English and comparative literature at Columbia University, where she teaches in nineteenth-century literature and the medical humanities. Her first book is *Romantic Autopsy: Literary Form and Medical Reading* (2022).

Roanne Kantor, PhD, is Assistant Professor of English at Stanford University. Her book, *South Asian Writers, Latin American Literature, and the Rise of Global English* (2022), was awarded the ACLA Helen Tartar First Book Subvention Prize in 2021. She is also a translator and the winner of the Susan Sontag Prize for Translation.

Travis Chi Wing Lau, PhD, is Assistant Professor of English at Kenyon College. His research and teaching focus on eighteenth- and nineteenth-century British literature and culture, health humanities, and disability studies. Alongside his scholarship, Lau frequently writes for venues of public scholarship like *Synapsis: A Journal of Health Humanities, Public Books, Lapham's Quarterly*, and the *Los Angeles Review of Books*. His poetry has appeared in *Barren Magazine, Wordgathering, Glass, South Carolina Review, Foglifter*, and the *New Engagement*, as well as in two chapbooks, *The Bone Setter* (2019) and *Paring* (2020).

Diana Rose Newby, PhD, is a lecturer in writing at Princeton University. She completed her PhD in English and comparative literature at Columbia University. Her research and teaching bring together studies of British literature with health and environmental humanities and the history of science.

Gabi Schaffzin, PhD, is Assistant Professor of Design Studies at York University. He completed his PhD in art history, theory, and criticism (art practice concentration) at UC San Diego. His work combines design history, information studies, and disability studies to look at the visual design of those tools that use numbers to communicate and measure pain in medical patients and trial subjects.

Livia Arndal Woods, PhD, is Assistant Professor of Literature at the University of Illinois at Springfield. Her work focuses on Victorian literature, gender and sexuality studies, and reading practices.

Index

able-bodied 11, 57, 61–2, 65, 70, 136
ableism 136, 138
About Time (Currie) 207
academic training 99. *See also* training
academy 191–5, 193 n.60, 201
Ackerknecht, Erwin 132
activism
   ACT-UP 156
   AIDS 156
   disability(ies) 6, 131, 136
   outspokenness and 142
   rights-based 132
   social justice 134
Adam Bede (Eliot) 25
aesthetic sensitivity 163, 165
   caregiver 170–5
affect
   of ableism 136
   computation and 105
   cultural ideas of 2
   of limb loss 61, 61 n.18
   subject and 119–21
Affect Imagery Consciousness (Tomkins) 120
Affordable Care Act 203
AIDS Coalition to Unleash Power (ACT-UP) 156
Aitken, R. C. B. 118
Allen, Martina 194
Altschuler, Sari 5 n.8, 6, 14, 158
   The Medical Imagination: Literature and Health in the Early United States 6, 129 n.3, 158 n.61
American College of Obstetricians and Gynecologists (ACOG) 51–2
American Psychological Association 106, 113
American Shakespeare Center 50
Americans with Disabilities Act of 1990 134
Amis, Martin
   Time's Arrow 207

Amorphophallus titanium (corpse flower) 188
amputee
   below-the-knee 57
   lived experience of being 61 n.17
   normal life 67, 70
   prosthesis 66
   transition from able-bodied to 11, 61–2, 70
   veteran 57, 62–4, 67–70
analgesic testing 122
Anatomy of a Soldier (Parker) 11, 19–20, 57–70
   amputee veteran 57, 62–4, 67–70
   limb loss 61–9
   military to civilian transition 58–9, 64, 70
   objectification of the injured body 59–60
   prosthetic gain 62–7
   social identity 63, 67–70
   sociocultural norms 67–70
   transitioning from able-bodied to amputee 61–2
Ann, Mary 151, 153–4
anthropology
   disciplinary vision 96
   medical 2, 13, 71, 94–6, 102, 212
anthropomorphized objects 57
anti-essentialism 1, 8
anti-gay campaign 149
The Argonauts (Nelson) 37
Aristotle 183
artificial intelligence 120
artistic aesthetics 171
assessing univocally 163–5, 170
Atkinson, Sarah
   The Edinburgh Companion to the Critical Medical Humanities 7
Atlas Shrugged (Rand) 198
attitudinal orientations 3, 7–9, 177

Atwood, Margaret
    The Handmaid's Tale 37, 198, 207
Auerbach, Nina 32
    Our Vampires, Ourselves 27
automated data importation 87
autotheory 182 n.5
azidothymidine (AZT) 156

Babycakes (Maupin) 149, 151, 153
Banner, Olivia
    Teaching Health Humanities 6
Barnes, Tom 57
Barrish, Phillip 198
Bates, David W. 91
Bayley, Ed 148
Beecher, Henry 115, 121
    Measurement of Subjective Responses 116
Benjamin, Regina 90
Benson, Peter 100
Berlant, Lauren 13, 96–7
    Cruel Optimism 96–7
Bernard, Claude 170
bias 4, 8, 10, 13, 19, 53, 88, 136
biocapitalism 183 n.9, 186, 193
bioethicists 16, 162, 198
bioethics. *See also* ethics
    disability 138
    discourses 164–5
    medical education and 201
    realist fiction in ethics 199
    training 207
biological sex 16, 183. *See also* sex
biomedicine/biomedical
    apparatus 77
    bias 4, 13
    biomedicalization 77, 92
    bodily realities 10, 13–14, 177
    cultural influence/norms 5, 6–7, 10, 12, 177
    discourse 136
    engineering 1
    frameworks 2, 10, 13
    history of 130
    hormonal 178
    ideas 2, 9
    institutions 10
    knowledge 1, 19, 125, 179
    matrix 178

    models 5, 133
    positivist science 2
    professional norms of 9
    sciences 1
biopolitics/biopolitical 121
Biss, Eula
    On Immunity 37
Black Mirror 208–9, 208 n.45
Black women
    in labor 52
    pregnancy complications 53
    reproductive bodies of 52
Blum, Michael 91
bodily identity 10, 65, 68, 70
bodily realities 10, 13–14, 125, 177
The Body in Pain (Scarry) 164
Bond, Michael 116–17
Bowker, Geoffrey
    Sorting Things Out 118
Bradley, Beatrice 41
Brandt, Allan 152
Brave New World (Huxley) 198–9
Breaking Dawn (Meyer) 10, 24, 31–5, 37
breathing tube 58 n.1, 60
British Medical Journal 114, 202
British Parliament
    First Reform Bill 145
Brody, Lauren Smith
    The Fifth Trimester 55
Brontë, Emily
    Wuthering Heights 25, 32
Brooker, Charlie 208
Browning, Jimmy D. 159
Brown-Séquard, Charles Édouard 183–4
Bryant, Anita 149
bureaucratic 202
    aspects of EHR 79
    authority 76
    forces 12, 75
Butler, Judith
    Notes toward a Performative Theory of Assembly 163

Caddick, Nick 65, 68–9
calculating machines 119
Callard, Felicity 130
Canguilhem, Georges 162
    The Normal and the Pathological 170
caregiver 161–76

aesthetic sensitivity 170–5
cultural relations 165–9
death 165–9
disease 165–9
end-of-life pain 175–6
ethical norms 170–5
experiencing equivocally 163–5
physicians and 137
suffering 165–9
Carlin, Nathan
  Teaching Health Humanities 6
Carmilla (Le Fanu) 11, 24, 27, 29–30, 32–3
Carr, David 143–4
catheter 57 n.1, 60
Centers for Disease Control and Prevention 155
Chambers, Tod 198–9
Chaney, Sarah 152
Charise, Andrea 3
Charon, Rita 85 n.61, 129, 130 n. 4, 158 n. 63
chart biopsy 88
A Chaste Maid in Cheapside (Middleton) 47
chemotherapy 138, 204–5
Chi, Jeffrey 89
childbirth 23, 26
  horrors of 20
  institutionalization of 53
  medicalization of 53
  narration of 26
  and pregnancy 20, 23–4, 34, 43
child displacements 53
"Christabel" (Coleridge) 24, 27–28, 29–30, 32–3
Claeys, Gregory
  Dystopia: A Natural History 201
clinical communication 91
clinical competencies 100
clinical efficiency 76
clinical pain 13
clinical performance 89
clinical procedure 60
clinical psychiatry 212
clinical research 72
clinical spaces 7
clinical trials 13
Cole, Thomas R.
  Teaching Health Humanities 6

Coleridge, Samuel Taylor 20
  "Christabel" 24, 27–28, 29–30, 32–3
collective diary-keeping 192
combat-related injury 69
The Compassion Protocol (Guibert) 172
competency education 93–103
  anthropology in medical education 94–6
  desiring social medicine 101–3
  social medicine pedagogy 96–101
computation 105
computerization 77
Comte, Auguste 170
Concerto for the Left Hand: Disability and the Defamiliar Body (Davidson) 213
Confessions of the Fox (Rosenberg) 181–95, 189 n.41
Cooper, Linda 58, 61, 64
Cree, Alice 68
cripistemologies 139
crip lives 135–8
crip theory 126, 135–8
crip time 125, 137, 139, 178, 213
crip turn 125, 134
CRISPR 138
critical consciousness 12–13, 97, 99
critical dystopia 209. *See also* dystopia
critical medical humanities 3, 130–1, 140
critical pedagogy 99
critical race studies 130
critical race theory 101
critical thinking 86, 90, 125
critique
  anthropological 93, 102, 212
  biocapitalist 186
  of biomedical models 5
  carceral 182
  cultural 3, 100
  defined 8
  discursive 191
  Foucault 19
  of hormonal teleology 178
  of ideology/ideological 1, 4–5
  of medicine 95, 101, 134
  political 4
  technoscientific object 72
Cruel Optimism (Berlant) 13, 96–7, 100
cultural competence 12, 72, 95, 97, 100, 102

cultural crisis in postpartum care 54
cultural relations 165–9
curative violence 126, 138
cure. *See also* diagnosis
   diagnosis and 134
   and medicalization 140
   medicine's fixation 137
   teleology 6, 126
   unforeseen harms 138
   violent effects of 137
Curran, Kelley 50
Currie, Mark
   About Time 207
Cvetkovich, Ann 145
cybernetics 105
Czernik, Zuzanna 85

David Copperfield (Dickens) 25–6
Davidson, Michael
   Concerto for the Left Hand: Disability and the Defamiliar Body 213
Dawn Pepita Langley Hall 148
Day, DeDe Halcyon 150
death 125
   apprehension of 164
   caregiver 165–9
   chosen and dignified 15, 161
   due to AIDS-related complications 153
   metaphorical 43
   physical 25
   physician-assisted 15
   postpartum 42 n.18
   suffering and 165, 167
Death with Dignity Act 204
decision-making
   cognitive bias in 88
   machine learning-based 90
   shared 91
   Visual Analogue Scale (VAS) 117–19
Deleuze, Gilles 189 n.41
   A Thousand Plateaus 189
Desjarlais, Robert
   Shelter Blues 93
Detsky, Allan S. 90
Dhaliwal, Gurpreet 90
diagnosis 117
   codes 84
   medical 93
   physician identities 86
   pre-populated differential 87
   VAS use in pain 73
Díaz, Junot 202
Dickens, Charles 146
   David Copperfield 25–6
DiGangi, Mario 46, 46 n.40
disability 99, 125
   activism 125
   challenges 125
   contingency 133
   historian 132, 134
   individualizing 135
   living with 68, 126
   medicalization of 136
   narratives 9
   revaluation of 138
   studies 131–2, 134–6, 139–40
   violence against people with 138
discrimination
   in employment 147
   institutional 133
   against people with AIDS 156
   systemic 134
   systemic against disabled people 134
disease 4
   among workers 114
   biomedical 132–3
   caregiver 165–9
   chronic 204
   effects of 153
   inherited 77
   venereal 152
doctor-assisted suicide/physician-assisted dying 15, 161, 176, 204. *See also* death
Doctoring. *See* Introduction to Medicine and Society (course)
doctor–patient relationship 12, 72, 76
documentation. *See* electronic documentation
Dolmage, Jay 137
Dorwart, Laura 54
Douglass, Frederick 192, 193
Dracula (Stoker) 11, 24, 27, 30–3
Dror, Otniel E. 14, 130
Duvall, Paula R. 86
dystopia 178–9, 197–209
   critical 209
   imagination *vs.* redescription 203–6

imagining real worlds 200–3
impulse to restore order 206–9

East India Company 184, 186–7
Eddington, Patrick 202
Edelman, Elazer R. 81, 88
The Edinburgh Companion to the Critical Medical Humanities (Atkinson, Macnaughton, Richards, Whitehead and Woods) 7
education. *See* competency education
electronic documentation/record-keeping 71, 81
electronic health record (EHR) 12, 72, 75–92
  bureaucratic aspects of 79
  to determine situation 78
  influence on clinical care 75
  methods 79
  physician as detective 86–91
  physician identity 79–80
  physician-storyteller 80–6
  as technoscientific object 76–7
Eliot, George
  Adam Bede 25
  Middlemarch 25, 145
The Empathy Exams (Jamison) 6
empathy training 10, 12, 71
endochronology 178, 181–95
  academy 191–5
  endocrinology 183–6
  vagrant 186–91
endocrinology 183–6
end-of-life pain/suffering 162–7, 171, 174, 175–6
The English Husbandman (Markham) 47
Engward, Hilary 59, 61, 64, 66
estrogen 183
ethical norms 163, 170–5
ethics 8, 170
  fiction in 199
Ethics in the Gutter: Empathy and Historical Fiction in Comics (Polak) 6
ethnic minorities 151
euthanasia 204 n.29, 206. *See also* doctor-assisted suicide/physician-assisted dying
evidence-based discourse 164–5
evidence-based practice 165

exclusion 4, 8, 19, 135, 166
exhaustion, postpartum 39–55
Exhaustion: A History (Schaffner) 42

Fanestil, Bradley D. 84
feedback
  on clinicians' electronic notes 86
  mechanisms 98
  from students 98–100
Feldman, Ellen 86
female vampire 27–31
femininity 25
Fenlands 191 n.49
Fielding, Jon 153–4
field's crip future 138–40
The Fifth Trimester (Brody) 55
Fifty Shades Freed (James) 10–11, 24, 35–6, 37
Fifty Shades of Grey (James) 11, 24, 32–6
Filippaki, Iro 199, 213
First Reform Bill (British Parliament) 145
First World War 13
flipside 206, 206 n.35
Floyd, George 166
forced sterilization 53
forced transition 57, 61. *See also* transitioning
Fossey, Matt
  Traumatic Limb Loss and the Needs of the Family 63 n.27
Foucauldian panopticon 77
Foucault, Michel 19, 162, 169 n.20, 171, 175
  History of Sexuality: The Will to Knowledge 169
Freud, Sigmund 162, 166–7, 171, 175
Frey, John J. 80, 83
Freyd, Max 108, 111–12, 117
Friedman, Lester D. 90, 195
  The Health Humanities Reader 4, 6–7
Further Tales of the City (Maupin) 149, 151, 153

Gabbe, Steven G.
  Obstetrics: Normal and Problem Pregnancies 40
Ganzini, Linda 176
Garland-Thomson, Rosemarie 138–9

gay
  civil rights 149
  community 146–9, 153–5, 157–8
  and lesbian 147, 149
  man/men 141, 150–1, 154–5
  readers 148
Gélis, Jacques 44
gender
  communal 181
  diversity 93
  hierarchies 99
  identity 94, 147
  nonnormative 94
  normative 93
  studies 101
gene editing 138
Gidde, Anson 157
Goldfarb, Stanley 96
Good, Byron J. 94
Good, Mary-Jo DelVecchio 94
Goroll, Allan H. 86
Gowing, Laura 40
Graber, Mark L. 89
Grace Cathedral 147
Gramophone, Film, Typewriter (Kittler) 78
Graphic Rating Scale (GRS) 106–12
Groopman, Jerome 81–2, 88, 91
Guattari, Felix 189 n.41
  A Thousand Plateaus 189
Guibert, Hervé 15, 161, 162, 165, 166–8, 169 n.20, 171, 175
  about death 169 n.20, 173
  The Compassion Protocol 172
  To the Friend Who Did Not Save My Life 169 n.20
  La Mort propagande 168
  literary work 169
Guillain-Barré syndrome 153
gynecological manuals 40, 43, 45, 52

Halamka, John D. 80
Halcyon, Edgar 148, 150, 152–3
The Handmaid's Tale (Atwood) 37, 198, 207
handwriting 81–2
Hansen, Helena 95
Harney, Stefano
  The Undercommons 193, 193 n.60
Hartzband, Pamela 80–2, 88, 91

Hawkins, Brian 155
Hayes, Mary 106
Hayles, N. Katherine 105, 122
  How We Became Posthuman 117
Hayward, Jennifer 146
health and HIV/AIDS 152–7
health humanities 3–9, 71, 195. *See also* medical humanities
  ambiguity and uncertainty 13
  biomedical sciences 1
  interdisciplinarity 212
  politics of 140
  transdisciplinary work 195
  transformation 129
The Health Humanities Reader (Jones, Wear and Friedman) 4, 6–7
Health Information Technology for Economic and Clinical Health Act (HITECH) 12, 75
Helms, Jesse 156
Herndl, Diane Price 14, 131–3, 140
heterosexuals 147–8, 154–5, 159. *See also* homosexuals
heterotopia 77
Hipes, Crosby 69
Hirschtick, Robert E. 84
historians 14, 44, 54, 132–4, 143–6, 152
historical imagination 143
History of Sexuality: The Will to Knowledge (Foucault) 169
HIV/AIDS 14, 152–7
Hoffman, Dustin 155
Holmes, Martha 140
Holmes, Seth 100
Home, Sir Everard 183 n.12
homeless drug users 99
homosexuals 149, 158. *See also* gay and lesbian
hormone
  creative reimagination of 178
  sex 16, 178, 181–6
horror reproduction (nineteenth century) 23–37
  female vampire 27–31
  reproductive bodies 24–31
  in *Twilight* and *Fifty Shades of Grey* 32–6
Howell, Elizabeth 53
How to Die in Oregon 204

How We Became Posthuman (Hayles) 117
Hudson, Rock 156
Hughes, Jamie Hacker
 Traumatic Limb Loss and the Needs of the Family 63 n.27
Hunter, John 183, 183 n.12
Hunter, Kelly 50
Huxley, Aldous
 Brave New World 198–9
hybridity 194
hypervisibility 31

ICD-10 Clinical Modification (International Statistical Classification of Diseases and Related Health Problems) 84
illness as metaphor 171
improvised explosive device (IED) 57, 63 n.27
incontinence 50
industrialization 146
Industrial Personnel of Philadelphia 106
inequality 8
 economic 95
 power and 99
 social 13
 structural 4
injured body, objectification of 59–60
institutional discrimination 133
intersex 178, 181, 191, 191 n.48, 192, 194
intervention 5–7
 curative 132, 136
 ethical 126
 humanistic 97
 medical 59 n.13, 136
 military 208
 tangible 3
 violent 41
intimate relationships 89. *See also* relationships
Introduction to Medicine and Society (course) 97–8, 97 n.11
inyenzi (cockroaches) 208 n.42
irreconcilable differences 131–4

James, E. L. 20
 Fifty Shades Freed 10–11, 24, 35–6, 37
 Fifty Shades of Grey 11, 24, 32–6

Jamison, Leslie
 The Empathy Exams 6
Jankowski, Theodora 44–6
Java Sea 187
Jones, Jim 142
Jones, Therese
 The Health Humanities Reader 4, 6–7
Jordan-Young, Rebecca M. 184
Journal of Educational Psychology 108
Journal of the American Medical Association (JAMA) 79
Joyce, James 207
Jutel, Annemarie 117

Kafer, Alison 136–7, 139–40
Kahn, Michael W. 85–6
Kanetaka, Bambi 151
Karkazis, Katrina Alicia 184
Kasparov, Gary 119
Keeling, Mary 58, 68
Kenan, Larry 151
Kendal, Evie 198–9
Khan, Bess 186, 191, 193
Khanna, Raman R. 91
Kim, Eunjung 137–8
Kittler, Friedrich A. 72, 77–8, 81, 83–5
 Gramophone, Film, Typewriter 78
Kleinman, Arthur 100
Kleykamp, Meredith 69
Kommer, Curtis G. 82
Kruger, Steven F. 142
Kudlick, Catherine 133–4

La Mort propagande (Guibert) 168
Lee, Thomas H. 91
Le Fanu, Sheridan 20
 Carmilla 11, 24, 27, 29, 32–3
legal discourses 15, 163, 165
Lepore, Jill 201
lesbian
 bookstores 150
 civil rights 149
 and gay 147, 149
 relationships 46
Lettow, Susanne 183 n.9
Levinas, Emmanuel 162, 173
Levy, Ariel
 The Rules Do Not Apply 37
life change 61

life-threatening complications 53
life with disability 68, 138
Lifflander, Anne Lucy 81, 88
limb loss 11, 57, 60–7, 63 n.27, 69–70
line-based scale 105, 122
Linebaugh, Peter
 The Many-Headed Hydra: Sailors, Slaves, Commoners, and the Hidden History of the Revolutionary Atlantic 192
Linker, Beth 132–3, 137
Linotype machine 110–11
literary aesthetics 171
Litvin, Cara B. 87
Livingston, Julie 133–4
living with disability 68
Longhurst, Christopher A. 90
lying-in 40
 ceremony 43–4, 47–9
 rights 11, 20, 41–2

Macnaughton, Jane
 The Edinburgh Companion to the Critical Medical Humanities 7
Madrigal, Anna 147–8, 153
The Many-Headed Hydra (Linebaugh and Rediker) 193
marginalized students 98
Markham, Gervase 47
 The English Husbandman 47
mastectomies 138
master diagnostician 90
maternity 23–24, 27, 34, 37, 46
Maupin, Armistead
 Babycakes 149, 151, 153
 Further Tales of the City 149, 151, 153
 Michael Tolliver Lives 142
 More Tales of the City 148–9, 153
 Significant Others 155
 Sure of You 142, 149, 156–7
 Tales of the City 126, 141–59
May, Molly Caro 50
McAlear, Rob 16, 167, 203–4, 206
McCain, John 203
McCoy, Richard 49
McLuhan, Marshall 72, 78
Measurement of Subjective Responses (Beecher) 116

medical anthropology 2, 13, 71, 94–6, 102, 212. *See also* anthropology
Medical Assistance in Dying (MAID) 126, 162–4
medical curricula 95–6, 100
medical discourses 70, 136, 174
medical documentation 86
medical education 91, 94–6
medical humanities 3–9, 71–2, 129–40
 crip lives 135–8
 crip theory 135–8
 field's crip future 138–40
 irreconcilable differences 131–4
The Medical Imagination: Literature and Health in the Early United States (Altschuler) 6, 129 n.3, 158 n.61
medical instruments 60, 70
medical insurance 54
medicalization
 of childbirth 53
 and cure 140
 of disability 136
 of human experience 77
medical knowledge 77
medically assisted death 126
medical students 88, 97, 100–2, 132, 158, 202, 208
medical training 5 n.8, 93–5, 97, 99, 102, 212
medical transition 11, 59, 67
medical triumphalism 134
Medicine and Empathy in Contemporary British Fiction: An Intervention in Medical Humanities (Whitehead) 6
medico-legal discourses 163
Melville, Herman
 Moby Dick 192
menstrual cycle 93
metaphor as disease 171
Metzl, Jonathan 95
Meyer, Stephenie 20
 Breaking Dawn 10, 24, 31, 33 n.25, 35, 37
 Twilight 11, 19, 24, 32–6, 33 n.25, 33 n.30
Michael Tolliver Lives (Maupin) 142
Middlemarch (Eliot) 25, 145
Middleton, Thomas
 A Chaste Maid in Cheapside 47

midwifery 46, 48
Midwives Book (Sharp) 52
military
   conflict 57
   identity 59, 62
   legacy 59
   life 58
   organization 59
   to civilian transition 58–9, 64, 70
   transitions 11, 58 n.1, 58–9, 61, 64, 70
Minot, Leslie Anne 30–1
Moby Dick (Melville) 192
More Tales of the City (Maupin) 148–9, 153
Morris, Rosemary 45
Moten, Fred
   The Undercommons 193, 193 n.60
motherhood
   burden of 48
   ideologies failing women 20, 39
   and pregnancy 42–3
motivation 151, 184, 198, 205
Muñoz, José Esteban 54
Munroe, Jennifer 47
My Life My Story program 86

Nadesan, Majia Holmer 122
Nass, Clifford 119
Nelson, Maggie
   The Argonauts 37
neoliberal society 102
neonatal testing 138
Nethercot, Arthur H. 29
New England Journal of Medicine (NEJM) 79
new normal 62, 66
Nineteen Eighty-Four (Orwell) 198, 209
nonnormative
   families 49
   gender 94
   sexuality 37
The Normal and the Pathological (Canguilhem) 170
normative gender 93
novel 146–52
   archive 145
   narrative perspectives 70
   Victorian 25
Nozick, Robert 208 n.45

Obama, Barack 12, 75
Obermeyer, Ziad 91
objectification of injured body 59–60
Obstetrics: Normal and Problem Pregnancies (Gabbe) 40
O'Connell, Meaghan 50
Oldfield, Benjamin J. 86
On Immunity (Biss) 37
OpenNotes 86
Oregon Health Plan (OHP) 204–5
Orgel, Stephen 39 n.7
orientations, attitudinal 3, 7–9, 177
Orwell, George
   Nineteen Eighty-Four 198, 209
O'Sullivan, Sean 146
Our Bodies, Ourselves 27
OurNotes 86
Our Vampires, Ourselves (Auerbach) 27
Oxford English Dictionary 119

Pacific Sun 144
Pageler, Natalie M. 90
pain
   analogic event 120
   analogue scale 12
   clinical studies 13
   diagnosis 73
   end-of-life 162–6, 171, 174, 175–6
   experience of 165
   management 33, 105, 122
   measurement of 116–17, 123
   medication during labor 34
   normalization of 66
   studies 116
   subjective nature of 115
   trials 105
Palin, Sarah 203–4
palliative care 138, 161, 167, 204
Parker, Harry
   Anatomy of a Soldier 11, 19–20, 57–70
Pasman, Roeline 164, 175
Patel, Jayshil J. 81
Paterson, Donald 106–8, 110, 112, 121
patient
   and caregiver 126, 165
   consultations 90
   dying 173
   narrative 14, 82, 84–5, 100
   safety 76, 82

satisfaction 75
testimony 6
transcribe 80
transcribing 84
transformation 77
patient–physician communication 79
patriarchal tyranny 45
Pease, Donald E. 102
pedagogy
  critical 99
  of critical consciousness 97
  social medicine 95–6, 100–1, 103
  social science 95
Peterson, Kaara L. 42, 42 n.18
physical capability 62
physician-diagnostician 90
physician–physician teamwork 79
physicians
  adapting to EHR 85
  as detective 86–91
  dissatisfaction 76
  education 3
  expression 81, 83
  identity 76, 79–80, 86, 90
physician-storyteller 80–6
Piercy, Marge
  Woman on the Edge of Time 199
Pilowsky, Issy 116–17
Pitts, Walter 119
Polak, Kate
  Ethics in the Gutter: Empathy and Historical Fiction in Comics 6
political/relational model 137
Pollard, Tanya 41
Ponte, Maya 100
posthumanism 105
postpartum
  bodies 40, 51, 54–55
  cultural crisis in 54
  discrimination against women after 52
  exhaustion 39–55
  life-threatening complications 53
  period 42, 52
  recovery 50
  rituals and care 45
  role of parents after 51
power and the judge 121–3
practitioner-in-training 72
Preciado, Paul B. 182

pregnancy 23, 26
  and childbirth 20, 23–24, 34, 43
  fear in 24
  and motherhood 42
  and postpartum period 42
pregnancy-related deaths 51
pregnant women 25, 41, 41 n.14
prejudice
  promoting 134
  social 133
Price, Margaret 137
prosthesis 64–7
prosthetics
  gain 62–7
  leg 58 n.1, 64–5, 67
  limb 11, 19–20, 64–6
Psychological Bulletin 106
Psychology Today 197

Queen Elizabeth II 142
queer studies 130–1

race/racial 99
  assumptions based on 1
  critical race theory 101
  and ethnic diversity 150
  and ethnicity 151
  faking of 151
  hierarchies 99
  identity 194
  tensions 166
RAF Institute of Aviation 114
Ramsey, Mona 151
Rand, Ayn
  Atlas Shrugged 198
Randy Stroup 204–6
Ratcliffe, Matthew 162
Reading for Health: Medical Narratives and the Nineteenth-Century Novel (Wright) 6
Reagan, Ronald 155
Rediker, Marcus
  The Many-Headed Hydra: Sailors, Slaves, Commoners, and the Hidden History of the Revolutionary Atlantic 192
Reeves, Byron 119
rehabilitation 57–8, 65–6, 70
relationships 189

interdisciplinary 42
intimate 89
personal 154
of physicians with patients, peers, and communities 97
professional 77
reproductive bodies 24–31, 48. *See also* horror reproduction (nineteenth-century)
reproductive justice for women of color 53
resilience 64
respiratory diseases 114
Reynolds, Paige Martin 41 n.14
rhetorical analysis 19, 125
Richards, Jennifer
 The Edinburgh Companion to the Critical Medical Humanities 7
Ricoeur, Paul
 Time and Narrative 207
rights-based activism 132. *See also* activism
rituals and care, postpartum 45
Rosenbaum, Lisa 82–4
Rosenberg, Jordy 15–16. *See also* endochronology
 Confessions of the Fox 181–95, 189 n.41
 intersex anatomy 191 n.48
Rosenfield, Kirstie Gulick 46
Rosenthal, David I. 80, 88–90
Rothman, David J. 162, 166, 168, 171, 175
Royal Shakespeare Company 50
The Rules Do Not Apply (Levy) 37
Ruml, Beardsly 113

sacrifice 52
Safder, Taimur 80, 85
Salam, Maya 53
Samuels, Ellen 137
San Francisco Chronicle 142, 144
San Quentin Prison 185
Savage, Dan 141
Save Our Children campaign 149
Scarry, Elaine 162, 170
 The Body in Pain 164
Schaffner, Anna Katharina 44
 Exhaustion: A History 42
Scheper-Hughes, Nancy 94
Schiff, Gordon D. 91
scientific discourse 165

Scott, Walter Dill 112–14
 The Theory of Advertising 114
Scott Company Engineers and Consultants 106, 117
Second International Conference on End of Life Law, Ethics, Policy and Practice 176
self-consciousness 67
self-identity 58, 62, 64
self-mutilation 152
serial format 146–52
serialization. *See Tales of the City* (Maupin)
serum 178, 181, 187, 192
 alchemical 182
 market of 185
 original creators 181
 of pirates 184, 186–7, 189, 191
sex
 biological 16, 183
 defined 2
 dualism 184, 185, 191
 education 156
 and feelings 145
 hormones 16, 178, 181–6
 life 35
 magazine 154–5
 workers 1
sexuality 24, 46. *See also Tales of the City* (Maupin)
 explicit 24
 female 24
 identity and 154
 nonnormative 37
 overt 31
 and reproductive bodies 34
 studies 16, 182
 urban 147
sexual play 181
Shakespeare, William
 Titus Andronicus 49
 The Winter's Tale 11, 19–20, 39–55
Shapin, Steven 9
shared decision-making 91. *See also* decision-making
Sharp, Jane
 Midwives Book 52
Sheffield, Elisabeth 192
Shelter Blues (Desjarlais) 93

Sheppard, Jack 181, 185–6, 191
Siebers, Tobin 136
Sigerist, Henry 132
Significant Others (Maupin) 155
Singer, Jeffrey A. 202
Singh, Hardeep 89
Singleton, Mary Ann 151, 152
Smith, Brett 65
social change 101, 135
social connectedness 68–9
social equity 187
social expectations 63, 70
social identity 58, 63, 67–70
social inferiority 52
social isolation 134
social justice 1, 13, 101, 134
social medicine
    desiring 101–3
    pedagogy 96–101
    purpose of training 96
social prejudice 133
sociocultural norms 67–70
Sontag, Susan 171
Sorting Things Out (Bowker and Star) 118
Stack, Sharon 147
Stanley, Leo L. 185
Star, Susan Leigh
    Sorting Things Out 118
Steedman, Carolyn 145
STEM 129–30
steroid chemistry 183
Stoker, Bram
    Dracula 11, 24, 27, 30–3
Stretches 192
structural competence 98, 102
    education 10, 12–13, 71–2
subjectivity and sex hormones 181
Sure of You (Maupin) 142, 149, 156–7
Suvin, Darko 206 n.37
Swift, Graham
    Waterland 207
Synapsis: A Health Humanities Journal 2
systemic discrimination 134

Tales of the City (Maupin) 126, 141–59, 211
    health 152–7
    historians 143–6
    historical method 143–6

HIV/AIDS 152–7
    novel 146–52
    serial format 146–52
Teaching Health Humanities (Banner, Carlin, Cole) 6
technoscientific. *See also* electronic health record (EHR)
    identities 92
    innovation 77, 92
    object 72, 76–7
technoscientization 77
teleology 6, 126, 178
Temkin, Owsei 132
terminal illness 125–6, 177
testis transplantation 183 n.12
testosterone 16, 171, 181–4, 186
The Theory of Advertising (Scott) 114
A Thousand Plateaus (Guattari and Deleuze) 189
Time and Narrative (Ricoeur) 207
Time's Arrow (Amis) 207
Titus Andronicus (Shakespeare) 49
Tolliver, Michael 146, 148, 150, 151, 153, 157
Tomkins, Sylvan
    Affect Imagery Consciousness 120
Tosh, John
    The Pursuit of History 145
To the Friend Who Did Not Save My Life (Guibert) 169 n.20
tourniquet 58–60, 60 n.13
Tousignant, Noémi 115
training
    academic 99
    basic 59
    empathy 10, 12, 71
    extracurricular 85
    hierarchies 99
    medical 93–5, 97, 99, 102
    physicians 3, 86
transcribing patient 80, 84, 86
transcription 81, 168
transgender
    boy 93
    characters 153
    community 153
    man 178, 181
    medicine 94
    memoirs 186

transitioning
  from able-bodied to amputee 61–2
  civilian 58–9
  defined 58
  military 58–9
transphobia 147
Traub, Valerie 44
Traumatic Limb Loss and the Needs of the Family (Fossey and Hughes) 59 n.10, 63 n.27
trauma/traumatic
  comedy and 146
  emotion and 159
  front-line techniques 63 n.27
  limb loss 57, 61
  reproductive 11
  and sacrifice 52
  sexual 27–28
Tripathi, Micky 80
Trump, Donald 198
Turing, Alan 119
Turnbull, Cadwell 205 n.33
Turner, Bryan S. 67
Twilight (Meyer) 11, 19, 24, 31–6, 33 n.25, 33 n.30

urbanization 146
urban landscapes. *See Tales of the City* (Maupin)
utopia 200–1, 206 n.37
  critical 209
  defined 200
  feminist 199
  gesture 191
  literary 201
  project 201
  society 201
  utopianism 201

Vadeboncoeur, Alain 176
vagrant 186–91
valued resource 91
Verghese, Abraham 78, 80, 88–90
veterans
  identity 68
  portrayals in US media 69
  social attitudes toward 69
  victimization of 69

Veterans' Affairs
  My Life My Story program 86
  victimization of veterans 69
Viney, William 130
Visual Analogue Scale (VAS) 13, 73, 105–23
  affect and the subject 119–21
  decision-making 117–19
  Graphic Rating Scale (GRS) 106–12
  power and the judge 121–3
  Scott's Wundtian Lineage 112–14

Wachter, Robert M. 91
Wall Street Journal 96
Wear, Delease
  The Health Humanities Reader 4, 6–7
Weizenbaum, Joseph 120
Wen, Leana 16, 197–8, 200, 203, 206
Wendell, Susan 137
Whitehead, Anne
  The Edinburgh Companion to the Critical Medical Humanities 7
  Medicine and Empathy in Contemporary British Fiction: An Intervention in Medical Humanities 6
Wiegman, Robyn 96, 101–2
Williams, Serena 53
Williams, William Carlos 80, 199
Wilson, Adrian 54, 120
Wilson, D'orothea 151
The Winter's Tale (Shakespeare) 11, 19–20, 39–55
Wolpaw, Daniel R. 80 n.25, 89
Woman on the Edge of Time (Piercy) 199
women 35 n.34, 55
  of color 20, 52
  community 48
  exposure of 25
  health classic 27
  life-threatening complications postpartum 53
  pregnant 41 n.14
  representation of 24
  reproductive bodies 11, 24, 31, 37, 52
  unsuspecting 29
Wong, Lionel 150
Woods, Angela 130
  The Edinburgh Companion to the Critical Medical Humanities 7

Wright, Erika
  Reading for Health: Medical Narratives and the Nineteenth-Century Novel 6
Wundt, Wilhelm 105, 113–14

Wuthering Heights (Brontë) 25, 32

Zulman, Donna M. 88, 90
Zwartjes, Arianne 182 n.5

www.ingramcontent.com/pod-product-compliance
Lightning Source LLC
Chambersburg PA
CBHW062129300426
44115CB00012BA/1859